Table of Contents — PDR® Pharmacopoeia Pocket Dosing Guide 2005

Foreword

Welcome to the PDR Pharmacopoeia Pocket Dosing Guide, now in its fourth edition. This convenient little book is designed to be at your fingertips whenever you need to double-check dosage recommendations, review available forms and strengths, or confirm a pregnancy rating. For 2005, it has been completely updated to include all the latest new drugs, forms, strengths, and indications.

To aid quick lookups and comparisons, PDR Pharmacopoeia is organized by major drug category and specific indication. Under each indication, you'll find applicable drugs sorted by class and listed alphabetically by generic name. For combination products, generic ingredients are listed alphabetically, with the strengths of the ingredients presented in the same order.

The book's major sections are listed on the Contents Page. The location of entries for specific brands, generics, and indications can be found in the index at the end of the book. For drugs with multiple uses, the index lists the page of each indication separately.

The PDR Pharmacopoeia also offers you a variety of quick-reference tables listing frequently used formulas and comparative prescribing information. For the exact location of these convenient resources, check the index at the end of the book.

Unlike other dosing guides, the PDR Pharmacopoeia is drawn almost exclusively from the FDA-approved drug labeling published in *Physicians' Desk Reference®*. Although diligent efforts have been made to ensure the accuracy of this information, please remember that this book is sold without warranties, express or implied, and that the publisher and editors disclaim all liability in connection with its use.

Remember, too, that this book deals only with dosage for the typical patient, and includes little information on usage in special populations and circumstances. The need for dosage adjustments in the presence of hepatic or renal insufficiency is signaled in the Comments column of the entries. For details regarding these adjustments, as well as complete pediatric and geriatric dosage guidelines, consult the latest edition of PDR®. Be sure to check PDR, too, whenever contraindications, warnings, or precautions may be an issue.

Throughout the book, you will find a drug's Controlled Substances Category (if any) immediately following its name. The drug's pregnancy rating and breastfeeding status appear in the Comments column of the entry. Keys to the symbols can be found below:

Controlled Substances Categories

CII. High potential for abuse, leading to severe psychological or physical dependence. **CIII.** Abuse may lead to moderate or low physical dependence or high psychological dependence. **CIV.** Abuse may lead to limited physical dependence or psychological dependence. **CV.** Consequences of abuse are more limited than those of drugs in Category CIV.

❷ Use-In-Pregnancy Ratings

A. Controlled studies shown no risk. **B.** No evidence of risk in humans. **C.** Risk cannot be ruled out. **D.** Positive evidence of risk: Use only when no safer alternative exists for a serious problem. **X.** Contraindicated in pregnancy. **N.** Not rated.

❀ Breastfeeding Safety

^ May be used in breastfeeding. > Caution advised or effect undetermined. v Contraindicated or not recommended.

H Dosage adjustment required for hepatic insufficiency.
R Dosage adjustment required for renal insufficiency.

Dosage Forms

A key to the abbreviations may be found on page 4.

PDR® PHARMACOPOEIA POCKET DOSING GUIDE 2005

Editor: Tammy Chernin, RPh
Managing Editor: Greg Tallis, RPh
Associate Editors: Min Ko, PharmD; Sheila Talatala, PharmD
Clinical Content Operations Manager: Thomas Fleming, PharmD
Senior Electronic Publishing Designer: Livio Udina
Production Editor: Gwynned Kelly
Project Manager: Lynn S. Wilhelm

Executive Vice President, PDR: David Duplay
Vice President, PDR Services: Brian Holland
Senior Director, Brand and Product Management: Valerie Berger
Director, Brand and Product Management: Carmen Mazzatta
Vice President, Sales and Marketing: Dikran N. Barsamian
Director of Operations: Robert Klein
Director of Trade Sales: Bill Gaffney
Senior Director, Publishing Sales and Marketing: Michael Bennett
Promotion Manager: Linda Levine

ABBREVIATIONS

ABBREVIATIONS & DESCRIPTIONS

CAP	community-aquired pneumonia
Cap	capsule
Cap,ER	extended release capsule
CI	contraindicated
Cnt	concentrate
conc	concentration
Cre	cream
d	day
D/C	discontinue
Eli	elixir
Foa	foam
Gel	gel/jelly
gm	gram
h	hour
hs	at bedtime
IM	intramuscular
inj	injection
IU	international units
IV	intravenous

ABBREVIATIONS & DESCRIPTIONS

ml	milliliter
mth	month
NTE	not to exceed
Oint	ointment
Pkt	packet
PO	by mouth
Pow	powder
prn	as needed
q	every
qd	once daily
qid	four times daily
qod	every other day
qow	every other week
SC	subcutaneous
Sl	sublingual
Sol	solution
Sol,Neb	solution, nebulized
Spr	spray
Sup	suppository

Kg	kilogram		**Susp**	*suspension*
Liq	liquid		**Syr**	syrup
Lot	lotion		**Tab**	tablet
Loz	lozenge		**Tab,ER**	extended release tablet
mcg	microgram		**tid**	3 times daily
MDI	metered dose inhaler		**tiw**	3 times weekly
mEq	milli-equivalent		**U**	units
mg	milligram		**w/a**	while awake
min	minute		**wk**	week
MIU	million international units		**yo**	years old

WEIGHTS & MEASURES; CONVERSIONS & FORMULAS

METRIC WEIGHT

1 kilogram (kg)	=	1,000 gram
1 gram (g)	=	1,000 mg
1 milligram (mg)	=	0.001 gm

U.S. FLUID MEASURE

1 fluidrachm	=	60 minim (min)
1 fluidounce	=	8 fld drachm
	=	480 min

METRIC WEIGHT

1 microgram (mcg)	=	0.001 mg
1 gamma	=	1 mcg

U.S. FLUID MEASURE

1 pint (pt)	=	16 fl oz
	=	7,680 min
1 quart (qt)	=	2 pt
	=	32 fl oz
1 gallon (gal)	=	4 qts
	=	128 fl oz

APOTHECARY WEIGHT

1 scruple	=	20 grains (gr)
1 drachm	=	3 scruples
	=	60 gr
1 ounce (oz)	=	8 drachms
	=	24 scruples
	=	480 gr
1 pound (lb)	=	12 oz
	=	96 drachms
	=	288 scruples
	=	5,760 gr

AVOIRDUPOIS WEIGHT

1 ounce	=	437.5 gr
1 pound	=	16 oz

CONVERSION FACTORS

1 gram	=	15.4 gr
1 grain	=	64.8 mg
1 ounce (AV)	=	28.35 gm
	=	437.5 gr
1 ounce (Ap)	=	31.1 gm
	=	480 gr
1 pound (Av)	=	453.6 gm
1 kilogram	=	2.68 pound Ap
	=	2.2 lbs Av
1 fluidounce	=	29.57 ml
1 fluidrachm	=	3.697 ml
1 minim	=	0.06 ml

COMMON MEASURES

1 teaspoonful	=	5 ml
	=	1/6 fl oz
1 tablespoonful	=	15 ml
	=	1/2 fl oz
1 wineglassful	=	60 ml
	=	2 fl oz
1 teacupful	=	120 ml
	=	4 fl oz

TEMPERATURE

For °F to °C, the formula is: 5/9 (°F minus 32) = °C
For °C to °F, the formula is: 9/5 °C plus 32 = °F
1 kelvin (K)   =   9/5 °F

COCKCROFT/GAULT CREATININE CLEARANCE FORMULA

$$Cl_{Cr\ (males^*\ ml/min)} = \frac{(140 - Age)(Body\ Weight\ in\ kg)}{(SrCr)(72\ kg)}$$

*For females multiply result by 0.85

BODY SURFACE AREA [BSA (M²)]

$$BSA = (\ [Ht\ (cm) \bullet Wt\ (kg)\ ]/\ 3600\ )^{1/2}$$

ANION GAP (AG)

$$AG = (Na^+ + K^+) - (Cl^- + HCO_3^-)\ or\ AG = Na^+ - (Cl^- + HCO_3^-)$$

NEUTROPENIA CALCULATION

$$ANC = (\%\ segs + \%\ bands) \times total\ WBC$$

ANALGESICS

Arthritis Therapy

SEE ALSO NSAIDS

NAME	FORM/STRENGTH	DOSAGE	COMMENTS
Adalimumab (Humira)	Inj: 40 mg/0.8 ml	**Adults: RA:** 40 mg SC qowk. Patients not taking MTX may derive additional benefit by increasing to 40 mg qwk.	●B ❀v TB & other opportunistic infections reported.
Anakinra (Kineret)	Inj: 100 mg/0.67 ml	≥**18 yo: RA:** 100 mg SC qd.	●B ❀>
Auranofin (Ridaura)	Cap: 3 mg	**Adults: RA: Usual:** 3 mg bid or 6 mg qd. **Max:** 9 mg/d.	●C ❀v May cause gold toxicity.
Aurothioglucose (Solganal)	Inj: 50 mg/ml	**Adults: RA: Initial:** 1st wk 10 mg IM. **Titrate:** 2nd & 3rd wk 25 mg IM, 4th & subsequent wks 50 mg IM until 0.8-1 gm given; continue 50 mg IM q3-4wks. **6-12 yo: JRA:** 1/4 of adult dose IM. **Max:** 25 mg/dose.	●C ❀v Possible toxic reactions.
Azathioprine (Imuran, Azasan)	(Imuran) Tab: 50mg; Inj:100 mg; (Azasan) Tab: 25 mg, 50 mg, 75 mg, 100 mg	**Adults: RA: Initial:** 1 mg/kg/d given qd-bid. **Titrate:** Increase by 0.5 mg/kg/d after 6-8 wks & then q4wks. **Max:** 2.5 mg/kg/d. **Maint:** Decrease by 0.5 mg/kg/d or 25 mg/d q4wks until lowest effective dose.	●D ❀v R Neoplasia. Mutagenesis. Hematologic toxicity.
Celecoxib (Celebrex)	Cap: 100 mg, 200 mg	**Adults: OA:** 200 mg qd or 100 mg bid. **RA:** 100-200 mg bid.	●C ❀v H

Drug	Form	Dosage	Ratings
Cyclosporine (Neoral)	**Cap:** 25 mg, 100 mg; **Sol:** 100 mg/ml	**≥18 yo: RA: Initial:** 2.5 mg/kg/d, taken bid. **Titrate:** Increase by 0.5-0.75 mg/kg/d after 8 wks & again after 12 wks. **Max:** 4 mg/kg/d. Decrease by 25%-50% to control adverse events. **Combo with MTX: Maint:** 3 mg/kg/d or less. **Max:** 15 mg/kg.	◐C ✿v Infection. Neoplasia. Nephrotoxicity. Malignancy risk w/certain psoriasis therapies.
Etanercept (Enbrel)	**Inj:** 25 mg	**Adults: RA/Psoriatic Arthritis/Ankylosing Spondylitis:** 50 mg/wk SC. Give as two 25 mg SC inj at separate sites on same day or 3-4 days apart. **4-17 yo: JRA:** 0.8 mg/kg/wk SC. **Max:** 50 mg/wk and 25 mg/inj site. **≤31 kg:** One SC inj once weekly. **>31 kg:** Two SC inj on same day or 3-4 days apart.	◐B ✿v
Gold Sodium Thiomalate (Aurolate)	**Inj:** 50 mg/ml	**Adults: RA: Usual:** 10 mg IM 1st wk, 20 mg 2nd wk, 25-50 mg IM wkly until cumulative dose of 1 gm, toxicity, or clinical improvement. **Maint:** 25-50 mg every other wk. **Pediatrics: JRA: Initial:** Test dose of 10 mg. **Maint:** 1 mg/kg IM wkly. **Max:** 50 mg/single inj.	◐C ✿v Possible toxic reactions.
Hydroxychloroquine Sulfate (Plaquenil)	**Tab:** 200 mg	**Adults: RA: Initial:** 400-600 mg/d with food or glass of milk. Increase dose in 5-10d until optimum response. **Maint:** After 4-12 wks, 200-400 mg/d.	◐N ✿>
Infliximab (Remicade)	**Inj:** 100 mg	**Adults: RA In Combination With MTX:** 3 mg/kg IV, repeat at 2 & 6 wks, then q8wks. **Incomplete Response:** Increase to 10mg/kg or give q4wks.	◐B ✿v TB, fungal, & other opportunistic infections reported.

NAME	FORM/STRENGTH	DOSAGE	COMMENTS
Leflunomide (Arava)	**Tab:** 10 mg, 20 mg	**Adults: RA: LD:** 100 mg qd x 3 d. **Maint:** 20 mg qd. **Max:** 20 mg/d. **If dose not tolerated or ALT elevations >2 but ≤3X UNL:** Reduce dose to 10 mg/d. If elevations persist or ALT >3X UNL, discontinue.	⊕X ❄v **H** CI in pregnancy. Hepato-toxicity. Immuno-suppression.
Meloxicam (Mobic)	**Tab:** 7.5 mg, 15 mg	≥18 yo: OA: **Initial/Maint:** 7.5 mg qd. **Max:** 15 mg/d.	⊕C ❄v
Methotrexate Sodium (Rheumatrex)	**Tab:** 2.5 mg, 5 mg, 7.5 mg, 15 mg	**Adults: RA: Initial:** 7.5 mg once weekly or 2.5 mg q12h x 3 doses once weekly. **Max:** 20 mg/wk. Reduce to lowest effective dose. **JRA: 2-16 yo:** 10 mg/m² once weekly. Adjust dose to optimal response.	⊕X ❄v CI in pregnancy & nursing. [19]
Penicillamine (Cuprimine)	**Cap:** 125 mg, 250 mg	**Adults: RA: Initial:** 125 mg-250 mg qd; increase q1-3mths by 125 mg-250 mg/d. **Maint:** 500-750 mg/d.	⊕N ❄v CI in pregnancy, renal insufficiency & agranulocytosis.
Penicillamine (Depen)	**Tab:** 250 mg	**Adults: RA: Initial:** 125 mg-250 mg qd; increase q1-3mths by 125 mg-250 mg/d. **Maint:** 500-750 mg/d.	⊕N ❄v CI in pregnancy, renal insufficiency & agranulocytosis.
Rofecoxib (Vioxx)	**Susp:** 12.5 mg/5 ml, 25 mg/5 ml; **Tab:** 12.5 mg, 25 mg, 50 mg	**Adults: OA: Initial:** 12.5 mg qd. **Max:** 25 mg qd. **RA:** 25 mg qd.	⊕C ❄v **H**
Sulfasalazine (Azulfidine EN-tabs)	**Tab, Enteric:** 500 mg	**Adults: RA: Initial:** 0.5-1 gm qd. **Usual:** 1 gm bid. **Max:** 3 gm/d. **6-16 yo: JRA:** 30-50 mg/kg/d given bid. **Max:** 2 gm/d.	⊕B ❄>

| Valdecoxib (Bextra) | Tab: 10 mg, 20 mg | ≥18 yo: OA/RA: 10 mg qd. | ●C ❄v |

Narcotics

Drug	Form	Dosage	Rating
Codeine CII	(Phosphate) Inj: 15 mg/ml, 30 mg/ml; Sol: 15 mg/5 ml; Tab: 30 mg, 60 mg; (Sulfate) Tab: 15 mg, 30 mg, 60 mg	Adults: 15-60 mg PO/IM/SC q4-6h. Peds: ≥1 yo: 0.5 mg/kg PO q4-6h or 0.5 mg/kg IM/SC q4h, up to 3 mg/kg/d IM/SC in divided doses.	●C ❄>
Codeine Phosphate/ APAP CIII (Tab) CV (Eli) (Tylenol w/Codeine)	Eli: 12-120 mg/5 ml; Tab: (#3) 30-300 mg, (#4) 60-300 mg	Tab: Adults: 15 mg-60 mg codeine/dose & 300 mg-1 gm APAP/dose up to q4h prn. Max: 360 mg codeine and 4 gm APAP per 24h. Peds: 0.5 mg/kg of codeine. Eli: Adults: 15 ml q4h prn. Peds: 3-6 yo: 5 ml tid-qid. 7-12 yo: 10 ml tid-qid.	●C ❄>
Fentanyl CII (Duragesic)	Patch: 25 mcg/h, 50 mcg/h, 75 mcg/h, 100 mcg/h	Adults: Individualize dose. Dose based on opioid tolerance. Initial: 25 mcg/h for 72h. Titrate: Adjust based on daily supplementary opioid dose; use ratio of 90 mg/24h of oral morphine to a 25 mcg/h increase in Duragesic dose. May take 6d to reach equilibrium after dose change.	●C ❄v CI in acute or post-op pain, mild/ intermittent pain & initial dose >25 mcg/h.
Fentanyl Citrate CII (Actiq)	Loz (unit): 0.2 mg, 0.4 mg, 0.6 mg, 0.8 mg, 1.2 mg, 1.6 mg	≥16 yo: Breakthrough Pain: Initial: 0.2 mg for pain (consume over 15 min). Titrate: Increase to next strength if pain episodes require >1 unit/pain episode. Maint: 1 unit/pain episode. Max: 2 units/pain episode or 4 units/d.	●C ❄v CI in acute or post-op pain, non-opioid tolerant patients.

[19] Monitor for bone marrow, lung, liver & kidney toxicities. Serious toxic reactions.

NAME	FORM/STRENGTH	DOSAGE	COMMENTS
Hydrocodone Bitartrate/ Ibuprofen CIII (Reprexain, Vicoprofen)	**Tab:** (Reprexain) 5 mg-200 mg, (Vicoprofen) 7.5 mg-200 mg	**≥16 yo: Usual:** 1 tab q4-6h prn. **Max:** 5 tabs/d.	▣C ❄v
Hydrocodone Bitartrate/APAP CIII (Lortab, Maxidone, Vicodin, Vicodin ES, Vicodin HP)	**Sol:** (Lortab) 7.5-500 mg/ 15 ml; **Tab:** 2.5-500 mg, 5-500 mg, 7.5-500 mg, 10-500 mg; **Tab:** (Maxidone) 10-750 mg, (Vicodin) 5-500 mg, (Vicodin ES) 7.5-750 mg, (Vicodin HP) 10-660 mg	**Adults: Pain: Vicodin:** 1-2 tabs q4-6h prn. **Max:** 8 tabs/d. **Vicodin HP:** 1 tab q4-6h prn. **Max:** 6 tabs/d. **Vicodin ES/Maxidone:** 1 tab q4-6h prn. **Max:** 5 tabs/d. **Lortab:** (2.5-500 mg tab, 5-500 mg tab) 1-2 tabs q4-6h prn. **Max:** 8 tabs/d. (7.5-500 mg tab, 10-500 mg tab) 1 tab q4-6h prn. **Max:** 6 tabs/d. (Sol) 15 ml q4-6h prn. **Max:** 90 ml/d. **≥2 yrs: Lortab: Sol:** **12-15 kg:** 3.75 ml. **16-22 kg:** 5 ml. **23-31 kg:** 7.5 ml. **32-45 kg:** 10 ml. **≥46 kg:** 15 ml. May repeat q4-6h.	▣C ❄v
Hydromorphone HCl CII (Dilaudid, Dilaudid HP)	**Inj:** 1 mg/ml, 2 mg/ml, 4 mg/ml, (HP form) 10 mg/ml; **Liq:** 1 mg/ml; **Sup:** 3 mg; **Tab:** 2 mg, 4 mg, 8 mg	**Adults: Usual: Inj:** 1-2 mg IM/IV/SC q4-6h prn. **HP Inj:** 1-14 mg IM/SQ. **Liq:** 2.5-10 mg PO q3-6h prn. **Tab:** 2-4 mg q4-6h PO prn. **Sup:** 1 sup PR q6-8h prn.	▣C ❄v
Levorphanol Tartrate CII (Levo-Dromoran)	**Inj:** 2 mg/ml; **Tab:** 2 mg	**≥18 yo: IV: Usual:** Up to 1 mg, in divided doses q3-6h prn. **Max:** 4-8 mg/24h. **IM/SC: Usual:** 1-2 mg q6-8h prn. **Max:** 3-8 mg/24h. **PO: Usual:** 2-3 mg q6-8h prn. **Max:** 6-12 mg/24h.	▣C ❄v
Meperidine HCl CII (Demerol)	**Inj:** 25 mg/ml, 50 mg/ml, 75 mg/ml, 100 mg/ml; **Syr:** 50 mg/5 ml; **Tab:** 50 mg, 100 mg	**Adults: Usual:** 50-150 mg PO/IM/SC q3-4h prn. **Peds: Usual:** 0.5 mg/lb-0.8 mg/lb PO/IM/SC, up to adult dose, q3-4h prn. Mix syrup in 1/2 glass of water to prevent topical anesthetic effect on mucous membranes.	▣N ❄> H R Cl with MAOI use within 14 days.

Meperidine/ Promethazine CII	**Cap:** 50 mg-25 mg	**Adults:** 1 cap q4-6h prn.	◐N ❄️> **H R CI** with MAOI use within 14 days.
Methadone HCl CII (Dolophine)	**Inj:** 10 mg/ml; **Sol:** 5 mg/5 ml, 10 mg/5 ml; **Tab:** 5 mg, 10 mg, 40 mg	**Adults: Pain: Usual:** 2.5-10 mg PO/IM/SC q3-4h prn. Special dosing for detoxification/maintenance treatment.	◐N ❄️>
Morphine Sulfate CII (Astramorph/PF, Duramorph)	**Inj:** 0.5 mg/ml, 1 mg/ml, 5 mg/ml	**Adults: IV: Initial:** 2-10 mg/70 kg. **Epidural: Initial:** 5 mg in lumbar region, increase by 1-2 mg if needed. **Max:** 10 mg/24h. **Continuous Epidural: Initial:** 2-4 mg/24h, give additional 1-2 mg if needed. **Max:** 10 mg/24h. **Intrathecal:** 0.2-1 mg single inj.	◐C ❄️>
Morphine Sulfate CII (Avinza)	**Cap,ER:** 30 mg, 60 mg, 90 mg, 120 mg	**Adults: ≥18 yo: Conversion from PO Morphine:** Give total daily morphine dose as a single dose q24h. **Conversion from Parenteral Morphine: Initial:** Give about 3x previous daily parenteral morphine requirement. **Conversion from Other Parenteral or PO** **Non-Morphine Opioids: Initial:** Give 1/2 of estimated daily morphine requirement q24h. May supplement with immediate-release morphine or short-acting analgesics. **Titrate:** Adjust as frequently as qod. **Non-Opioid Tolerant:** 30 mg q24h. **Titrate:** Increase by no more than 30 mg q4d. **Max:** 1600 mg/d.	◐C ❄️v Swallow whole or sprinkle contents on applesauce. Do not crush, chew, or dissolve cap beads. The 60, 90, & 120 mg caps are for opioid-tolerant patients.

NAME	FORM/STRENGTH	DOSAGE	COMMENTS
Morphine Sulfate CII (Kadian, MS Contin, Oramorph SR)	**Cap,ER:** (Kadian) 20 mg, 30 mg, 50 mg, 60 mg, 100 mg; **Tab,ER:** (MS Contin, Oramorph SR) 15 mg, 30 mg, 60 mg, 100 mg, (MS Contin) 200 mg	**Adults: Conversion to MS Contin/Oramorph SR:** Give 1/2 of the 24h immediate-release oral morphine dose q12h. May give 1/3 of daily oral morphine dose q8h with MS Contin. **Conversion to Kadian:** Give 1/2 of the total daily oral morphine dose as Kadian q12h or total daily oral morphine dose as q24h.	◐C ❄v Swallow whole. MS Contin 200 mg tab is only for opioid-tolerant patients.
Morphine Sulfate CII (MSIR)	**Cap:** 15 mg, 30 mg; **Cnt:** 20 mg/ml; **Sol:** 10 mg/5 ml, 20 mg/5 ml; **Tab:** 15 mg, 30 mg	**Adults: Usual:** 5-30 mg q4h.	◐C ❄v
Oxycodone HCl CII (Oxycontin)	**Tab,ER:** 10 mg, 20 mg, 40 mg, 80 mg, 160 mg	**Adults: ≥18 yrs: Opioid Naive:** 10 mg q12h. **Titrate:** Increase to 20 mg q12h, then increase total daily dose by 25-50% of current dose. Increase q1-2d. **Conversion from Oxycodone:** Divide 24h oxycodone dose by 50% to obtain q12h dose. Round down to appropriate strength. **Opioid Tolerant:** May use 80 mg or 160 mg tabs. D/C other around-the-clock opioids. High-fat meals increase peak levels of 160 mg tab. **With CNS Depressants:** Reduce by 1/3 or 1/2.	◐B ❄v For continuous analgesia. Abuse potential. 80 mg & 160 mg tabs are only for opioid-tolerant patients. Swallow whole.
Oxycodone HCl CII (OxyFast, OxyIR, Roxicodone)	**(OxyFast) Sol:** 20 mg/ml; **(OxyIR) Cap:** 5 mg; **(Roxicodone) Sol:** 5 mg/5 ml, 20 mg/ml; **Tab:** 5 mg, 15 mg, 30 mg	**Adults: Pain: OxyFast, OxyIR:** 5 mg q6h prn. **Roxicodone:** 5-30 mg q4-6h prn.	◐B ❄v

Oxycodone HCl/APAP CII (Percocet, Roxicet, Tylox)	**(Percocet) Tab:** 2.5-325 mg, 5-325 mg, 7.5-325 mg, 7.5-500 mg, 10-325 mg, 10-650 mg; **(Roxicet) Sol:** 5-325 mg/5 ml; **Tab:** 5-325 mg; 5-500 mg; **(Tylox) Cap:** 5-500 mg	**Adults: Pain:** Percocet (2.5-325 mg tab) 1-2 tabs q6h prn. (5-325 mg tab) 1 tab q6h prn. (7.5-500 mg tab) 1 tab q6h. (10-650 mg tab) 1 tab q6h. (7.5-325 mg tab) 1 tab q6h prn. **Max:** 8 tabs/d. (10-325 mg tab) 1 tab q6h prn. **Max:** 6 tabs/d. Do not exceed 4 gm APAP/d. **Roxicet:** (5-325 mg tab or 5-500 mg tab) 1 tab q6h prn. (5 mg-325 mg/5 ml) 5 ml q6h prn. **Tylox:** 1 cap q6h prn.	⊙C ✿>
Oxycodone HCl/Oxycodone Terephthalate/ASA CII (Percodan, Endodan)	**Tab:** 4.5 mg-0.38 mg-325 mg	**Adults: Pain: Usual:** 1 tab q6h prn. **Max:** 12 tabs/d.	⊙N ✿>
Pentazocine HCl/ASA CIV (Talwin Compound)	**Tab:** 12.5 mg-325 mg	**Adults & Peds:** ≥12 yo: **Pain: Usual:** 2 tabs tid-qid.	⊙N ✿>
Pentazocine/Naloxone HCl CIV (Talwin NX)	**Tab:** 50 mg-0.5 mg	**Adults & Peds:** ≥12 yo: **Pain: Initial:** 1 tab q3-4h. **Titrate:** Increase to 2 tabs prn when needed. **Max:** 12 tabs/d.	⊙C ✿> Not for injection.
Propoxyphene HCl/Caffeine/ASA CIV (Darvon Compound 32, Darvon Compound 65)	**Cap:** 32 mg-32.4 mg-389 mg; 65 mg-32.4 mg-389 mg	**Adults:** 1 cap q4h prn. **Max:** 390 mg propoxyphene HCl/d. **Elderly:** Increase dose interval.	⊙N ✿> H R
Propoxyphene Napsylate CIV (Darvon-N)	**Tab:** 100 mg	**Adults: Pain: Usual:** 100 mg q4h prn. **Max:** 600 mg/d.	⊙N ✿> H R

NAME	FORM/STRENGTH	DOSAGE	COMMENTS
Propoxyphene Napsylate/ APAP CIV (Darvocet A500)	**Tab:** 100 mg-500 mg	**Adults: Usual:** 1 tab q4h prn. **Max:** 6 tabs/24 hrs. **Elderly:** Increase dosing interval.	⊙N ❄> H R
Propoxyphene Napsylate/ APAP CIV (Darvocet-N 50, Darvocet-N 100)	**Tab:** 50 mg-325 mg; 100 mg-650 mg	**Adults: Pain: Usual:** 100 mg propoxyphene & 650 mg APAP q4h prn. **Max:** 600 mg/d of propoxyphene.	⊙N ❄> H R

NSAIDs

NAME	FORM/STRENGTH	DOSAGE	COMMENTS
Celecoxib (Celebrex)	**Cap:** 100 mg, 200 mg, 400 mg	**Adults: Acute Pain: Day 1:** 400 mg, then 200 mg if needed. **Maint:** 200 mg bid prn. **OA:** 200 mg qd or 100 mg bid. **RA:** 100-200 mg bid. **FAP:** 400 mg bid.	⊙C ❄v H
Diclofenac Potassium (Cataflam)	**Tab:** 50 mg	**Adults: Pain:** 50 mg tid or 100 mg x 1 dose, then 50 mg tid. **Max:** 150 mg/d (200 mg/d on d1). **OA:** 50 mg bid-tid. **Max:** 200 mg/d. **RA:** 50 mg tid-qid. **Max:** 225 mg/d.	⊙B ❄v
Diclofenac Sodium (Voltaren, Voltaren-XR)	**Tab,Enteric:** 25 mg, 50 mg, 75 mg; **Tab,ER:** 100 mg	**Adults: OA: Voltaren:** 50 mg bid-tid or 75 mg bid. **Voltaren-XR:** 100 mg qd. **RA: Voltaren:** 50 mg tid-qid or 75 mg bid. **Voltaren-XR:** 100 mg qd-bid. **Max:** 225 mg/d.	⊙B ❄v
Diclofenac Sodium/ Misoprostol (Arthrotec)	**Tab,Enteric:** 50 mg-0.2 mg, 75 mg-0.2 mg	**Adults: OA:** 50 mg tid. **RA:** 50 mg tid-qid. If intolerable, give 50-75 mg bid for OA or RA.	⊙X ❄v Misoprostol is an abortifacient.
Diflunisal (Dolobid)	**Tab:** 250 mg, 500 mg	**≥12 yo: Pain: Initial:** 1 gm, then 500 mg q8-12h. **OA/RA: Usual:** 250-500 mg bid. **Max:** 1500 mg/d.	⊙C ❄v

Etodolac (Lodine, Lodine XL)	(Lodine) Cap: 200 mg, 300 mg; Tab: 400 mg, 500 mg; (Lodine XL) Tab,ER: 400 mg, 500 mg, 600 mg	Adults: Lodine: Pain: Usual: 200-400 mg q6-8h. Max: 1200 mg/d. OA/RA: Usual: 300 mg bid-tid, or 400-500 mg bid. Max: 1200 mg/d. Lodine XL: OA/RA: Usual: 400-1000 mg qd. Max: 1200 mg/d.	◐C ✿v
Fenoprofen Calcium (Nalfon)	Cap: 200 mg, 300 mg; Tab: 600 mg	Adults: Pain: Usual: 200 mg q4-6h prn. OA/RA: Usual: 300-600 mg tid-qid. Max: 3200 mg/d.	◐N ✿>
Flurbiprofen (Ansaid)	Tab: 50 mg, 100 mg	Adults: OA/RA: 200-300 mg/d given as bid, tid, or qid. Max: 300 mg/d or 100 mg/dose.	◐B ✿v R
Ibuprofen (Infants' Motrin, Children's Motrin, Junior Strength Motrin, Motrin IB)	Drops: (Infants') 50 mg/1.25 ml; Susp: (Children's) 100 mg/5 ml; Tab: (Junior) 100 mg; Tab, Chewable: (Children's) 50 mg, (Junior) 100 mg; Tab: (Motrin IB) 200 mg	Infants': 6-11 mths (12-17 lbs): 1.25 ml (50 mg) q6-8h prn. 12-23 mths (18-23 lbs): 1.875 ml (75 mg) q6-8h prn. Children's/Junior: 2-3 yo (24-35 lbs):100 mg q6-8h prn. 4-5 yo (36-47 lbs): 150 mg q6-8h prn. 6-8 yo (48-59 lbs): 200 mg q6-8h prn. 9-10 yo (60-71 lbs): 250 mg q6-8h prn. 11 yo (72-95 lbs): 300 mg q6-8h prn. Max: 6 mths-11 yo: 4 doses/d. Motrin IB: ≥12 yo: 200 mg q4-6h while symptoms persist, may increase to 400 mg q4-6h. Max: 1200 mg/24h.	◐N ✿>
Ibuprofen (Motrin)	Susp: 100 mg/5 ml; Tab: 400 mg, 600 mg, 800 mg	Adults: OA/RA: 300 mg qid or 400-800 mg tid-qid. Pain: 400 mg q4-6h. ≥6 mths: JRA: 30-40 mg/kg/d given tid-qid. 20 mg/kg/d w/ milder disease. 6 mth-12 yo: Pain: 10 mg/kg q6-8h. Max: 40 mg/kg/d.	◐B ✿v R Avoid use during late pregnancy.

NAME	FORM/STRENGTH	DOSAGE	COMMENTS
Indomethacin (Indocin, Indocin SR)	**Cap:** 25 mg, 50 mg; **Cap,ER:** 75 mg; **Sup:** 50 mg; **Susp:** 25 mg/5 ml	**≥14 yo: Indocin: RA/OA: Initial:** 25 mg PO bid-tid. **Titrate:** Increase by 25-50 mg/d wkly. **Max:** 200 mg/d. **Bursitis/Tendinitis:** 75-150 mg/d given tid-qid x 7-14d. **Acute Gouty Arthritis:** 50 mg PO tid until tolerable, then d/c. **Indocin SR: RA/OA: Initial:** 75 mg qd. **Maint:** 75 mg bid. Take w/food.	●N ❄v
Ketoprofen (Oruvail)	**Cap:** 50 mg, 75 mg; **Cap,ER:** (Oruvail) 100 mg, 150 mg, 200 mg	**Adults: Cap: Pain:** 25-50 mg q6-8h prn. **Max:** 300 mg/d. **OA/RA:** 75 mg tid or 50 mg qid. **Max:** 300 mg/d. **Oruvail: OA/RA:** 200 mg qd.	●B ❄v H R
Ketorolac Tromethamine (Toradol)	**Inj:** 15 mg/ml, 30 mg/ml; **Tab:** 10 mg	**16 to <65 yo: Single Dose:** 60 mg IM or 30 mg IV. **Multiple Dose:** 30 mg IV/IM q6h. **Max:** 120 mg/d. **Transition from IV/IM to PO:** 20 mg PO, then 10 mg PO q4-6h. **Max:** 40 mg/24h. **≥65 yo or <50 kg: Single Dose:** 30 mg IM or 15 mg IV. **Multiple Dose:** 15 mg IV/IM q6h. **Max:** 60 mg/d. **Transition from IV/IM to PO:** 10 mg PO q4-6h. **Max:** 40 mg/24h. Max duration is 5d.	●C ❄v R CI in PUD, hx of GI bleeding, advanced renal impairment, cerebrovascular bleeding, hemorrhagic diathesis, incomplete hemostasis, intrathecal/epidural use, labor/delivery & nursing & with ASA/NSAIDs.
Meclofenamate Sodium	**Cap:** 50 mg, 100 mg	**≥14 yo: Pain: Usual:** 50-100 mg q4-6h. **Max:** 400 mg/d. **RA/OA:** 200-400 mg/d as tid-qid.	●N ❄v

Drug	Form	Dosage	
Mefenamic Acid (Ponstel)	**Cap:** 250 mg	**≥14 yo: Pain:** 500 mg, then 250 mg q6h prn, up to 1 wk.	⊕C ❄v
Meloxicam (Mobic)	**Tab:** 7.5 mg	**≥18 yo: OA: Initial/Maint:** 7.5 mg qd. **Max:** 15 mg/d.	⊕C ❄v
Nabumetone (Relafen)	**Tab:** 500 mg, 750 mg	**Adults: OA/RA: Initial:** 1 gm qd. **Usual:** 1.5-2 gm/d as qd-bid. **Max:** 2 gm/d.	⊕C ❄v
Naproxen (Naprosyn, EC-Naprosyn)	**Susp:** 25 mg/ml; **Tab:** 250 mg, 375 mg, 500 mg; **Tab,Enteric:** 375 mg, 500 mg	**Adults: RA/OA/Ankylosing Spondylitis: Naprosyn:** 250-500 mg bid. **EC-Naprosyn:** 375-500 mg bid. **Acute Gout: Naprosyn: Initial:** 750 mg, then 250 mg q8h. **JRA:** ≥2 yo: 5 mg/kg of naproxen bid.	⊕B ❄v
Naproxen Sodium (Anaprox, Anaprox DS, Naprelan)	**Tab:** (Anaprox) 275 mg; (Anaprox DS) 550 mg; **Tab,ER:** (Naprelan) 375 mg, 500 mg	**Adults: RA/OA/Ankylosing Spondylitis: Tab:** 275 mg-550 mg bid. **Tab,ER:** 750-1000 mg qd. **Max:** 1500 mg/d. **Pain/Tendinitis/Bursitis: Tab: Initial:** 550 mg, then 550 mg q12h or 275 mg q6-8h prn. **Max:** 1100 mg/d for maint. **Tab,ER: Intial:** 1000-1500 mg qd. **Max:** 1000 mg/d for maint. **Acute Gout: Tab:** 825 mg, then 275 mg q8h. **Tab,ER:** 1000-1500 gm on day 1, then 1000 mg qd. **JRA:** ≥2 yo: **Tab:** 5 mg/kg of naproxen bid.	⊕B ❄v
Oxaprozin (Daypro)	**Tab:** 600 mg	**Adults: OA:** 600-1200 mg qd. **Max:** 1800 mg/d. **RA:** 1200 mg qd. **Max:** 1800 mg/d. **Peds: 6-16 yo: JRA:** ≥55 kg: 1200 mg qd. **32-54 kg:** 900 mg qd. **22-31 kg:** 600 mg qd.	⊕C ❄> R
Piroxicam (Feldene)	**Cap:** 10 mg, 20 mg	**Adults: OA/RA:** 20 mg qd or 10 mg bid.	⊕C ❄v

NAME	FORM/STRENGTH	DOSAGE	COMMENTS
Rofecoxib (Vioxx)	Susp: 12.5 mg/5 ml, 25 mg/5 ml; Tab: 12.5 mg, 25 mg, 50 mg	≥18 yo: Acute Pain: 50 mg qd prn up to 5d. OA: Initial: 12.5 mg qd. Max: 25 mg/d. RA: 25 mg qd.	◑C ❄v H
Sulindac (Clinoril)	Tab: 150 mg, 200 mg	Adults: Pain/Gouty Arthritis: 200 mg bid. OA/RA: 150 mg bid. Max: 400 mg/d.	◑N ❄v
Tolmetin Sodium (Tolectin DS, Tolectin)	Cap: (Tolectin DS) 400 mg; Tab: (Tolectin) 600 mg	Adults: OA/RA: 400 mg tid. Max: 1800 mg/d. Peds: ≥2 yo: JRA: Initial: 20 mg/kg/d given tid-qid. Usual: 15-30 mg/kg/d given tid-qid.	◑C ❄v
Valdecoxib (Bextra)	Tab: 10 mg, 20 mg	≥18 yo: OA/RA: 10 mg qd.	◑C ❄v

Salicylates

NAME	FORM/STRENGTH	DOSAGE	COMMENTS
Aspirin (Bayer Aspirin)	Chewtab: 81 mg; Tab: 81 mg, 325 mg, 500 mg; Tab,Enteric: 81 mg, 325 mg	≥12 yo: Pain: 325-1000 mg q4-6h prn. Max: 4 gm/d.	◑N ❄> H R Avoid use during 3rd trimester.
Choline Magnesium Trisalicylate (Trilisate)	Liq: 500 mg/5 ml; Tab: 500 mg, 750 mg, 1000 mg	Adults: Pain: OA/RA: 1500 mg bid or 3000 mg qhs (not including elderly). Peds: 12-37 kg: 50 mg/kg/d as bid. >37 kg: 2250 mg/d as bid.	◑C ❄> R
Salsalate (Disalcid, Salflex)	Tab: 500 mg, 750 mg	Adults: Usual: 1000 mg tid or 1500 mg bid.	◑C ❄>

Miscellaneous

Acetaminophen (Tylenol Children's, Tylenol Extra Strength, Tylenol Infants', Tylenol Junior, Tylenol Regular Strength)	**Drops:** (Infants') 80 mg/0.8 ml; **Sol:** (Extra Strength) 500 mg/15 ml; **Susp:** (Children's) 160 mg/5 ml; **Tab:** (Regular Strength) 325 mg, (Extra Strength) 500 mg; **Tab, Chewable:** (Children's) 80 mg, (Junior) 160 mg	**Pediatric: Max:** 5 doses/d. **0-3 mths (6-11 lbs):** 40 mg q4h prn. **4-11 mths (12-17 lbs):** 80 mg q4h prn. **12-23 mths (18-23 lbs):** 120 mg q4h prn. **2-3 yo (24-35 lbs):** 160 mg q4h prn. **4-5 yo (36-47 lbs):** 240 mg q4h prn. **6-8 yo (48-59 lbs):** 320 mg q4h prn. **9-10 yo (60-71 lbs):** 400 mg q4h prn. **11 yo (72-95 lbs):** 480 mg q4h prn. **12 yo:** 640 mg q4h prn. **Older Children/Adults: Regular Strength: 6-11 yo:** 325 mg q4-6h prn. **Max:** 1625 mg/d. **≥12 yo:** 650 mg q4-6h prn **Max:** 3900 mg/d. **Extra Strength: ≥12 yo:** 1000 mg q4-6h prn. **Max:** 4000 mg/d.	◐N ✿>
Gabapentin (Neurontin)	**Cap:** 100 mg, 300 mg, 400 mg; **Sol:** 250 mg/5 ml; **Tab:** 600 mg, 800 mg	**Postherpetic Neuralgia: Adults:** 300 mg single dose on d1, then 300 mg bid on d2, and 300 mg tid on d3. Increase further prn pain. **Max:** 600 mg tid.	◐C ✿> R
Tramadol HCl (Ultram)	**Tab:** 50 mg	**Chronic Pain: ≥17 yo: Initial:** 25 mg qam. **Titrate:** Increase by 25 mg/d q3d to 25 mg qid, then by 50 mg/d q3d to 50 mg qid. **Maint:** 50-100 mg q4-6h prn. **Max:** 400 mg/d.	◐C ✿v H R
Tramadol HCl/APAP (Ultracet)	**Tab:** 37.5-325 mg	**≥16 yo: Acute Pain:** 2 tabs q4-6h, up to 5d. **Max:** 8 tabs/d.	◐C ✿v H R

NAME	FORM/STRENGTH	DOSAGE	COMMENTS

ANTI-INFECTIVES

AIDS Therapy

FUSION INHIBITORS

Name	Form/Strength	Dosage	Comments
Enfuvirtide (Fuzeon)	**Inj:** 90 mg/ml	**Adults:** 90 mg SC bid. **Peds: 6-16 yo:** 2 mg/kg SC bid. **Max:** 90 mg bid. Inject into the upper arm, anterior thigh, or abdomen.	◨B ❄v

NON-NUCLEOSIDE REVERSE TRANSCRIPTASE INHIBITORS

Name	Form/Strength	Dosage	Comments
Delavirdine Mesylate (Rescriptor)	**Tab:** 100 mg, 200 mg	**≥16 yo:** 400 mg tid.	◨C ❄v
Efavirenz (Sustiva)	**Cap:** 50 mg, 100 mg, 200 mg; **Tab:** 600 mg	**Adults:** 600 mg qd. **≥3 yo: 10-40 kg:** 200-600 mg qd. **>40 kg:** 600 mg qd.	◨C ❄v Avoid high fat meals.
Nevirapine (Viramune)	**Tab:** 200 mg; **Susp:** 50 mg/5 ml	**Adults: Initial:** 200 mg qd x 14d. **Maint:** 200 mg bid. **Peds: 2 mths-8 yo: Initial:** 4 mg/kg qd x 14d. **Maint:** 7 mg/kg qd. **≥8 yo: Initial:** 4 mg/kg qd x 14d. **Maint:** 4 mg/kg bid.	◨C ❄v H Severe hypersensitivity & skin reactions. Hepatotoxicity.

NUCLEOSIDE REVERSE TRANSCRIPTASE INHIBITORS

Name	Form/Strength	Dosage	Comments
Abacavir Sulfate (Ziagen)	**Sol:** 20 mg/ml; **Tab:** 300 mg	**Adults:** 300 mg bid. **Peds: 3 mths-16 yo: Usual:** 8 mg/kg bid. **Max:** 300 mg bid.	◨C ❄v Fatal hypersensitivity reactions. Lactic acidosis. Hepatomegaly.

Abacavir/Lamivudine/ Zidovudine (Trizivir)	**Tab:** 300 mg-150 mg-300 mg	**>40 kg:** 1 tab bid. Avoid in patients <40 kg.	◉C ❄v R Fatal hypersensitivity reactions. Hematologic toxicity. Lactic acidosis. Hepatomegaly.
Didanosine (Videx, Videx EC, Videx Pediatric)	**(Videx) Chewtab:** 25 mg, 50 mg, 100 mg, 150 mg, 200 mg; **Sol (powder in pkt):** 100 mg, 167 mg, 250 mg; **(Videx EC) Cap,Delay:**125 mg, 200 mg, 250 mg, 400 mg; **(Videx Pediatric) Sol:** 10 mg/ml	**Adults: ≥60 kg: Videx: Chewtab:** 200 mg bid or 400 mg qd. **Sol:** 250 mg bid. **Videx EC:** 400 mg qd. **<60 kg: Chewtab:** 125 mg bid or 250 mg qd. **Sol:** 167 mg bid. **Videx EC:** 250 mg qd. **Peds:** 120 mg/m² bid. Take on empty stomach.	◉B ❄v R Pancreatitis. Peripheral neuropathy. Lactic acidosis. Hepatomegaly.
Emtricitabine (Emtriva)	**Cap:** 200 mg	**Adults: ≥18 yrs:** 200 mg qd.	◉B ❄v R Lactic acidosis. Hepatomegaly.
Lamivudine (Epivir)	**Sol:** 10 mg/ml; **Tab:** 150 mg, 300 mg	**Adults:** 150 mg bid or 300 mg qd. **Peds: 3 mth-16 yo: Usual:** 4 mg/kg bid. **Max:** 150 mg bid.	◉B ❄v R Lactic acidosis. Hepatomegaly.

NAME	FORM/STRENGTH	DOSAGE	COMMENTS
Lamivudine/Zidovudine (Combivir)	**Tab:** 150 mg-300 mg	≥**12 yo:** 1 tab bid.	⊙C ❄v H R Lactic acidosis. Hepatomegaly. Hematologic toxicity. Symptomatic myopathy.
Stavudine (Zerit)	**Cap:** 15 mg, 20 mg, 30 mg, 40 mg; **Sol:** 1 mg/ml	**Adults:** <60 kg: 30 mg bid. ≥**60 kg:** 40 mg bid. **Peds: Birth-13d:** 0.5 mg/kg q12h. ≥**14d and <30 kg:** 1 mg/kg q12h. >**30 kg:** Adult dose.	⊙C ❄v R Lactic acidosis. Hepatomegaly. Pancreatitis.
Zalcitabine (Hivid)	**Tab:** 0.375 mg, 0.75 mg	≥**13 yo:** 0.75 mg q8h.	⊙C ❄v H R Peripheral neuropathy. Pancreatitis. Lactic acidosis. Hepatomegaly.
Zidovudine (Retrovir)	**Cap:** 100 mg; **Tab:** 300 mg; **Syr:** 50 mg/5 ml; **Inj:** 10 mg/ml	**Adults:** 600 mg/d PO in divided doses or 1 mg/kg IV 5-6x/d. **Peds: 6 wks-12 yo:** 160 mg/m² PO q8h. **Maternal-Fetal Transmission:** 100 mg PO 5x/d until labor, then 2 mg/kg IV, then 1 mg/kg/h until umbilical cord clamped. **Neonatal:** 2 mg/kg PO or 1.5 mg/kg IV q6h until 6 wks old. Start 12h after birth.	⊙C ❄v H R Hematologic toxicity. Symptomatic myopathy. Lactic acidosis. Hepatomegaly.

NUCLEOTIDE REVERSE TRANSCRIPTASE INHIBITORS

Tenofovir Disoproxil (Viread)	**Tab:** 300 mg	**Adults:** 300 mg qd with a meal.	⊕B ❀v

PROTEASE INHIBITORS

Amprenavir (Agenerase)	**Cap:** 50 mg, 150 mg; **Sol:** 15 mg/ml	**≥13 yo or ≥50kg: Cap** 1200 mg bid. **Sol:** 1400 mg bid. **4-12 yo or <50 kg: Cap:** 20 mg/kg bid or 15 mg/kg tid. **Sol:** 22.5 mg/kg bid or 17 mg/kg tid. **Max:** 2400 mg/d. **Sol:** 22.5 mg/kg bid or 17 mg/kg tid. **Max:** 2800 mg/d. Sol & cap are not interchangeable. Avoid high fat meals and Vitamin E.	⊕C (Cap) Sol CI in pregnancy. ❀v **H R** (Sol) Sol contains propylene glycol.
Atazanavir Sulfate (Reyataz)	**Cap:** 100 mg, 150 mg, 200 mg	**Adults:** 400 mg qd with food. **Concomitant Efavirenz:** Give atazanavir 300 mg and ritonavir 100 mg with efavirenz 600 mg qd with food. **Concomitant Buffered Didanosine:** Give atazanavir 2 hrs before or 1 hr after didanosine.	⊕B ❀v **H**
Fosamprenavir Calcium (Lexiva)	**Tab:** 700 mg	**Adults: Therapy-naive:** 1400 mg bid OR 1400 mg qd + ritonavir 200 mg qd OR 700 mg bid + ritonavir 100 mg bid. **PI-Experienced:** 700 mg bid + ritonavir 100 mg bid.	⊕C ❀v **H**
Indinavir Sulfate (Crixivan)	**Cap:** 100 mg, 200 mg, 333 mg, 400 mg	**Adults:** 800 mg q8h with water. Hydrate to prevent nephrolithiasis/urolithiasis.	⊕C ❀v **H**

NAME	FORM/STRENGTH	DOSAGE	COMMENTS
Lopinavir/Ritonavir (Kaletra)	**Cap:** 133.3-33.3 mg; **Sol:** 80-20 mg/ml	**Adults: Caps/Sol:** 3 caps or 5 ml bid w/ food. **Peds: Sol: 6 mths-12 yo: 7 to <15 kg:** 12 mg/kg bid. **15-40 kg:** 10 mg/kg bid. **>12 yo or >40 kg:** Adult dose. Dose based on lopinavir. **Concomitant efavirenz or nevirapine: Adults: Caps/Sol:** 4 caps or 6.5 ml bid. **Peds: Sol: 6 mths-12 yo: 7 to <15 kg:** 13 mg/kg bid. **15-45 kg:** 11 mg/kg bid. **>12 yo or >45 kg:** Adult dose. Take w/ food. Dose based on lopinavir.	◑C ✿v
Nelfinavir Mesylate (Viracept)	**Powder (susp):** 50 mg/gm; **Tab:** 250 mg, 625 mg	**Adults:** 1250 mg bid or 750 mg tid. **2-13 yo:** 20-30 mg/kg tid. Take with food.	◑B ✿v
Ritonavir (Norvir)	**Cap:** 100 mg; **Sol:** 80 mg/ml	**Adults: Initial:** 300 mg bid & increase q2-3d by 100 mg bid. **Maint:** 600 mg bid. **Concomitant Saquinavir:** Better tolerated with 400 mg bid. **Peds: ≥2 yo: Initial:** 250 mg/m² bid & increase q2-3d by 50 mg/m². **Maint:** 400 mg/m² bid. **Max:** 600 mg bid. Take with food.	◑B ✿v Avoid certain antihistamines, sedative hypnotics, antiarrhythmics, or ergot alkaloids.
Saquinavir (Fortovase)	**Cap:** 200 mg	≥16 yo: 1200 mg tid with food or up to 2h after a meal.	◑B ✿v
Saquinavir Mesylate (Invirase)	**Cap:** 200 mg	>16 yo: 1000 mg bid with ritonavir 100 mg bid. Take within 2h after full meal.	◑B ✿v Invirase and Fortovase are not bioequivalent.

Antiviral Agents

ANTI-CYTOMEGALOVIRUS AGENTS

Drug	Formulation	Dosing	Notes
Cidofovir (Vistide)	**Inj:** 75 mg/ml	**Adults & Peds: CMV Retinitis: Induction:** 5 mg/kg qwk x 2wks. **Maint:** 5 mg/kg q2wks. Patients must receive hydration and probenecid with each dose.	⊕C ❀v R Neutropenia. Renal impairment. Carcinogenic, teratogenic & hypospermia in animal studies.
Fomivirsen Sodium (Vitravene)	**Inj:** 6.6 mg/ml	**Adults: CMV Retinitis: Induction:** 330 mcg (0.05 ml) intravitreal every other wk x 2 doses. **Maint:** 330 mcg (0.05 ml) intravitreal q4wks.	⊕C ❀v
Foscarnet Sodium (Foscavir)	**Inj:** 24 mg/ml	**Adults & Peds: CMV Retinitis: Induction:** 90 mg/kg q12h or 60 mg/kg q8h. **Maint:** 90-120 mg/kg/d. Should hydrate patient.	⊕C ❀> R Renal impairment. Seizures.
Ganciclovir (Cytovene)	**Cap:** 250 mg, 500 mg	**Adults & Peds: CMV Disease Prevention in Advanced HIV (at risk) or Transplant Patients:** 1000 mg tid. **Alternative to IV for CMV Retinitis Treatment in Immunocompromised Patients:** 1000 mg tid or 500 mg 6x/d q3h. Take with food.	⊕C ❀v R [12]

[12] Granulocytopenia. Anemia. Thrombocytopenia. Carcinogenic, teratogenic & aspermatogenic in animal studies.

NAME	FORM/STRENGTH	DOSAGE	COMMENTS
Ganciclovir Sodium (Cytovene-IV)	**Inj:** 500 mg/10 ml	**Adults & Peds: Treatment of CMV Retinitis in Immunocomprimised Patients: Induction:** 5 mg/kg q12h x 14-21d. **Maint:** 5 mg/kg qd x 7d/wk or 6 mg/kg qd x 5d/wk. **Prevention of CMV Disease in Transplant Patients (at risk): Initial:** 5 mg/kg q12h x 7-14d. **Maint:** 5 mg/kg qd x 7d/wk or 6 mg/kg qd x 5d/wk.	●C ❀v R [12]
Ganciclovir (Vitrasert)	**Implant:** 4.5 mg	**≥9 yo: CMV Retinitis: Treatment:** Each implant releases the drug over 5-8 mths; may remove or replace after depletion.	●C ❀v
Valganciclovir (Valcyte)	**Tab:** 450 mg	**Adults: CMV Retinitis: Induction:** 900 mg bid x 21d. **Maint:** 900 mg qd. **Prevention of CMV Disease in High-Risk Kidney, Heart, & Kidney-Pancreas Transplant Patients:** 900 mg qd within 10 days of transplant until 100 days posttransplant. Take with food.	●C ❀v R Follow exact dosing guidelines. [12]

HEPATITIS

NAME	FORM/STRENGTH	DOSAGE	COMMENTS
Adefovir Dipivoxil (Hepsera)	**Tab:** 10 mg	**Adults:** 10 mg qd.	●C ❀v R Monitor hepatic function after D/C. Monitor for nephrotoxicity if, or at risk of, renal dysfunction. HIV resistance. Lactic Acidosis. Hepatomegaly

Hepatitis A Inactivated/ Hepatitis B Recombinant (Twinrix)	**Inj:** 720 U-20 mcg	**Adults:** 1 ml IM at 0-, 1- and 6-mth schedule.	◐C ✿>
Hepatitis B Vaccine, Recombinant (Engerix-B, Recombivax HB)	**Inj:** (Engerix-ped) 10 mcg/0.5 ml, (Recombivax HB-ped) 5 mcg/0.5 ml, (Engerix-adult) 20 mcg/ml, (Recombivax HB adult) 10 mcg/ml	**Engerix: >19 yo:** 20 mcg/ml IM at 0, 1, 6 mths. **≤19 yo:** 10 mcg/0.5ml IM at 0, 1, 6 mths. **Booster: ≥11 yo:** 20 mcg IM. **≤10 yo:** 10 mcg IM. **Recombivax: ≥20 yo:** 10 mcg IM at 0, 1, 6 mths. **0-19 yo:** 5 mcg IM at 0, 1, 6 mths.	◐C ✿>
Interferon alfa-2a (Roferon-A)	**Inj:** 3 MIU, 6 MIU, 9 MIU, 36 MIU	**HCV: ≥18 yo:** IM/SC: 3 MIU TIW x 12 mths or 6 MIU TIW x 3 mths, then 3 MIU TIW x 9 mths.	◐C ✿v [13]
Interferon alfa-2b (Intron-A)	**Inj:** 10 MIU/0.2 ml, 3 MIU/0.2 ml, 5 MIU/ 0.2 ml, 10 MIU/ml, 6 MIU/ml, 3 MIU/0.5 ml, 5 MIU/0.5 ml, 3 MIU, 5 MIU, 10 MIU, 18 MIU, 25 MIU, 50 MIU	**HCV: Adults:** 3 MIU IM/SC TIW x 18-24 mths. **HBV: Adults:** 5 MIU IM/SC qd or 10 MIU TIW x 16 wks. **Peds:** 3 MIU/m² IM/SC TIW x 1 wk, then 6 MIU/m² TIW x 15-23 wks. **Max:** 10 MIU/m² TIW. Adjust based on WBC, granulocyte, and/or platelet counts.	◐C ✿v [13]
Interferon alphacon-1 (Infergen)	**Inj:** 30 mcg/ml	**HCV: ≥18 yo:** 9 mcg SC TIW x 24 wks, then 15 mcg SC TIW x 6 mths if needed.	◐C ✿>

[12] Granulocytopenia. Anemia. Thrombocytopenia. Carcinogenic, teratogenic & aspermatogenic in animal studies.
[13] May cause or aggravate neuropsychiatric, autoimmune, ischemic, & infectious disorders.

NAME	FORM/STRENGTH	DOSAGE	COMMENTS
Lamivudine (Epivir HBV)	**Sol:** 5 mg/ml; **Tab:** 100 mg	**Adults: HBV:** 100 mg qd. **Peds: 2-17 yo:** 3 mg/kg qd. **Max:** 100 mg/d.	●C ❉v R Lactic acidosis. Hepatomegaly.
Peginterferon alfa-2a (Pegasys)	**Inj:** 180 mcg/0.5 ml, 180 mcg/ml	**HCV:** ≥18 yo: **Monotherapy:** 180 mcg SC once wkly x 48 wks. Adjust dose by neutrophils, platelets, severity of depression, and renal or hepatic function. **With Copegus:** ≥18 yo: 180 mcg SC once wkly x 48 wks for genotypes 1,4; x 24 wks for genotypes 2,3.	●C ❉v H R [13]
Peginterferon alfa-2b (Peg-Intron)	**Inj:** 100 mcg/ml, 160 mcg/ml, 240 mcg/ml, 300 mcg/ml	**HCV:** ≥18 yo: Administer SC once wkly x 1 yr. **Monotherapy: 50 mcg/0.5 ml vial: ≤45 kg:** 40 mcg (0.4 ml); **46-56 kg:** 50 mcg (0.5 ml). **80 mcg/0.5 ml vial: 57-72 kg:** 64 mcg (0.4 ml); **73-88 kg:** 80 mcg (0.5 ml). **120 mcg/0.5 ml vial: 89-106 kg:** 96 mcg (0.4 ml); **107-136 kg:** 120 mcg (0.5 ml). **150 mcg/0.5 ml vial: 137-160 kg:** 150 mcg (0.5 ml). **With Rebetol: 50 mcg/0.5 ml vial: <40 kg:** 50 mcg (0.5 ml). **80 mcg/0.5 ml vial: 40-50 kg:** 64 mcg (0.4 ml); **51-60 kg:** 80 mcg (0.5 ml). **120 mcg/0.5 ml vial: 61-75 kg:** 96 mcg (0.4 ml); **76-85 kg:** 120 mcg (0.5 ml). **150 mcg/0.5 ml vial: >85 kg:** 150 mcg (0.5 ml). Dose varies based on weight, WBC, platelets, neutrophils and/or severity of depression .	●C ❉v [13]

Ribavirin (Copegus)	Tab: 200 mg	HCV: ≥18 yo With PEGASYS: Genotypes 1,4: <75 kg: 500 mg bid x 48 wks. ≥75 kg: 600 mg bid x 48 wks. Genotypes 2,3: 400 mg bid x 24 wks. Dosage adjustment/discontinuation based on cardiovascular status, Hgb, renal function.	⊗X ✿v R CI in pregnancy, male partners of pregnant females, & significant cardiac disease. Hemolytic anemia.
Ribavirin (Rebetol)	Cap: 200 mg; Sol: 40 mg/ml	Adults: With INTRON A: ≤75 kg: 400 mg qam and 600 mg qpm. >75 kg: 600 mg qam & 600 mg qpm. Treat x 24-48 wks if no prior interferon (IFN) therapy and x 24 wks if prior IFN therapy. With PEG-INTRON: 400g bid, qam & qpm with food. Dose based on Hgb and cardiac history. Peds: ≥3 yrs: 15 mg/kg/day in divided doses qam and qpm. Use sol if =25 kg or cannot swallow caps. With INTRON A: 25-36 kg: 200 mg bid, qam & qpm. 37-49 kg: 200 mg qam and 400 mg qpm. 50-61kg: 400 mg bid, qam and qpm. >61kg: Dose as adult. Genotype 1: Treat for 48 wks. Genotype 2/3: Treat for 24 wks.	⊗X ✿v R CI in pregnancy, male partners of pregnant females, & significant cardiac disease. Hemolytic anemia.
Ribavirin/Interferon alfa-2b (Rebetron)	KIT (Inj-Cap): 200 mg-3 MIU/0.2 ml, 200 mg-3 MIU/0.5 ml	HCV: ≥18 yo: ≤75 kg: 3 MIU SC TIW with 400 mg PO qam & 600 mg PO qpm. >75 kg: 3 MIU SC TIW with 600 mg PO bid. Adjust based on cardiac history, Hgb, neutrophil, platelet and/or WBC count.	⊗X ✿v R CI in pregnancy & male partners of pregnant females.

[13] May cause or aggravate neuropsychiatric, autoimmune, ischemic, & infectious disorders.

NAME	FORM/STRENGTH	DOSAGE	COMMENTS
HERPES INFECTION			
Acyclovir Sodium (Zovirax)	**Inj:** 25 mg/ml, 50 mg/ml	**Herpes Simplex:** <12 yo: 10 mg/kg IV q8h x 7d. **Genital Herpes:** 5 mg/kg IV q8h x 5d. **Encephalitis:** >12 yo: 10 mg/kg IV q8h x 10d. <12 yo: 20 mg/kg IV q8h x 10d. **Zoster:** >12 yo: 10 mg/kg IV q8h x 7d. <12 yo: 20 mg/kg IV q8h x 7d. **Birth-3 mths:** 10 mg/kg IV q8h x 7d.	⊞B ✿ < R
Acyclovir (Zovirax)	**Cap:** 200 mg; **Tab:** 400 mg, 800 mg; **Susp:** 200 mg/5 ml	**Zoster:** 800 mg 5x/d x 7-10d. **Genital Herpes: Initial:** 200 mg 5x/d x 10d. **Maint:** 400 mg bid or 200 mg 3-5x/d x 1yr or 200 mg 5x/d x 5d. **Recurrent:** 200 mg 5x/d x 5d. **Varicella:** ≥2 yo: <40 kg: 20 mg/kg qid x 5d. >40 kg: 800 mg qid x 5d.	⊞B ✿ < R
Acyclovir (Zovirax)	**Oint:** 5%	**Adults: Herpes Genitalis/Herpes Labialis:** Apply q3h, 6x/d x 7d. Initiate with 1st sign/symptom.	⊞B ✿ <
Famciclovir (Famvir)	**Tab:** 125 mg, 250 mg, 500 mg	≥18 yo: **Zoster:** 500 mg q8h x 7d. **Genital Herpes: Recurrent:** 125 mg bid x 5d. **Suppression:** 250 mg bid up to 1yr. **Recurrent Orolabial or Genital Herpes in HIV Patients:** 500 mg bid x 7d.	⊞B ✿ < R
Valacyclovir HCl (Valtrex)	**Tab:** 500 mg, 1 gm	**Adults & Post-Pubertal Peds: Zoster:** 1 gm tid x 7d. **Genital Herpes: Initial:** 1 gm bid x 10d. **Recurrent:** 500 mg bid x 3d. **Suppressive:** (≤9 episodes/yr) 500 mg qd or (>9 episodes/yr) 1000 mg qd, up to 1yr. **Suppressive Therapy with HIV and CD4 ≥100cells/mm³:** 500 mg bid, up to 6 mths. **Labialis:** 2 g q12h x 1d. Start at earliest symptom.	⊞B ✿ < R

Drug	Formulation	Dosing	Ratings
Amantadine HCl (Symmetrel)	**Tab:** 100 mg; **Syr:** 50 mg/5 ml	**Influenza A Prophylaxis & Treatment: Adults** 200 mg qd or 100 mg bid. **≥65 yo:** 100 mg qd. **Peds: 9-12 yo:** 100 mg bid. **1-9 yo:** 4.4-8.8 mg/kg/d. **Max:** 150 mg/d.	●C ❀v R
Oseltamivir Phosphate (Tamiflu)	**Cap:** 75 mg; **Susp:** 12 mg/ml	**Treatment: ≥13 yo: Cap/Susp:** 75 mg bid x 5d, begin within 2d of symptom onset. **≥1 yo: Susp: ≤15 kg:** 30 mg bid x 5d. **>15-23 kg:** 45 mg bid x 5d. **>23-40 kg:** 60 mg bid x 5d. **>40 kg:** 75 mg bid x 5d. **Prophylaxis: ≥13 yo: Cap/Susp:** Begin within 2d of exposure. 75 mg qd for at least 7d, up to 6 wks in community outbreak.	●C ❀> R
Rimantadine HCl (Flumadine)	**Tab:** 100 mg; **Syr:** 50 mg/5 ml	**Influenza A: Prophylaxis: ≥10 yo:** 100 mg bid. **<10 yo:** 5 mg/kg qd. **Max:** 150 mg/d. **Treatment: Adults:** 100 mg bid; begin within 48h of symptom onset & treat x 7d from initial symptom onset.	●C ❀v H R
Zanamivir (Relenza)	**Disk:** 4 mg/inh	**Adults & Peds: ≥7 yo: Treatment:** 2 inh q12h x 5d.	●C ❀>

Bone and Joint Infection

AMINOGLYCOSIDES

Drug	Formulation	Dosing	Ratings
Amikacin Sulfate (Amikin)	**Inj:** 50 mg/ml, 250 mg/ml	**IM/IV: Adults, Children & Older Infants:** 7.5 mg/kg q12h or 5 mg/kg IM/IV q8h. **Max:** 1.5 gm/d **Newborns: LD:** 10 mg/kg. **Maint:** 7.5 mg/kg q12h.	●D ❀v R [1]

[1] Potential neurotoxicity, ototoxicity & neuromuscular blockade. Avoid concurrent use with neurotoxic/nephrotoxic agents & diuretics.

NAME	FORM/STRENGTH	DOSAGE	COMMENTS
Gentamicin Sulfate (Garamycin)	**Inj:** 40 mg/ml	**IM/IV: Adults:** 3 mg/kg/d given q8h. **Max:** 5 mg/kg/d in 3-4 doses. Reduce to 3 mg/kg/d as soon as clinically indicated. **Peds:** 2-2.5 mg/kg q8h. **Infants/Neonates:** 2.5 mg/kg q8h. **≤1 wk:** 2.5 mg/kg q12h.	⬛N ✽> R [1]
Tobramycin Sulfate (Nebcin)	**Inj:** 10 mg/ml, 40 mg/ml, 1.2 gm	**IM/IV: Adults:** 3 mg/kg/d given q8h. **Max:** 5 mg/kg/d in 3-4 doses. Reduce to 3 mg/kg/d as soon as clinically indicated. **Peds: >1 wk:** 2-2.5 mg/kg q8h or 1.5-1.89 mg/kg q6h. **≤1 wk:** Up to 2 mg/kg q12h.	⬛D ✽> R [1]

CEPHALOSPORINS

NAME	FORM/STRENGTH	DOSAGE	COMMENTS
Cefamandole Nafate (Mandol)	**Inj:** 1 gm, 2 gm	**IM/IV: Adults:** 1 gm q4-6h. **Max:** 12 gm/d. **Infants & Peds:** 50-100 mg/kg/d given q4-8h. **Max:** 150 mg/kg/d, not to exceed 12 gm/d.	⬛B ✽> R
Cefazolin (Ancef, Kefzol)	**Inj:** 500 mg/50 ml, 1 gm/50 ml, 500 mg, 1 gm, 10 gm, 20 gm	**IM/IV: Adults: Usual:** 500 mg-1 gm q6-8h. **Peds: Usual:** 25-50 mg/kg/d given as tid-qid. **Max:** 100 mg/kg/d.	⬛B ✽> R Safety in prematures & neonates not known.
Cefotaxime Sodium (Claforan)	**Inj:** 500 mg, 1 gm, 2 gm, 10 gm	**IM/IV: Adults & Peds ≥50kg:** 1-2 gm q8h. **Max:** 12 gm/d. **1 mth-12 yo: <50 kg:** 50-180 mg/kg/d divided into 4-6 doses. **1-4 wks:** 50 mg/kg IV q8h. **0-1 wk:** 50 mg/kg IV q12h.	⬛B ✽> R
Cefotetan Disodium (Cefotan)	**Inj:** 1 gm, 1 gm/50 ml, 2 gm, 2 gm/50 ml, 10 gm	**IM/IV: Adults:** 1-2 gm q12h. **Max:** 6 gm/d.	⬛B ✽> R

Cefoxitin (Mefoxin)	Inj: 1 gm, 1 gm/50 ml, 2 gm, 2 gm/50 ml, 10 gm	IV: Adults: 1 gm q4h or 2 gm q6-8h. Peds: ≥3 mths: 80-160 mg/kg/d given as q4-6h. Max: 12 gm/d.	B ❄> R
Ceftazidime (Ceptaz, Fortaz, Tazicef)	Inj: 500 mg, 1 gm, 2 gm, 6 gm, 10 gm	IV: Fortaz/Tazicef: Adults: 2 gm q12h. Peds: 1 mth-12 yo: 30-50 mg/kg q8h, up to 6 gm/d. 0-4 wks: 30 mg/kg q12h. Ceptaz: Adults & Peds ≥12 yo: 2 gm q12h.	B ❄> (Fortaz, Tazicef) ❄v (Ceptaz) R
Ceftizoxime (Cefizox)	Inj: 500 mg, 1 gm, 2 gm, 10 gm	IM/IV: Adults: 1-2 gm q8-12h. Max: 6 gm/d. Peds: ≥6 mths: 50 mg/kg q6-8h, not to exceed adult dose.	B ❄> R
Ceftriaxone Sodium (Rocephin)	Inj: 1 gm/50 ml, 2 gm/50 ml, 250 mg, 500 mg, 1 gm, 2 gm, 10 gm	IM/IV: Adults: Usual: 1-2 gm qd (or in equally divided doses bid.) Max: 4 gm/d.	B ❄>
Cefuroxime (Kefurox, Zinacef)	Inj: 750 mg, 1.5 gm, 7.5 gm	IM/IV: Adults: 1.5 gm q8h. Peds: >3 mths: 50 mg/kg q8h. Max: 4.5 gm/d.	B ❄> R
Cephalexin (Keflex)	Cap: 250 mg, 500 mg; Susp: 125 mg/5 ml, 250 mg/5 ml; Tab: 250 mg, 500 mg	Adults: Usual: 250 mg q6h. Max: 4 gm/d. Peds: Usual: 25-50 mg/kg/d in divided doses.	B ❄>

PENICILLINS

Piperacillin Sodium	Inj: 2 gm, 3 gm, 4 gm	IM/IV: Adults & Peds: ≥12 yo: 3-4 gm q4-6h. Max: 24 gm/d.	B ❄> R

[1] Potential neurotoxicity, ototoxicity & neuromuscular blockade. Avoid concurrent use with neurotoxic/nephrotoxic agents & diuretics.

NAME	FORM/STRENGTH	DOSAGE	COMMENTS
Ticarcillin Disodium/ Clavulanate Potassium (Timentin)	**Inj:** 3 gm-100 mg, 3 gm-100 mg/100 ml, 30 gm-1 gm	**IV: Adults: ≥60 kg:** 300 mg/kg/d ticarcillin given q4h. **<60 kg:** 200-300 mg/kg/d ticarcillin given q4-6h. **Peds: ≥3 mths & <60 kg:** 50 mg/kg/d ticarcillin given q4-6h. **≥3 mths & ≥60 kg:** 3.1 gm q4-6h.	▣B �> R

QUINOLONES

Ciprofloxacin (Cipro)	**Inj:** 10 mg/ml, 200 mg/ 100 ml, 400 mg/200 ml; **Susp:** 250 mg/5 ml, 500 mg/5 ml; **Tab:** 100 mg, 250 mg, 500 mg, 750 mg	**≥18 yo: Mild-Moderate:** 500 mg PO q12h or 400 mg IV q12h x ≥4-6 wks. **Severe:** 750 mg PO q12h or 400 mg IV q8h x ≥4-6 wks.	▣C �464v R

MISCELLANEOUS

Clindamycin (Cleocin)	**Cap:** 75 mg, 150 mg, 300 mg; **Susp:** 75 mg/ 5 ml; **Inj:** 150 mg/ml, 300 mg/50 ml, 600 mg/ 50 ml, 900 mg/50 ml	**IM/IV: Adults:** 600-2700 mg/d in 2-4 doses (max 600 mg IM single dose). **Peds: <1 mth:** 15-20 mg/kg/d in 3-4 doses. **1 mth-16 yo:** 20-40 mg/kg/d in 3-4 doses. **PO: Adults:** 150-450 mg q6h. **Peds:** 8-20 mg/kg/d given 3-4 doses.	▣B �464v (IV) �> (PO) Associated with severe, fatal colitis.
Imipenem/Cilastatin Sodium (Primaxin IV)	**Inj:** 250-250 mg, 500-500 mg	**IV: Adults: ≥70 kg: Mild:** 250-500 mg q6h. **Moderate:** 500 mg q6-8h or 1 gm q8h. **Severe:** 500 mg q6h or 1 gm q6-8h. **Max:** 50 mg/kg/d or 4 gm/d, whichever is lower. **Peds: ≥3 mths:** 15-25 mg/kg q6h. **Max:** 4 gm/d. **4 wks-3 mths & ≥1500 gm:** 25 mg/kg q6h. **1-4 wks & ≥1500 gm:** 25 mg/kg q8h. **<1 wk & ≥1500 gm:** 25 mg/kg q12h.	▣C �> R

| Metronidazole (Flagyl) | Cap: 375 mg; Inj: 500 mg/100 ml; Tab: 250 mg, 500 mg | Adults: PO: 7.5 mg/kg q6h. IV: LD: 15 mg/kg. Maint: After 6h, 7.5 mg/kg q6h. Max: 4 gm/d. | ●B ❄v H CI in 1st trimester. |

Fungal Infection

Amphotericin B Lipid Complex (Abelcet)	Inj: 5 mg/ml	Adults & Peds: Invasive Fungal Infections: 5 mg/kg as a single IV infusion at 2.5 mg/kg/h. If infusion time >2h, mix contents by shaking infusion bag q2h.	●B ❄v R
Amphotericin B Liposome (Ambisome)	Inj: 50 mg; Susp: 100 mg/ml	Adult & Peds: Give over 120 min & reduce to 60 min if well tolerated. Emperic Therapy in Febrile, Neutropenic Patients: 3 mg/kg/d IV. Aspergillosis/Candida/Cryptococcus: 3-5 mg/kg/d IV. Visceral Leishmaniasis: (Immunocompetent) 3 mg kg/d IV for days 1-5, 14, 21. (Immunocompromised) 4 mg/kg/d IV for days 1-5, 10, 17, 24, 31, 38. Cryptococcal Meningitis in HIV Patients: 6 mg/kg/d IV.	●B ❄v
Amphotericin B (Amphocin, Fungizone)	Inj: 50 mg	Life-Threatening Fungal Infections: Adults: 0.25-1 mg/kg/d IV. Peds: Limit to smallest effective dose.	●B ❄v R Not for noninvasive disease.
Caspofungin Acetate (Cancidas)	Inj: 50 mg, 70 mg	Adults: Invasive Aspergillosis: LD: 70 mg IV on day 1. Maint: 50 mg/d IV. Esophageal Candidiasis: 50 mg/d IV. Candidemia/Candida Infections (intra-abdominal abscesses, peritonitis, & pleural space infection): LD: 70 mg IV on day 1. Maint: 50 mg/d IV.	●C ❄> H

NAME	FORM/STRENGTH	DOSAGE	COMMENTS
Fluconazole (Diflucan)	**Inj:** 200 mg/100 ml, 400 mg/200 ml; **Susp:** 50 mg/5 ml, 350 mg/5 ml; **Tab:** 50 mg, 100 mg, 150 mg, 200 mg	**Adults: PO: Vaginal Candidiasis:** 150 mg single dose. **IV/PO: Oropharyngeal Candidiasis:** 200 mg on d1, then 100 mg qd x min 2 wks. **Esophageal Candidiasis:** 200 mg on d1, then 100 mg qd x min 3 wks & 2 wks after symptoms resolve. **Max:** 400 mg/d. **Systemic Candida Infections:** 400 mg/d. **UTI & Peritonitis:** 50-200 mg/d. **Cryptococcal Meningitis:** 400 mg on d1, then 200 mg qd x 10-12 wks after negative CSF culture. **Relapse Suppression in AIDS:** 200 mg qd. **Prophylaxis in BMT:** 400 mg qd. **Peds: IV/PO: Oropharyngeal Candidiasis:** 6 mg/kg on d1, then 3 mg/kg/d x min 2 wks. **Esophageal Candidiasis:** 6 mg/kg on d1, then 3 mg/kg/d x min 3 wks & 2 wks after symptoms resolve. **Max:** 12 mg/kg/d. **Systemic Candida Infections:** 6-12 mg/kg/d. **Cryptococcal Meningitis:** 12 mg/kg on d1, then 6 mg/kg/d x 10-12 wks after negative CSF culture. **Relapse Suppression in AIDS:** 6 mg/kg/d.	◑C ✼ ≈v R
Flucytosine (Ancobon)	**Cap:** 250 mg, 500 mg	**Adults: Candida/Cryptococcus:** 50-150 mg/kg/d in divided doses at 6h intervals.	◑C ✼ ≈v R Extreme caution with renal dysfunction. Monitor hematologic, renal and hepatic status.

Griseofulvin, Microcrystalline (Grifulvin V)	**Susp:** 125 mg/5 ml; **Tab:** 500 mg	**Adults: Tinea Corporis, Cruris & Capitis:** 500 mg qd; **Tinea Pedis, Unguium:** 1 gm qd. **Peds: 30-50 lbs:** 125-250 mg qd. **>50 lbs:** 250-500 mg qd. Treat capitis x 4-6 wks, corporis x 2-4 wks, pedis x 4-8 wks, unguium x min 4 mths (fingernails) or 6 mths (toenails).	●N ❄> CI in pregnancy.
Griseofulvin, Ultramicrocrystalline (Gris-Peg)	**Tab:** 125 mg, 250 mg	**Adults: Tinea Corporis, Cruris & Capitis:** 375 mg/d as single or divided doses. **Tinea Pedis, Unguium:** 375 mg bid. **>2 yo: Usual:** 3.3 mg/lb/d. **35-60 lb:** 125-187.5 mg qd. **>60 lb:** 187.5-375 mg qd. Treat capitis x 4-6 wks, corporis x 2-4 wks, pedis x 4-8 wks, unguium x min 4 mths (fingernails) or 6 mths (toenails).	●N ❄> CI in pregnancy.
Itraconazole (Sporanox)	**Cap:** 100 mg; **Sol:** 10 mg/ml; **Inj:** 10 mg/ml	**Adults: Cap:** Take w/full meal. **Blastomycosis/ Histoplasmosis:** 200 mg qd. Increase by 100 mg if no improvement. **Max:** 400 mg/d. **Aspergillosis:** 200-400 mg/d. **Life-threatening Infection: LD:** 200 mg tid x 1st 3d. Continue x min 3 mths & until infection subsides. **Onychomycosis: Toenails:** 200 mg qd x 12 wks. **Fingernails:** 200 mg bid x 1 wk, stop therapy x 3 wks, then repeat. **Inj: Febrile, Neutropenic Patients:** 200 mg IV bid x 4 doses, then 200 mg IV qd up to 14d. Continue w/sol 200 mg PO bid up to 28d. **Blastomycosis/ Histoplasmosis/Aspergillosis:** 200 mg bid x 4 doses, then 200 mg qd, up to 14d. Continue w/caps for min 3 mths & until infection subsides. **Sol:** Take on empty stomach. Swish 10 ml at a time for several sec, then swallow. **Oropharyngeal Candidiasis:** 200 mg/d x 1-2 wks. **Esophageal Candidiasis:** 100-200 mg qd x min 3 wks. Continue x 2 wks after symptoms resolve.	●C ❄v CI w/cisapride, pimozide, quinidine, dofetilide. Serious cardiovascular events reported w/ CYP450 3A4 inhibitors. Avoid inj w/CrCl <30 ml/min. Do not interchange cap & sol.

NAME	FORM/STRENGTH	DOSAGE	COMMENTS
Ketoconazole (Nizoral)	**Tab:** 200 mg	**Adults: Initial:** 200 mg qd. **Titrate:** May increase to 400 mg qd. **≥2 yo:** 3.3-6.6 mg/kg qd. For topical, see under Skin & Mucous Membrane Antifungals.	⬤C ❄v Hepatotoxicity. CI w/terfenadine, astemizole, cisapride.
Nystatin (Bio-Statin)	**Cap:** 500,000 U, 1,000,000 U; **Powder:** 150,000,000 U	**Intestinal Moniliasis:** 300,000-1,000,000 U tid-qid. Continue for min 48h after cure.	⬤N ❄>
Nystatin (Mycostatin)	**Loz:** 200,000 U; **Susp:** 100,000 U/ml; **Tab:** 500,000 U	**Oral Candidiasis: Adults & Peds: Loz:** 200,000-400,000 U 4-5x/d up to 14d. **Susp:** 4-6 ml qid. Continue x 48h after relief of symptoms. **Infants: Susp:** 2 ml qid. **GI Candidiasis: Tab:** 500,000-1,000,000 U tid. Continue x min 48h after cure.	⬤C ❄>
Terbinafine HCl (Lamisil)	**Tab:** 250 mg	**Adults: Fingernail Onychomycosis:** 250 mg qd x 6 wks. **Toenail Onychomycosis:** 250 mg qd x 12 wks.	⬤B ❄v
Voriconazole (Vfend)	**Inj:** 200 mg/30 ml; **Susp:** 40 mg/ml; **Tab:** 50 mg, 200 mg	**Adults & Peds: ≥12 yo: Invasive Aspergillosis/** *Scedosporium apiospermum* **or** *Fusarium* **Infection: LD:** 6 mg/kg IV q12h x 2 doses. **Maint:** 4 mg/kg IV q12h. Switch to PO when appropriate. **Maint: >40 kg:** 200 mg PO q12h; increase to 300 mg PO q12h if needed. **<40 kg:** 100 mg PO q12h; increase to 150 mg PO q12h if needed. **Esophageal Candidiasis: (Tab) >40 kg:** 200 mg PO q12h. **<40 kg:** 100 mg PO q12h. Treat for minimum of 14d and at least 7d following resolution of	⬤D ❄v H R

symptoms. **Intolerant to Treatment:** Decrease IV maint dose to 3 mg/kg q12h, and PO maint dose by 50 mg steps to 200 mg q12h (or 100 mg q12h for <40 kg). Take PO 1h before or after a meal.

Lower Respiratory Tract Infection

AMINOGLYCOSIDES

Amikacin Sulfate (Amikin)	**Inj:** 50 mg/ml, 250 mg/ml	**IV: Adults, Children & Older Infants:** 7.5 mg/kg q12h or 5 mg/kg IM/IV q8h. **Max:** 1.5 gm/d **Newborns: LD:** 10 mg/kg. **Maint:** 7.5 mg/kg q12h.	◐D ❄v R [1]
Gentamicin Sulfate (Garamycin)	**Inj:** 40 mg/ml	**IV: Adults:** 3 mg/kg/d given q8h. **Max:** 5 mg/kg/d in 3-4 doses. Reduce to 3 mg/kg/d as soon as clinically indicated. **Peds:** 2-2.5 mg/kg q8h. **Infants/Neonates:** 2.5 mg/kg q8h. ≤1 wk: 2.5 mg/kg q12h.	◐N ❄> R [1]
Tobramycin Sulfate (Nebcin)	**Inj:** 10 mg/ml, 40 mg/ml, 1.2 gm	**IV: Adults:** 3 mg/kg/d given q8h. **Max:** 5 mg/kg/d in 3-4 doses. Reduce to 3 mg/kg/d as soon as clinically indicated. **Peds: >1 wk:** 2-2.5 mg/kg q8h or 1.5-1.89 mg/kg q6h. **<1 wk:** Up to 2 mg/kg q12h.	◐D ❄> R [1]

CARBAPENEM

Ertapenem Sodium (Invanz)	**Inj:** 1 gm	**Adults:** 1 gm qd x 10-14d. May give IV up to 14d; IM up to 7d.	◐B ❄> R

[1] Potential neurotoxicity, ototoxicity & neuromuscular blockade. Avoid concurrent use with neurotoxic/nephrotoxic agents & diuretics.

NAME	FORM/STRENGTH	DOSAGE	COMMENTS
CEPHALOSPORINS			
Cefaclor (Ceclor, Ceclor CD)	**Cap:** 250 mg, 500 mg; **Susp:** 125 mg/5 ml, 187 mg/5 ml, 250 mg/ 5 ml, 375 mg/5 ml; **Tab,ER:** (CD) 375 mg, 500 mg	**Adults: Cap/Susp:** 500 mg q8h. **Tab,ER:** 500 mg q12h x 7d. **Peds:** ≥1 mth: **Cap/Susp:** 40 mg/kg/d given q8h. **Max:** 1 gm/d.	■B ❄>
Cefdinir (Omnicef)	**Cap:** 300 mg	**≥13 yo: CAP:** 300 mg q12h x 10d. **Acute Exacerbations of Chronic Bronchitis:** 300 mg q12h x 5-10d or 600 mg q24h x 10d.	■B ❄> R
Cefditoren Pivoxil (Spectracef)	**Tab:** 200 mg	**≥12 yo: Bronchitis Exacerbation:** 400 mg bid x 10d. **Pneumonia:** 400 mg bid x 14d.	■B ❄> R
Cefepime HCl (Maxipime)	**Inj:** 500 mg, 1 gm, 2 gm	**Adults: Moderate-Severe:** 1-2 gm IV q12h x 10d. **Peds: 2 mths-16 yo:** ≤40 kg: 50 mg/kg IV q12h. **Max:** Do not exceed adult dose.	■B ❄> R
Cefixime (Suprax)	**Susp:** 100 mg/5 ml; **Tab:** 200 mg, 400 mg	**>12 yo or >50 kg: Tab/Susp:** 400 mg qd or 200 mg bid. **≤50 kg or >6 mths: Susp:** 8 mg/kg qd or 4 mg/kg bid.	■B ❄v R
Cefpodoxime Proxetil (Vantin)	**Susp:** 50 mg/5 ml, 100 mg/5 ml; **Tab:** 100 mg, 200 mg	**≥12 yo:** 200 mg q12h x 10-14d.	■B ❄v R
Cefprozil (Cefzil)	**Susp:** 125 mg/5 ml, 250 mg/5 ml; **Tab:** 250 mg, 500 mg	**Adults & Peds ≥13 yo:** 500 mg q12h x 10d.	■B ❄v R

Ceftibuten (Cedax)	Cap: 400 mg; Susp: 90 mg/5 ml	≥12 yo: 400 mg qd x 10d. ≥6 mths: 9 mg/kg qd x 10d. Max: 400 mg/d.	⬤B ❄> R
Ceftriaxone Sodium (Rocephin)	Inj: 1 gm/50 ml, 2 gm/50 ml, 250 mg, 500 mg, 1 gm, 2 gm, 10 gm	IM/IV: Adults: Usual: 1-2 gm qd (or in equally divided doses bid). Max: 4 gm/d.	⬤B ❄>
Cefuroxime Axetil (Ceftin)	Tab: 125 mg, 250 mg, 500 mg	Adults & Peds ≥13 yo: 250-500 mg bid x 5-10d.	⬤B ❄v R
Cephalexin (Keflex)	Cap: 250 mg, 500 mg; Susp: 125 mg/5 ml, 250 mg/5 ml; Tab: 250 mg, 500 mg	Adults: Usual: 250 mg q6h. Max: 4 gm/d. Peds: Usual: 25-50 mg/kg/d in divided doses.	⬤B ❄>
Cephradine (Velosef)	Cap: 250 mg, 500 mg; Susp: 250 mg/5 ml	Pneumonia: Adults: 500 mg q6h or 1 gm q12h. Peds: >9 mths: 25-50 mg/kg/d given q6h or q12h (up to adult dose).	⬤B ❄> R

KETOLIDES

Telithromycin (Ketek)	Tab: 400 mg	Adults: Bronchitis Exacerbation: 800 mg qd x 5d. CAP: 800 mg qd x 7-10d.	⬤C ❄>

MACROLIDES

Azithromycin (Zithromax)	Inj: 500 mg; Susp: 100 mg/5 ml, 200 mg/5 ml, 1 gm/pkt; Tab: 250 mg, 600 mg	CAP: ≥16 yo: PO: 500 mg qd x 1d, then 250 mg qd on d2-5. IV: 500 mg qd x 2d, then 250 mg bid x 5-8d. ≥6 mths: Susp: 10 mg/kg qd x 1d, then 5 mg/kg on d2-5. Acute Exacerbation of COPD: PO: Adults: 500 mg qd x 3d. ≥16 yo: 500 mg qd x 1d, then 250 mg qd on d2-5.	⬤B ❄>

NAME	FORM/STRENGTH	DOSAGE	COMMENTS
Clarithromycin (Biaxin)	**Susp:** 125 mg/5 ml, 250 mg/5 ml; **Tab:** 250 mg, 500 mg; **Tab,ER:** 500 mg	**Adults: Acute Exacerbation of Chronic Bronchitis: Susp/Tab:** 250-500 mg q12h x 7-14d. **Tab,ER:** 1 gm qd x 7d. **CAP: Susp/Tab:** 250 mg q12h x 7-14d. **Tab,ER:** 1 gm qd x7d. **Peds: ≥6 mths: CAP: Susp/Tab:** 7.5 mg/kg q12h x 10d.	⬤C ❅> R
Dirithromycin (Dynabac)	**Tab,Delay:** 250 mg	**Adults & Peds ≥12 yo:** 500 mg qd x 7-14d.	⬤C ❅>
Erythromycin Base	**Tab:** 250 mg	**Adults: Usual:** 250 mg q6h or 500 mg q12h. **Peds: Usual:** 30-50 mg/kg/d in divided doses. **Max:** 4 gm/d.	⬤B ❅>
Erythromycin Ethylsuccinate (E.E.S., EryPed)	**Chewtab:** (EryPed) 200 mg; **Sus:** (EryPed) 100 mg/2.5 ml, 200 mg/5 ml, 400 mg/5 ml, (E.E.S.) 200 mg/5 ml, 400 mg/5 ml; **Tab:** (E.E.S.) 400 mg	**Adults: Usual:** 1600 mg/d given q6h, q8h, or q12h. **Max:** 4 gm/d. **Peds: Usual:** 30-50 mg/kg/d in divided doses q6h, q8h, or q12h. Double dose for more severe infections.	⬤B ❅>
Erythromycin (Ery-Tab, PCE)	**Tab,Enteric:** (Ery-Tab) 250 mg, 333 mg, 500 mg; **Tab,ER:** (PCE) 333 mg, 500 mg	**Adults: Usual:** 250 mg qid, 333 mg q8h, or 500 mg q12h. **Peds: Usual:** 30-50 mg/kg/d in divided doses. **Max:** 4 gm/d.	⬤B ❅>
Erythromycin Stearate (Erythrocin)	**Tab:** 250 mg, 500 mg	**Adults: Usual:** 250 mg q6h or 500 mg q12h. **Peds: Usual:** 30-50 mg/kg/d in divided doses. **Max:** 4 gm/d.	⬤B ❅>
Troleandomycin (TAO)	**Cap:** 250 mg	**Adults:** 250-500 mg qid. **Peds:** 125-250 mg or 6.6-11 mg/kg q6h.	⬤N ❅>

MONOBACTAMS

Loracarbef (Lorabid)	**Cap:** 200 mg, 400 mg; **Susp:** 100 mg/5 ml, 200 mg/5 ml	**Adults & Peds ≥13 yo: Bronchitis:** 200-400 mg q12h x 7d. **Pneumonia:** 400mg q12h x 14d.	▣B ❄> R

OXAZOLIDINONE

Linezolid (Zyvox)	**Inj:** 2 mg/ml; **Susp:** 100 mg/5 ml; **Tab:** 600 mg	**Usual:** Treat x 10-14d. **Adults & Peds ≥12 yo:** 600 mg IV/PO q12h. **Birth-11 yo:** 10 mg/kg IV/PO q8h.	▣C ❄>

PENICILLINS

Amoxicillin (Amoxil, DisperMox, Trimox)	**Cap:** (Amoxil, Trimox) 250 mg, 500 mg; **Chewtab:** (Amoxil) 200 mg, 400 mg; **Susp:** (Amoxil) 50 mg/ml, 125 mg/5 ml, 200 mg/5 ml, 250 mg/5 ml, 400 mg/5 ml, (Trimox) 125 mg/5 ml, 250 mg/5 ml; **Tab:** (Amoxil) 500 mg, 875 mg; **Tab, Dispersible:** (DisperMox) 200 mg, 400 mg, 600 mg	**Adults & Peds >40 kg:** 875 mg q12h or 500 mg q8h. **>3 mths & <40 kg:** 45 mg/kg/d given q12h or 40 mg/kg/d given q8h. **≤3 mths: Usual/Max:** 15 mg/kg q12h.	▣B ❄> R

NAME	FORM/STRENGTH	DOSAGE	COMMENTS
Amoxicillin/Clavulanate (Augmentin)	**Chewtab:** 125-31.25 mg, 200-28.5 mg, 250-62.5 mg, 400-57 mg; **Susp:** (per 5 ml) 125-31.25 mg, 200-28.5 mg, 250-62.5 mg, 400-57 mg; **Tab:** 250-125 mg, 500-125 mg, 875-125 mg	Dose based on amoxicillin component. **Adults & Peds ≥40 kg: Tab:** 875 mg q12h or 500 mg q8h. May use 125 mg/5 ml or 250 mg/5 ml susp in place of 500 mg tab & 200 mg/5 ml susp or 400 mg/5 ml susp in place of 875 mg tab. **Chewtab/Susp:** ≥12 wks: 45 mg/kg/d given q12h or 40 mg/kg/d given q8h. **<12 wks:** 15 mg/kg q12h (use 125 mg/5 ml susp).	▣B ❄> H R 2-250 mg tabs are not equivalent to 1-500 mg tabs. Only use 250 mg tab if peds ≥40 kg. Chewtab & tab not interchangeable.
Amoxicillin/Clavulanate (Augmentin XR)	**Tab,ER:** 1000 mg-62.5 mg	**≥16 yo:** 2 tabs q12h x 7-10d.	▣ B ❄>
Ampicillin (Principen)	**Cap:** 250 mg, 500 mg; **Susp:** 125 mg/5ml, 250 mg/5ml	**Adults & Peds: >20 kg:** 250 mg qid. **Peds: ≤20 kg:** 50 mg/kg/d given tid-qid.	▣B ❄v
Dicloxacillin Sodium (Dynapen)	**Cap:** 250 mg, 500 mg; **Susp:** 62.5 mg/5 ml	**Adults & Peds ≥40 kg: Mild-Moderate:** 125 mg q6h. **Severe:** 250 mg q6h. **Peds: <40 kg: Mild-Moderate:** 3.125 mg/kg q6h. **Severe:** 6.25 mg/kg q6h.	▣B ❄>
Penicillin V Potassium (Penicillin VK, Veetids)	**Susp:** 125 mg/5 ml, 250 mg/5 ml; **Tab:** 250 mg, 500 mg	**Adults & Peds ≥12 yo: Pneumococcal:** 250-500 mg q6h til afebrile x 2d.	▣B ❄>
Piperacillin Sodium/ Tazobactam (Zosyn)	**Inj:** 40-5 mg/mL, 60-7.5 mg/mL, 2-0.25 gm, 3-0.375 gm, 4-0.5 gm, 4-0.5 gm/100 mL, 36-4.5 gm	**Adults: Usual:** 3.375 gm IV q6h x 7-10d. **Nosocomial Pneumonia:** 4.5 gm IV q6h x 7-14d plus aminoglycoside.	▣B ❄> R

QUINOLONES

Drug	Formulations	Dosing	Ratings
Ciprofloxacin (Cipro)	**Inj:** 10 mg/ml, 200 mg/ 100 ml, 400 mg/200 ml; **Susp:** 250 mg/5 ml, 500 mg/5 ml; **Tab:** 100 mg, 250 mg, 500 mg, 750 mg	**≥18 yo: Mild-Moderate:** 500 mg PO q12h or 400 mg IV q12h x 7-14d. **Severe:** 750 mg PO q12h or 400 mg IV q8h x 7-14d.	⊕C ✻v R
Gatifloxacin (Tequin)	**Inj:** 2 mg/ml; 10 mg/ml; **Tab:** 200 mg, 400 mg	**≥18 yo: Pneumonia:** 400 mg PO/IV x 7-14d. **Bronchitis Exacerbation:** 400 mg PO/IV qd x 5d.	⊕C ✻> R
Levofloxacin (Levaquin)	**Inj:** 5 mg/ml, 25 mg/ml; **Tab:** 250 mg, 500 mg, 750 mg	**≥18 yo: CAP** 500 mg IV/PO qd x 7-14d or 750 mg IV/PO qd x 5 days. **Nosocomial Pneumonia:** 750mg IV/PO qd x 7-14d.	⊕C ✻v R
Lomefloxacin (Maxaquin)	**Tab:** 400 mg	**≥18 yo:** 400 mg qd x 10d.	⊕C ✻v R
Moxifloxacin HCl (Avelox)	**Inj:** 400 mg/250 ml; **Tab:** 400 mg	**≥18 yo:** 400 mg PO/IV qd x 5d (for ABECB) or 7-14d (for CAP).	⊕C ✻v
Ofloxacin (Floxin)	**Tab:** 200 mg, 300 mg, 400 mg	**≥18 yo:** 400 mg q12h x 10d.	⊕C ✻v H R
Sparfloxacin (Zagam)	**Tab:** 200 mg	**≥18 yo: LD:** 400 mg on d1. **Maint:** 200 mg q24h x 9d.	⊕C ✻v R

SULFONAMIDES AND COMBINATIONS

Drug	Formulations	Dosing	Ratings
Sulfamethoxazole/ Trimethoprim (Bactrim, Bactrim DS, Septra, Septra DS, Sulfatrim Pediatric)	**Susp:** 200-40 mg/5 ml; **Tab:** (SS) 400-80 mg, (DS) 800-160 mg	**Adults:** 800 mg SMX & 160 mg TMP (1 DS tab, 2 SS tabs, or 20 ml) q12h x 14d.	⊕C ✻v R CI in pregnancy & nursing.

NAME	FORM/STRENGTH	DOSAGE	COMMENTS
TETRACYCLINES			
Doxycycline Hyclate (Vibramycin, Vibra-Tabs)	**Cap:** 50 mg, 100 mg; **Tab:** 100 mg	**Adults:** 100 mg q12h on d1, then 100 mg qd or 50 mg q12h. **Severe:** 100 mg q12h. **Peds:** >8 yo & ≤100 lbs: 1 mg/lb bid on d1, then 1 mg/lb qd or 0.5 mg/lb bid. **Severe:** 2 mg/lb. >100 lbs: Adult dose. **Inhalation Anthrax (Post-Exposure): Adults:** 100 mg bid x 60d. **Peds:** >8 yo & <100 lbs: 1 mg/lb bid x 60d. ≥**100 lbs:** Adult dose.	▣D ✿v
Doxycycline Monohydrate (Monodox, Vibramycin)	**Cap:** (Monodox) 50 mg, 100 mg; **Susp:** (Vibramycin) 25 mg/5 ml	**Adults:** 100 mg q12h or 50 mg q6h on d1, then 100 mg qd or 50 mg q12h. **Severe:** 100 mg q12h. **Peds:** >8 yo & ≤100 lbs: 1 mg/lb bid on d1, then 1 mg/lb qd or 0.5 mg/lb bid. **Severe:** 2 mg/lb. >100 lbs: Adult dose. **Inhalation Anthrax (Post-Exposure): Adults:** 100 mg bid x 60d. **Peds:** >8 yo & <100 lbs: 1 mg/lb bid x 60 d. ≥**100 lbs:** Adult dose.	▣D ✿v
Minocycline HCl (Dynacin, Minocin)	**Cap:** (Dynacin) 50 mg, 75 mg, 100 mg, (Minocin) 50 mg, 100 mg; **Tab:** (Dynacin) 75 mg, 100 mg; **Inj:** (Minocin) 100 mg	**Adults:** 200 mg PO/IV, then 100 mg q12h or 50 mg qid. >8 yo: 4 mg/kg PO/IV, then 2 mg/kg q12h.	▣D ✿v R
Tetracycline HCl (Sumycin)	**Cap:** 250 mg, 500 mg; **Susp:** 125 mg/5 ml	**Adults:** 250 mg qid or 500 mg bid. **Peds:** >8 yo: 25-50 mg/kg divided bid-qid.	▣D ✿v R

| Clindamycin (Cleocin) | Cap: 75 mg, 150 mg, 300 mg; Susp: 75 mg/5 ml; Inj: 150 mg/ml, 300 mg/50 ml, 600 mg/50 ml, 900 mg/50 ml | IM/IV: Adults: 600-2700 mg/d in 2-4 doses. Max: 600 mg IM single dose. Peds: <1 mth: 15-20 mg/kg/d in 3-4 doses. 1 mth-16 yo: 20-40 mg/kg/d in 3-4 doses. PO: Adults: 150-450 mg q6h. Peds: 8-20 mg/kg/d given 3-4 doses. | ⊞B ✿v (IV) ✿> (PO) Associated with severe, fatal colitis. |

Malaria

| Atovaquone/Proguanil (Malarone, Malarone Pediatric) | Tab: 250-100 mg; Tab, Ped: 62.5-25 mg | Acute Attack: Adults: 4 tabs qd x 3d. Peds: 5-8 kg: 2 ped tabs qd x 3 d. 9-10 kg: 3 ped tabs x 3 d. 11-20 kg: 1 tab qd x 3d. 21-30 kg: 2 tabs qd x 3d. 31-40 kg: 3 tabs qd x 3d. >40 kg: 4 tabs qd x 3d. Prophylaxis: Adults: 1 tab qd. Peds: 11-20 kg: 1 ped tab qd. 21-30 kg: 2 ped tabs qd. 31-40 kg: 3 ped tabs qd. >40 kg: 1 tab qd. Start 1-2d prior to endemic area exposure & continue x 7d after return. | ⊞C ✿> R |
| Chloroquine Phosphate (Aralen Phosphate) | Tab: 500 mg (500 mg tab = 300 mg chloroquine base) | Acute Attack: Adults: Initial: 1 gm, then 500 mg after 6-8h, then 500 mg qd x 2d. Infants & Peds: Total dose of 25 mg base/kg taken over 3d, as follows: 1st Dose: 10 mg base/kg (max 600 mg base single dose). 2nd Dose: 5 mg base/kg (max 300 mg base single dose) 6h after 1st dose. 3rd Dose: 5 mg base/kg 18h after 2nd dose. 4th Dose: 5 mg base/kg 24h after 3rd dose. Suppression: Adults: 500 mg qwk. Peds: 5 mg base/kg qwk (max 500 mg). Begin 2 wks prior to endemic area exposure & continue x 8 wks after return. | ⊞N ✿v Avoid during pregnancy. |

NAME	FORM/STRENGTH	DOSAGE	COMMENTS
Hydroxychloroquine Sulfate (Plaquenil)	**Tab:** 200 mg (equivalent to 155 mg base)	**Acute Attack: Adults: Initial:** 800 mg, then 400 mg after 6-8h, then 400 mg x 2d. **Infants & Peds:** Total dose of 25 mg base/kg taken over 3d, as follows: **1st Dose:** 10 mg base/kg (max 620 mg base single dose). **2nd Dose:** 5 mg base/kg (max 310 mg base single dose) 6h after 1st dose. **3rd Dose:** 5 mg base/kg 18h after 2nd dose. **4th Dose:** 5 mg base/kg 24h after 3rd dose. **Suppression: Adults:** 400 mg qwk. **Infants & Peds:** 5 mg base/kg qwk (max 400 mg). Begin 2 wks prior to endemic area exposure & continue x 8 wks after return.	●N ❄>
Mefloquine HCl (Lariam)	**Tab:** 250 mg	**Acute Attack: Adults:** 1250 mg single dose. **Peds: ≥6 mths:** 20-25 mg/kg. Split in 2 doses 6-8h apart. **Prophylaxis: Adults:** 250 mg qwk. **Peds: ≥3 mths:** 3-5 mg/kg qwk. **>45 kg:** 250 mg/wk. **>30-45 kg:** 3/4 tab/wk. **>20-30 kg:** 1/2 tab/wk. **5-20 kg:** 1/4 tab/wk. Begin 1 wk prior to endemic area exposure & continue x 4 wks after return.	●C ❄v
Primaquine Phosphate	**Tab:** 26.3 mg	**Adults: Usual:** 1 tab qd x 14d.	●N ❄>
Pyrimethamine (Daraprim)	**Tab:** 25 mg	**Acute Attack:** Use alternative as monotherapy. **Adults:** 25 mg qd with concomant sulfonamide x 2d or 50 mg qd (monotherapy) x 2d, then prophylaxis dose. **Peds: 4-10 yo:** 25 mg qd (monotherapy) x 2d, then prophylaxis dose. **Prophylaxis: Adults & Peds: >10 yo:** 25 mg qwk. **4-10 yo:** 12.5 mg qwk. **<4 yo:** 6.25 mg qwk.	●C ❄v

| Quinine Sulfate | Cap: 325 mg; Tab: 260 mg | Adults: 1-3 tabs or caps tid x 6-12d. | ⊞X ❄> |

Meningitis, Bacterial

AMINOGLYCOSIDES

Amikacin Sulfate (Amikin)	Inj: 50 mg/ml, 250 mg/ml	IV: Adults, Children & Older Infants: 7.5 mg/kg q12h or 5 mg/kg IM/IV q8h. Max: 1.5 gm/d Newborns: LD: 10 mg/kg. Maint: 7.5 mg/kg q12h.	⊞D ❄v R [1]
Gentamicin Sulfate (Garamycin)	Inj: 40 mg/ml	IV: Adults: 3 mg/kg/d given q8h. Max: 5 mg/kg/d in 3-4 doses. Reduce to 3 mg/kg/d as soon as clinically indicated. Peds: 2-2.5 mg/kg q8h. Infants/Neonates: 2.5 mg/kg q8h. ≤1 wk: 2.5 mg/kg q12h.	⊞N ❄> R [1]
Tobramycin Sulfate (Nebcin)	Inj: 10 mg/ml, 40 mg/ml, 1.2 gm	IV: Adults: 3 mg/kg/d given q8h. Max: 5 mg/kg/d in 3-4 doses. Reduce to 3 mg/kg/d as soon as clinically indicated. Peds: >1 wk: 2-2.5 mg/kg q8h or 1.5-1.89 mg/kg q6h. <1 wk: Up to 2 mg/kg q12h.	⊞D ❄> R [1]

CARBAPENEM

Meropenem (Merrem)	Inj: 500 mg, 1 gm	IV: Adults & Peds >50 kg: 1 gm q8h. ≥3 mths: <50 kg: 40 mg/kg q8h. Max: 2 gm q8h.	⊞B ❄> R

CEPHALOSPORINS

Cefotaxime Sodium (Claforan)	Inj: 500 mg, 1 gm, 2 gm, 10 gm	IV: Adults or >50 kg: 2 gm q6-8h. Max: 12 gm/d. 1 mth-12 yo: <50 kg: 50-180 mg/kg/d divided into 4-6 doses. 1-4 wks: 50 mg/kg IV q8h. 0-1 wk: 50 mg/kg IV q12h.	⊞B ❄> R

[1] Potential neurotoxicity, ototoxicity & neuromuscular blockade. Avoid concurrent use with neurotoxic/nephrotoxic agents & diuretics.

NAME	FORM/STRENGTH	DOSAGE	COMMENTS
Ceftazidime (Ceptaz, Fortaz, Tazicef)	**Inj:** 500 mg, 1 gm, 2 gm, 6 gm, 10 gm	**IV: Fortaz/Tazicef: Adults:** 2 gm q8h. **Peds: 1 mth-12 yo:** 30-50 mg/kg q8h, up to 6 gm/d. **0-4 wks:** 30 mg/kg q12h. **Ceptaz: Adults & Peds ≥12 yo:** 2 gm q8h.	◯B ❄> (Fortaz, Tazicef) ❄v (Ceptaz) **R**
Ceftizoxime (Cefizox)	**Inj:** 500 mg, 1 gm, 2 gm, 10 gm	**IV: Adults:** 3-4 gm q8h. **Peds: ≥6 mths:** 50 mg/kg q6-8h, not to exceed adult dose.	◯B ❄> **R**
Ceftriaxone Sodium (Rocephin)	**Inj:** 1 gm/50 ml, 2 gm/50 ml, 250 mg, 500 mg, 1 gm, 2 gm, 10 gm	**IV: Adults:** 1-2 gm qd (or in equally divided doses bid). **Max:** 4 gm/d. **Peds:** Initial of 100 mg/kg (NTE 4 gm), then 100 mg/kg qd or (in equally divided doses q12h) for 7-14d. **Max:** 4 gm/d.	◯B ❄>
Cefuroxime (Kefurox, Zinacef)	**Inj:** 750 mg, 1.5 gm, 7.5 gm	**IV: Adults:** 1.5 gm q6h. **Max:** 3 gm q8h. **Peds: >3 mths:** 200-240 mg/kg/d divided q6-8h.	◯B ❄> **R**
PENICILLINS			
Ampicillin Sodium	**Inj:** 125 mg, 250 mg, 500 mg, 1 gm, 2 gm, 10 gm	**IV: Adults & Peds:** 150-200 mg/kg/day given q3-4h.	◯B ❄>
Penicillin G Potassium (Pfizerpen)	**Inj:** 5 MU, 20 MU	**IV: Adults:** *Listeria:* 15-20 MU/d x 2 wks. *Pasteurella:* 4-6 MU/d x 2 wks. *Meningococcic:* 1-2 MU IM q2h or 20-30 MU/d continuous IV.	◯B ❄>

Mycobacterium Avium Complex

Azithromycin (Zithromax)	**Susp:** 100 mg/5 ml, 200 mg/5 ml, 1 gm/pkt; **Tab:** 600 mg	**Adults: Prevention:** 1200 mg qwk. **Treatment:** 600 mg qd with ethambutol 15 mg/kg/d.	◯B ❄>

Drug	Formulations	Dosage	
Clarithromycin (Biaxin)	**Susp:** 125 mg/5 ml, 250 mg/5 ml; **Tab:** 250 mg, 500 mg	**Prevention & Treatment: Adults:** 500 mg bid. **Peds:** ≥20 mths: 7.5 mg/kg bid. **Max:** 500 mg bid.	⊕C ❄> R
Rifabutin (Mycobutin)	**Cap:** 150 mg	**Adults:** 300 mg qd or 150 mg bid w/ food. Reduce dose w/ nelfinavir or indinavir.	⊕B ❄v R

Otitis Media, Acute
CEPHALOSPORINS

Drug	Formulations	Dosage	
Cefaclor (Ceclor)	**Cap:** 250 mg, 500 mg; **Susp:** 125 mg/5 ml, 187 mg/5 ml, 250 mg/ 5 ml, 375 mg/5 ml	**Peds:** ≥1 mth: 40 mg/kg/d given in divided doses. **Max:** 1 gm/d.	⊕B ❄>
Cefdinir (Omnicef)	**Susp:** 125 mg/5 ml	**6 mths-12 yo:** 7 mg/kg q12h x 5-10d or 14 mg/kg q24h x 10d.	⊕B ❄> R
Cefixime (Suprax)	**Susp:** 100 mg/5 ml; **Tab:** 200 mg, 400 mg	**>12 yo or >50 kg: Tab/Susp:** 400 mg qd or 200 mg bid. **Peds ≤50 kg or >6 mths: Susp:** 8 mg/kg qd or 4 mg/kg bid.	⊕B ❄v R
Cefpodoxime Proxetil (Vantin)	**Susp:** 50 mg/5 ml, 100 mg/5 ml; **Tab:** 100 mg, 200 mg	**2 mths-11 yo:** 5 mg/kg q12h x 5d.	⊕B ❄v R
Cefprozil (Cefzil)	**Susp:** 125 mg/5 ml, 250 mg/5 ml; **Tab:** 250 mg, 500 mg	**6 mths-12 yo:** 15 mg/kg q12h x 10d.	⊕B ❄v R
Ceftibuten (Cedax)	**Cap:** 400 mg; **Susp:** 90 mg/5 ml	**≥6 mths:** 9 mg/kg qd x 10d. **Max:** 400 mg/d.	⊕B ❄> R

NAME	FORM/STRENGTH	DOSAGE	COMMENTS
Ceftriaxone Sodium (Rocephin)	**Inj:** 1 gm/50 ml, 2 gm/50 ml, 250 mg, 500 mg, 1 gm, 2 gm, 10 gm	**Peds:** 50 mg/kg IM single dose. **Max:** 1 gm/dose.	▣B ✿>
Cefuroxime Axetil (Ceftin)	**Susp:** 125 mg/5 ml, 250 mg/5 ml; **Tab:** 125 mg, 250 mg, 500 mg	**3 mths-12 yo:** Susp: 15 mg/kg bid x 10d. **Max:** 1 gm/d. **Tab:** 250 mg bid x 10d.	▣B ✿v **R** Tabs & susp are not bioequivalent.
Cephalexin (Keflex)	**Cap:** 250 mg, 500 mg; **Susp:** 125 mg/5 ml, 250 mg/5 ml; **Tab:** 250 mg, 500 mg	**Peds:** 75-100 mg/kg/d given qid.	▣B ✿>
Cephradine (Velosef)	**Cap:** 250 mg, 500 mg; **Susp:** 250 mg/5 ml	**Peds:** >9 mths: *H.influenzae:* 75-100 mg/kg/d given q6h or q12h. **Max:** 4 gm/d.	▣B ✿> **R**
MACROLIDES			
Azithromycin (Zithromax)	**Susp:** 100 mg/5 ml, 200 mg/5 ml; 1 gm/pkt	**Peds:** ≥6 mths: 30 mg/kg x 1 dose; 10 mg/kg qd x 3d; or 10 mg/kg qd x 1d, then 5 mg/kg qd on d2-5.	▣B ✿>
Clarithromycin (Biaxin)	**Susp:** 125 mg/5 ml, 250 mg/5 ml; **Tab:** 250 mg, 500 mg	**Peds:** ≥6 mths: 7.5 mg/kg q12h x10d.	▣C ✿> **R**
MACROLIDES AND COMBINATIONS			
Erythromycin Ethylsuccinate/ Sulfisoxazole Acetyl (Pediazole)	**Susp:** 200-600 mg/5 ml	**≥2 mths:** Dose based on 50 mg/kg/d erythromycin or 150 mg/kg/d sulfisoxazole given tid-qid x 10d. **Max:** 6 gm/d of sulfisoxazole.	▣C ✿v

MONOBACTAMS

Loracarbef (Lorabid)	**Susp:** 100 mg/5 ml, 200 mg/5 ml	**6 mths-12 yo:** 15 mg/kg q12h x 10d.	◓B ❄> R

PENICILLINS

Amoxicillin (Amoxil, DisperMox, Trimox)	**Cap:** (Amoxil, Trimox) 250 mg, 500 mg; **Chewtab:** (Amoxil) 200 mg, 400 mg; **Susp:** (Amoxil) 50 mg/ml, 125 mg/5 ml, 200 mg/5 ml, 250 mg/5 ml, 400 mg/5 ml, (Trimox) 125 mg/5 ml, 250 mg/5 ml; **Tab:** (Amoxil) 500 mg, 875 mg; **Tab, Dispersible:** (DisperMox) 200 mg, 400 mg, 600 mg	**Peds: >40 kg:** 500-875 mg q12h or 250-500 mg q8h, depending on severity. **>3 mths:** 25-45 mg/kg/d divided q12h or 20-40 mg/kg/d divided q8h, depending on severity. **≤3 mths:** Usual/Max: 15 mg/kg q12h.	◓B ❄> R

NAME	FORM/STRENGTH	DOSAGE	COMMENTS
Amoxicillin/Clavulanate (Augmentin)	**Chewtab:** 125-31.25 mg, 200-28.5 mg, 250-62.5 mg, 400-57 mg; **Susp:** (per 5 ml) 125-31.25 mg, 200-28.5 mg, 250-62.5 mg, 400-57 mg; **Tab:** 250-125 mg, 500-125 mg, 875-125 mg	Dose based on amoxicillin component. **Peds: ≥40 kg: Tab:** 500 mg q12h or 250 mg q8h. May use 125 mg/5 ml or 250 mg/5 ml susp in place of 500 mg tab & 200 mg/5 ml susp or 400 mg/5 ml susp in place of 875 mg tab. **≥12 wks: Susp/Chewtab:** 45 mg/kg/d given q12h or 40 mg/kg/d given q8h. **<12 wks: Susp:** 15 mg/kg q12h (use 125 mg/5 ml susp).	▣B ❄> **H R** 2-250 mg tabs are not equivalent to 1-500 mg tab. Only use 250 mg tab if peds ≥40 kg. Chewtab & tab not interchangeable.
Amoxicillin/Clavulanate (Augmentin ES-600)	**Susp:** 600-42.9 mg/5 ml	**3 mths-12 yo: <40 kg:** 45 mg/kg q12h based on amoxicillin component x 10d. Not interchangeable with other Augmentin susp.	▣B ❄> **H R** Not interchangeable with other Augmentin susp.

SULFONAMIDES AND COMBINATIONS

Sulfamethoxazole/ Trimethoprim (Bactrim, Bactrim DS, Septra, Septra DS, Sulfatrim Pediatric)	**Susp:** 200-40 mg/5 ml; **Tab:** (SS) 400-80 mg, (DS) 800-160 mg	**≥2 mths:** 4 mg/kg TMP & 20 mg/kg SMX q12h x 10d.	▣C ❄v **R** CI in pregnancy & nursing.

Pneumocystis Carinii Pneumonia

Atovaquone (Mepron)	**Susp:** 750 mg/5 ml	**Adults & Peds: ≥13 yrs:** Take with food. **Prevention:** 1500 mg qd. **Treatment:** 750 mg bid x 21d.	▣C ❄>

Pentamidine Isethionate (Pentam, Nebupent)	**Inj:** (Pentam) 300 mg; **Sol,Neb:** (Nebupent) 300 mg	**Adults/Peds: Pentam:** ≥4 mths: Treatment: 4 mg/kg IM/IV qd x 14-21d. **Nebupent:** ≥16 yo: Prevention: 300 mg q4wks via nebulizer.	◐C ❖v
Sulfamethoxazole/ Trimethoprim (Bactrim, Bactrim DS, Septra, Septra DS, Sulfatrim Pediatric)	**Susp:** 200-40 mg/5 ml; **Tab:** (SS) 400-80 mg, (DS) 800-160 mg	**Treatment: Adults & Peds:** 15-20 mg/kg TMP & 75-100 mg/kg SMZ divided q6h x 14-21d. **Prophylaxis: Adults:** 1 DS tab qd. **Peds:** 150 mg/m² TMP & 750 mg/m² SMZ divided bid x 3 consecutive days/wk. **Max:** 320 mg TMP/1600 mg SMZ per d.	◐C ❖v R CI in pregnancy & nursing.
Trimetrexate Glucuronate (Neutrexin)	**Inj:** 25 mg/5 ml, 200 mg/30 ml	≥18 yo: 45 mg/m² qd x 21d.	◐D ❖v H R Leucovorin 20 mg/m² qid IV/PO x 24d must be given concomitantly.

Septicemia, Bacterial
AMINOGLYCOSIDES

| Amikacin Sulfate (Amikin) | **Inj:** 50 mg/ml, 250 mg/ml | **IV: Adults, Children & Older Infants:** 7.5 mg/kg q12h or 5 mg/kg IM/IV q8h. **Max:** 1.5 gm/d **Newborns: LD:** 10 mg/kg. **Maint:** 7.5 mg/kg q12h. | ◐D ❖v R [1] |
| Gentamicin Sulfate (Garamycin) | **Inj:** 40 mg/ml | **IV: Adults:** 3 mg/kg/d given q8h. **Max:** 5 mg/kg/d in 3-4 doses. Reduce to 3 mg/kg/d as soon as clinically indicated. **Peds:** 2-2.5 mg/kg q8h. **Infants/Neonates:** 2.5 mg/kg q8h. ≤1 wk: 2.5 mg/kg q12h. | ◐N ❖> R [1] |

[1] Potential neurotoxicity, ototoxicity & neuromuscular blockade. Avoid concurrent use with neurotoxic/nephrotoxic agents & diuretics.

NAME	FORM/STRENGTH	DOSAGE	COMMENTS
Tobramycin Sulfate (Nebcin)	**Inj:** 10 mg/ml, 40 mg/ml, 1.2 gm	**IV: Adults:** 3 mg/kg/d given q8h. **Max:** 5 mg/kg/d in 3-4 doses. Reduce to 3 mg/kg/d as soon as clinically indicated. **Peds: >1 wk:** 2-2.5 mg/kg q8h or 1.5-1.89 mg/kg q6h. **<1 wk:** Up to 2 mg/kg q12h.	⊞D ❄> R [1]

CEPHALOSPORINS

NAME	FORM/STRENGTH	DOSAGE	COMMENTS
Cefamandole Nafate (Mandol)	**Inj:** 1 gm, 2 gm	**IV: Adults:** Up to 2 gm q4h. **Infants & Peds:** 50-100 mg/kg/d given q4-8h. **Max:** 150 mg/kg/d, not to exceed 12 gm/d.	⊞B ❄> R
Cefazolin (Ancef, Kefzol)	**Inj:** 500 mg/50 ml, 1 gm/50 ml, 500 mg, 1 gm, 10 gm, 20 gm	**IV: Adults:** 1-1.5 gm q6h. **Peds:** 100 mg/kg/d given as tid-qid.	⊞B ❄> R Safety in neonates not known.
Cefoperazone (Cefobid)	**Inj:** 1 gm, 2 gm, 10 gm	**IV: Adults:** 6-12 gm given as bid-qid.	⊞B ❄>
Cefotaxime Sodium (Claforan)	**Inj:** 500 mg, 1 gm, 2 gm, 10 gm	**IV: Adults or >50 kg:** 2 gm q4h. **Max:** 12 gm/d. **1 mth-12 yo: <50 kg:** 50-180 mg/kg/d divided into 4-6 doses. **1-4 wks:** 50 mg/kg IV q8h. **0-1 wk:** 50 mg/kg IV q12h.	⊞B ❄> R
Cefoxitin (Mefoxin)	**Inj:** 1 gm, 1 gm/50 ml, 2 gm, 2 gm/50 ml, 10 gm	**IV: Adults:** 1 gm q4h or 2 gm q6-8h. **Peds: ≥3 mths:** 80-160 mg/kg/d given as q4-6h. **Max:** 12 gm/d.	⊞B ❄> R
Ceftazidime (Ceptaz, Fortaz, Tazicef)	**Inj:** 500 mg, 1 gm, 2 gm, 6 gm, 10 gm	**IV: Fortaz/Tazicef: Adults:** 2 gm q8h. **Peds: 1 mth-12 yo:** 30-50 mg/kg q8h, up to 6 gm/d. **0-4 wks:** 30 mg/kg q12h. **Ceptaz: Adults & Peds ≥12 yo:** 2 gm q8h.	⊞B ❄> (Fortaz, Tazicef) ❄v (Ceptaz) R

Ceftizoxime (Cefizox)	Inj: 500 mg, 1 gm, 2 gm, 10 gm	IV: Adults: 3-4 gm q8h. Peds: ≥6 mths: 50 mg/kg q6-8h, not to exceed adult dose.	⬤B ✿> R
Ceftriaxone Sodium (Rocephin)	Inj: 1 gm/50 ml, 2 gm/ 50 ml, 250 mg, 500 mg, 1 gm, 2 gm, 10 gm	IV: Adults: 1-2 gm qd (or in equally divided doses bid). Max: 4 gm/d. Peds: 50-75 mg/kg in divided doses q12h. Max: 2 gm/d.	⬤B ✿>
Cefuroxime (Kefurox, Zinacef)	Inj: 750 mg, 1.5 gm, 7.5 gm	IV: Adults: 1.5 gm q6-8h. Peds: >3 mths: 100 mg/kg/d given q6-8h. Max: 4.5 gm/d.	⬤B ✿> R
Cephalothin Sodium	Inj: 1 gm/50 ml, 2 gm/50 ml	IV: Adults: 1-2 gm q4h. Peds: 20-30 mg/kg q4h.	⬤B ✿> R

MONOBACTAMS

Aztreonam (Azactam)	Inj: 500 mg, 1 gm, 2 gm, 1 gm/50 ml, 2 gm/50 ml	IV: Adults: 2 gm q6-8h. Peds: 30 mg/kg q6-8h.	⬤B ✿v R

PENICILLINS

Nafcillin Sodium	Inj: 1 gm/50 ml, 1 gm, 2 gm, 10 gm	Adults: Usual: 0.5 gm IV q4-6h.	⬤N ✿>
Oxacillin Sodium	Inj: 1 gm/50 ml, 2 gm/50 ml, 1 gm, 2 gm, 10 gm	Adults: 1 gm IM/IV q4-6h. Peds: <40 kg: 100 mg/kg/d IM/IV divided q4-6h. Premature & Neonates: 25 mg/kg/d IM/IV.	⬤B ✿>
Piperacillin Sodium	Inj: 2 gm, 3 gm, 4 gm	IV: Adults & Peds: ≥12 yo: 200-300 mg/kg/d given as q4-6h or 3-4 gm q4-6h.	⬤B ✿> R

[1] Potential neurotoxicity, ototoxicity & neuromuscular blockade. Avoid concurrent use with neurotoxic/nephrotoxic agents & diuretics.

NAME	FORM/STRENGTH	DOSAGE	COMMENTS
Ticarcillin Disodium/ Clavulanate Potassium (Timentin)	**Inj:** 3 gm-100 mg, 3 gm-100 mg/100 ml, 30 gm-1 gm	**IV: Adults:** ≥60 kg: 300 mg/kg/d ticarcillin given q4h. <60 kg: 200-300 mg/kg/d ticarcillin given q4-6h. **Peds:** ≥3 mths & <60 kg: 50 mg/kg/d ticarcillin given q4h. ≥3 mths & ≥60 kg: 3.1 gm q4h.	●B ✿> R
Ticarcillin (Ticar)	**Inj:** 3 gm, 20 gm	**Adults & Peds:** 200-300 mg/kg/d IV given q4-6h. 0-7 days & <2000gm: 75 mg/kg IM/IV q12h. 0-7 days & >2000 gm or >7 days & <2000 gm: 75 mg/kg IM/IV q8h. >7 days & >2000 gm: 100 mg/kg IM/IV q8h.	●N ✿>

MISCELLANEOUS

NAME	FORM/STRENGTH	DOSAGE	COMMENTS
Chloramphenicol (Chloromycetin)	**Inj:** 1 gm	**IV: Adults & Peds:** 50-100 mg/kg/d given q6h. **Infants:** 25 mg/kg/d given q6h.	●N ✿v H R Serious, fatal blood dyscrasias.
Clindamycin (Cleocin)	**Inj:** 150 mg/ml, 300 mg/50 ml, 600 mg/50 ml, 900 mg/50 ml	**IV: Adults:** 1200-2700 mg/d given bid-qid. Up to 4800 mg/d. **Peds:** 1 mth-16 yo: 20-40 mg/kg/d given tid-qid. <1 mth: 15-20 mg/kg/d given tid-qid.	●B ✿v Associated with severe, fatal colitis.
Imipenem/Cilastatin Sodium (Primaxin IV)	**Inj:** 250-250 mg, 500-500 mg	**IV: Adults:** ≥70 kg: Mild: 250-500 mg q6h. Moderate: 500 mg q6-8h or 1 gm q8h. Severe: 500 mg q6h or 1 gm q6-8h. Max: 50 mg/kg/d or 4 gm/d, whichever is lower. **Peds:** ≥3 mths: 15-25 mg/kg q6h. Max: 4 gm/d. 4 wks-3 mths & ≥1500 gm: 25 mg/kg q6h. 1-4 wks & ≥1500 gm: 25 mg/kg q8h. <1 wk & ≥1500 gm: 25 mg/kg q12h.	●C ✿> R

| Vancomycin
(Vancocin, Vancoled) | Inj: 250 mg/5 ml,
500 mg/6 ml, 500 mg,
1 gm, 10 gm | IV: Adults: 500 mg q6h or 1 gm q12h.
Children: 10 mg/kg q6h. Infants & Neonates: 15 mg/kg
x 1 dose then 10 mg/kg q12h for 1st wk of life, & q8h
up to 1 mth of age. | ⊕C ✿v R |

Skin/Skin Structure Infections

CARBAPENEM

| Ertapenem Sodium
(Invanz) | Inj: 1 gm | Adults: 1 gm qd x 7-14d. May give IV up to 14d; IM up
to 7d. | ⊕B ✿> R |

CEPHALOSPORINS

Cefaclor (Ceclor, Ceclor CD)	Cap: 250 mg, 500 mg; Susp: 125 mg/5 ml, 187 mg/5 ml, 250 mg/ 5 ml, 375 mg/5 ml; Tab,ER: (CD) 375 mg, 500 mg	Adults: Cap/Susp: 250 mg q8h. Tab,ER: 375 mg q12h. Peds: ≥1 mth: Cap/Susp: 20 mg/kg/d given q8h. Max:1 gm/d.	⊕B ✿>
Cefadroxil (Duricef)	Cap: 500 mg; Susp: 250 mg/5 ml, 500 mg/5 ml; Tab: 1 gm	Adults: 1 gm qd or 500 mg bid. Peds: 15 mg/kg q12h (or 30 mg/kg qd for impetigo).	⊕B ✿> R
Cefdinir (Omnicef)	Cap: 300 mg; Susp: 125 mg/5 ml	≥13 yo: 300 mg cap q12h x 10d. 6 mths-12 yo: 7 mg/kg susp q12h x 10d.	⊕B ✿> R
Cefditoren Pivoxil (Spectracef)	Tab: 200 mg	≥12 yo: 200 mg bid x 10d.	⊕B ✿> R

NAME	FORM/STRENGTH	DOSAGE	COMMENTS
Cefepime HCl (Maxipime)	**Inj:** 500 mg, 1 gm, 2 gm	**Adults: Moderate-Severe:** 2 gm IV q12h x 10d. **Peds: 2 mths-16 yo:** ≤40 kg: 50 mg/kg IV q12h. **Max:** Do not exceed adult dose.	■B ❄> R
Cefpodoxime Proxetil (Vantin)	**Susp:** 50 mg/5 ml, 100 mg/5 ml; **Tab:** 100 mg, 200 mg	≥**12 yo:** 400 mg q12h x 7-14d.	■B ❄v R
Cefprozil (Cefzil)	**Susp:** 125 mg/5 ml, 250 mg/5 ml; **Tab:** 250 mg, 500 mg	**Adults & Peds ≥13 yo:** 250-500 mg q12h or 500 mg q24h x 10d. **2-12 mo:** 20 mg/kg q24h x 10d.	■B ❄v R
Ceftriaxone Sodium (Rocephin)	**Inj:** 1 gm/50 ml, 2 gm/ 50 ml, 250 mg, 500 mg, 1 gm, 2 gm, 10 gm	**IM/IV: Adults: Usual:** 1-2 gm qd (or in equally divided doses bid). **Max:** 4 gm/d. **Peds:** 50-75 mg/kg given qd (or in equally divided doses bid). **Max:** 2 gm/d.	■B ❄>
Cefuroxime Axetil (Ceftin)	**Susp:** 125 mg/5 ml, 250 mg/5 ml; **Tab:** 125 mg, 250 mg, 500 mg	**Adults & Peds ≥13 yo: Tab:** 250-500 mg bid x 10d. **3 mths-12 yo: Susp:** 15 mg/kg/d bid x 10d for impetigo.	■B ❄v R Tabs & susp are not bioequivalent.
Cephalexin (Keflex)	**Cap:** 250 mg, 500 mg; **Susp:** 125 mg/5 ml, 250 mg/5 ml; **Tab:** 250 mg, 500 mg	**Adults:** 500 mg q12h. **Peds:** 25-50 mg/kg/d given q12h.	■B ❄>
Cephradine (Velosef)	**Cap:** 250 mg, 500 mg; **Susp:** 250 mg/5 ml	**Adults:** 250 mg q6h or 500 mg q12h. **Peds: >9 mths:** 25-50 mg/kg/d given q6h or q12h (up to adult dose).	■B ❄> R
Loracarbef (Lorabid)	**Cap:** 200 mg, 400 mg; **Susp:** 100 mg/5 ml, 200 mg/5 ml	**Adults & Peds ≥13 yo:** 200 mg q12h x 7d. **6 mths-12 yo: Impetigo:** 7.5 mg/kg q12h x 7d.	■B ❄> R

MACROLIDES

Azithromycin (Zithromax)	**Susp:** 100 mg/5 ml, 200 mg/5 ml, 1 gm/pkt; **Tab:** 250 mg, 600 mg	**≥16 yo:** 500 mg qd x 1d, then 250 mg qd on d2-5.	⬛B ❄>
Clarithromycin (Biaxin)	**Susp:** 125 mg/5 ml, 250 mg/5 ml; **Tab:** 250 mg, 500 mg	**Adults:** 250 mg q12h x 7-14d. **Peds: ≥6 mths:** 7.5 mg/kg q12h x 10d.	⬛C ❄> R
Dirithromycin (Dynabac)	**Tab,Delay:** 250 mg	**Adults & Peds ≥12 yo:** 500 mg qd x 5-7d.	⬛C ❄>
Erythromycin Base	**Tab:** 250 mg	**Adults:** Usual: 250 mg q6h or 500 mg q12h. **Peds:** Usual: 30-50 mg/kg/d in divided doses. **Max:** 4 gm/d.	⬛B ❄>
Erythromycin Ethylsuccinate (E.E.S., EryPed)	**Chewtab:** (EryPed) 200 mg; **Sus:** (EryPed) 100 mg/2.5 ml, 200 mg/5 ml, 400 mg/ 5 ml, (E.E.S.) 200 mg/ 5 ml, 400 mg/5 ml; **Tab:** (E.E.S.) 400 mg	**Adults:** Usual: 1600 mg/d given q6h, q8h, or q12h. **Max:** 4 gm/d. **Peds:** Usual: 30-50 mg/kg/d in divided doses q6h, q8h, or q12h. Double dose for more severe infections.	⬛B ❄>
Erythromycin (Ery-Tab, PCE)	**Tab,Enteric:** (Ery-Tab) 250 mg, 333 mg, 500 mg; **Tab,ER:** (PCE) 333 mg, 500 mg	**Adults:** Usual: 250 mg qid, 333 mg q8h, or 500 mg q12h. **Peds:** Usual: 30-50 mg/kg/d in divided doses. **Max:** 4 gm/d.	⬛B ❄>
Erythromycin Stearate (Erythrocin)	**Tab:** 250 mg, 500 mg	**Adults:** Usual: 250 mg q6h or 500 mg q12h. **Peds:** Usual: 30-50 mg/kg/d in divided doses. **Max:** 4 gm/d.	⬛B ❄>

NAME	FORM/STRENGTH	DOSAGE	COMMENTS

OXAZOLIDINONE

Linezolid (Zyvox)	**Inj:** 2 mg/ml; **Susp:** 100 mg/5 ml; **Tab:** 600 mg	**Complicated: Treat x 10-14d.** Adults & Peds ≥12 yo: 600 mg IV/PO q12h. **Birth-11 yo:** 10 mg/kg IV/PO q8h. **Uncomplicated: Treat x 10-14d. Adults:** 400 mg PO q12h. **≥12 yo:** 600 mg PO q12h. **5-11 yo:** 10 mg/kg PO q12h. **<5 yo:** 10 mg/kg PO q8h.	◉C ❋>

PENICILLINS

Amoxicillin (Amoxil, DisperMox, Trimox)	**Cap:** (Amoxil, Trimox) 250 mg, 500 mg; **Chewtab:** (Amoxil) 200 mg, 400 mg; **Susp:** (Amoxil) 50 mg/ml, 125 mg/5 ml, 200 mg/5 ml, 250 mg/5 ml, 400 mg/5 ml, (Trimox) 125 mg/5 ml, 250 mg/5 ml; **Tab:** (Amoxil) 500 mg, 875 mg; **Tab, Dispersible:** (DisperMox) 200 mg, 400 mg, 600 mg	**Adults & Peds >40 kg:** 500-875 mg q12h or 250-500 mg q8h, depending on severity. **>3 mths:** 25-45 mg/kg/d divided q12h or 20-40 mg/kg/d divided q8h, depending on severity. **≤3 mths: Usual/Max:** 15 mg/kg q12h.	◉B ❋> R

Amoxicillin/Clavulanate (Augmentin)	**Chewtab:** 125-31.25 mg, 200-28.5 mg, 250-62.5 mg, 400-57 mg; **Susp:** (per 5 ml) 125-31.25 mg, 200-28.5 mg, 250-62.5 mg, 400-57 mg; **Tab:** 250-125 mg, 500-125 mg, 875-125 mg	Dose based on amoxicillin component. **Adults & Peds ≥40 kg: Tab:** 500-875 mg q12h or 250-500 mg q8h, depending on severity. May use 125 mg/5 ml or 250 mg/5 ml susp in place of 500 mg tab & 200 mg/5 ml susp or 400 mg/5 ml susp in place of 875 mg tab. **≥12 wks: Chewtab/Susp:** 25-45 mg/kg/d given q12h or 20-40 mg/kg/d given q8h, depending on severity. **<12 wks: Susp:** 15 mg/kg q12h (use 125 mg/5 ml susp).	◐B ❋> H R 2-250 mg tabs are not equivalent to 1-500 mg tabs. Only use 250 mg tab if peds ≥40 kg. Chewtab & tab not interchangeable.
Ampicillin Sodium/ Sulbactam Sodium (Unasyn)	**Inj:** 1-0.5 gm, 2-1 gm	**Adults & Peds ≥1 yo:** 1.5-3 gm IV/IM q6h. **Max:** 4 gm sulbactam/d.	◐B ❋> R
Dicloxacillin Sodium (Dynapen)	**Cap:** 250 mg, 500 mg; **Susp:** 62.5 mg/5 ml	**Adults & Peds ≥40 kg: Mild-Moderate:** 125 mg q6h. **Severe:** 250 mg q6h. **Peds <40 kg: Mild-Moderate:** 3.125 mg/kg q6h. **Severe:** 6.25 mg/kg q6h.	◐B ❋>
Penicillin V Potassium (Penicillin VK, Veetids)	**Susp:** 125 mg/5 ml, 250 mg/5 ml; **Tab:** 250 mg, 500 mg	**Adults & Peds ≥12 yo:** 250-500 mg q6-8h.	◐B ❋>
Piperacillin/Tazobactam (Zosyn)	**Inj:** 40-5 mg/mL, 60-7.5 mg/mL, 2-0.25 gm, 3-0.375 gm, 4-0.5 gm, 4-0.5 gm/100 mL, 36-4.5 gm	**Adults:** 3.375 gm IV q6h x 7-10d.	◐B ❋> R

NAME	FORM/STRENGTH	DOSAGE	COMMENTS
QUINOLONES			
Ciprofloxacin (Cipro)	**Inj:** 10 mg/ml, 200 mg/ 100 ml, 400 mg/200 ml; **Susp:** 250 mg/5 ml, 500 mg/5 ml; **Tab:** 100 mg, 250 mg, 500 mg, 750 mg	**≥18 yo: Mild-Moderate:** 500 mg PO q12h or 400 mg IV q12h x 7-14d. **Severe:** 750 mg PO q12h or 400 mg IV q8h x 7-14d.	◑C ✿v R
Gatifloxacin (Tequin)	**Inj:** 2 mg/ml; 10 mg/ml; **Tab:** 200 mg, 400 mg	**≥18 yo: Uncomplicated:** 400 mg PO/IV qd x 7-10d.	◑C ✿> R
Levofloxacin (Levaquin)	**Inj:** 5 mg/ml, 25 mg/ml; **Tab:** 250 mg, 500 mg, 750 mg	**≥18 yo: Uncomplicated:** 500 mg PO/IV qd x 7-10d. **Complicated:** 750 mg PO/IV qd x 7-14d.	◑C ✿v R
Moxifloxacin HCl (Avelox)	**Inj:** 400 mg/250 ml; **Tab:** 400 mg	**≥18 yo:** 400 mg PO/IV q24h x 7d.	◑C ✿v
Ofloxacin (Floxin)	**Tab:** 200 mg, 300 mg, 400 mg	**≥18 yo:** 400 mg q12h x 10d.	◑C ✿v H R
STREPTOGRAMIN AGENT			
Dalfopristin/Quinupristin (Synercid)	**Inj:** 350 mg-150 mg	**≥16 yo: Complicated:** 7.5 mg/kg IV q12h for at least 7d.	◑B ✿> H

TETRACYCLINES

Doxycycline Hyclate (Vibramycin, Vibra-Tabs)	**Cap:** 50 mg, 100 mg; **Tab:** 100 mg	**Adults:** 100 mg q12h on d1, then 100 mg qd or 50 mg q12h. **Severe:** 100 mg q12h. **Peds: >8 yo & ≤100 lbs:** 1 mg/lb bid on d1, then 1 mg/lb qd or 0.5 mg/lb bid. **>100 lbs:** Adult dose.	⬛D ❄v
Doxycycline Monohydrate (Monodox, Vibramycin)	**Cap:** (Monodox) 50 mg, 100 mg; **Susp:** (Vibramycin) 25 mg/5 ml	**Adults:** 100 mg q12h or 50 mg q6h on d1, then 100 mg qd or 50 mg q12h. **Severe:** 100 mg q12h. **Peds: >8 yo & ≤100 lbs:** 1 mg/lb bid on d1, then 1 mg/lb qd or 0.5 mg/lb bid. **Severe:** 2 mg/lb. **>100 lbs:** Adult dose.	⬛D ❄v
Minocycline HCl (Dynacin, Minocin)	**Cap:** 50 mg, 75 mg, 100 mg; **Inj:** 100 mg	**Adults:** 200 mg PO/IV, then 100 mg q12h or 50 mg qid. **>8 yo:** 4 mg/kg PO/IV, then 2 mg/kg q12h.	⬛D ❄v R

MISCELLANEOUS

Clindamycin (Cleocin)	**Cap:** 75 mg, 150 mg, 300 mg; **Susp:** 75 mg/5 ml; **Inj:** 150 mg/ml, 300 mg/50 ml, 600 mg/50 ml, 900 mg/50 ml	**IM/IV: Adults:** 600-2700 mg/d in 2-4 doses. Max 600 mg IM single dose. **Peds: <1 mth:** 15-20 mg/kg/d in 3-4 doses. **1 mth-16 yo:** 20-40 mg/kg/d in 3-4 doses. **PO: Adults:** 150-450 mg q6h. **Peds:** 8-20 mg/kg/d given 3-4 doses.	⬛B ❄v (IV) ❄> (PO) Associated with severe, fatal colitis.
Daptomycin (Cubicin)	**Inj:** 250 mg, 500 mg	**Adults: ≥18 yo:** 4 mg/kg IV infusion over 30 mins once every 24 hrs x 7-14d.	⬛B ❄> R

Tuberculosis

RECOMMENDED DRUGS FOR THE INITIAL TREATMENT OF TUBERCULOSIS IN CHILDREN* & ADULTS
DOSAGE SCHEDULE**

DRUG	DAILY DOSE (maximum dose)		TWO DOSES PER WEEK (maximum dose)		THREE DOSES PER WEEK (maximum dose)	
	CHILDREN	ADULTS	CHILDREN	ADULTS	CHILDREN	ADULTS
Isoniazid	10-15 mg/kg (300 mg)	5 mg/kg (300 mg)	20-30 mg/kg (900 mg)	15 mg/kg (900 mg)	—	15 mg/kg (900 mg)
Rifampin†	10-20 mg/kg (600 mg)	10 mg/kg (600 mg)	10-20 mg/kg (600 mg)	10 mg/kg (600 mg)	—	10 mg/kg (600 mg)
Pyrazinamide	15-30 mg/kg (2 gm)	18.2-26.8 mg/kg (2 gm)	50 mg/kg (2 gm)	36.4-53.6 mg/kg (4 gm)	—	27.3-44.6 mg/kg (3 gm)
Ethambutol‡	15-20 mg/kg (1 gm)	14.5-21.4 mg/kg (1.6 gm)	50 mg/kg (2.5 gm)	36.4-52.6 mg/kg (4 gm)	—	21.8-35.7 mg/kg (2.4 gm)

* Persons ≤14 yo and ≤40 kg.

Source: *Am J Respir Crit Care Med* 2003;167: 603-662.

** Based on ideal body weight except adult doses for pyrazinamide and ethambutol (estimated lean body weight).

† Adult dose may need to be adjusted with concomitant use of protease inhibitors or nonnucleoside reverse transcriptase inhibitors.

‡ Caution in children whose vision cannot be monitored (<5 yo). A dose of 15 mg/kg/d can be used in younger children with isoniazid or rifampin resistance.

NAME	FORM/STRENGTH	DOSAGE	COMMENTS
Aminosalicylic Acid (Paser)	**Granule:** 4 gm/pkt	**Adults:** 4 gm tid. Can sprinkle on apple sauce, yogurt, or swirl in tomato or orange juice.	◉C ✿>
Capreomycin Sulfate (Capastat Sulfate)	**Inj:** 1 gm	**Adults:** Usual: 1 gm IM/IV qd x 60-120d, then 1 gm x 2-3x/wk. **Max:** 20 mg/kg/d.	◉C ✿> R Caution with auditory or renal impairment. Avoid other ototoxic & nephrotoxic agents.
Cycloserine (Seromycin)	**Cap:** 250 mg	**Adults:** Usual: 250 mg bid x 2 wks. Usual: 500 mg-1 gm/d in divided doses. **Max:** 1 gm/d.	◉C ✿v
Ethambutol HCl (Myambutol)	**Tab:** 100 mg, 400 mg	**Adults & Peds:** ≥13 yo: Initial: 15 mg/kg q24h. **Retreatment:** 25 mg/kg q24h x 60d, then decrease to 15 mg/kg q24h.	◉N ✿> R
Ethionamide (Trecator-SC)	**Tab:** 250 mg	**Usual: Adults:** 15-20 mg/kg qd or in divided doses. **Max:** 1 gm/d. ≥**12 yo:** 10-20 mg/kg/d as bid-tid after meals or 15 mg/kg/qd.	◉C ✿>
Isoniazid (Nydrazid)	**Inj:** 100 mg/ml; **Syr:** 50 mg/5 ml; **Tab:** 100 mg, 300 mg	**Active TB: Adults:** 5 mg/kg, up to 300 mg qd. **Peds:** 10-20 mg/kg, up to 300-500 mg qd. **Prevention: Adults:** 300 mg qd. **Peds:** 10 mg/kg qd, up to 300 mg qd.	◉N ✿> 14

14 INH associated with hepatitis. Avoid in acute hepatic diseases

NAME	FORM/STRENGTH	DOSAGE	COMMENTS
Isoniazid/Pyrazinamide/Rifampin (Rifater)	Tab: 50 mg-300 mg-120 mg	Adults & Peds: ≥15 yo: Usual: ≤44 kg: 4 tabs qd, 45-54 kg: 5 tabs qd. ≥55 kg: 6 tabs qd. Take 1h before or 2h after a meal. Give pyridoxine to the malnourished, if predisposed to neuropathy, & adolescents.	⊙C ❀v [14]
Isoniazid/Rifampin (Rifamate)	Cap: 150 mg-300 mg	Adults: Usual: 2 caps qd, 1h before or 2h after a meal. Give pyridoxine to the malnourished, if predisposed to neuropathy, & adolescents.	⊙N ❀> [14]
Pyrazinamide	Tab: 500 mg	Adults & Peds: Usual: 15-30 mg/kg qd. Max: 3 gm/d. CDC recommends max 2 gm/d with daily regimen. Alternate Regimen: 50-70 mg/kg BIW. Continue x 2 mths.	⊙C ❀>
Rifampin (Rifadin, Rimactane)	Cap: 150 mg, 300 mg; Inj: 600 mg	PO/IV: Adults: 10 mg/kg qd. Max: 600 mg/d. Peds: 10-20 mg/kg qd. Max: 600 mg/d. Take PO 1h before or 2h after a meal with a full glass of water. Continue x 2 mths.	⊙C ❀v
Rifapentine (Priftin)	Tab: 150 mg	Adults & Peds: ≥12 yo: Intensive Phase: Initial: 600 mg BIW with an interval of not <72h between doses. Continue x 2 mths. Maint: 600 mg once wkly x 4 mths. Give pyridoxine to the malnourished, if predisposed to neuropathy, & adolescents.	⊙C ❀v

| Streptomycin Sulfate | Inj: 1 gm | **IM: Adults:** 15 mg/kg qd. **Max:** 1 gm. **Alternate Schedule:** 25-30 mg/kg BIW-TIW. **Max:** 1.5 gm. **Peds:** 20-40 mg/kg qd. **Max:** 1 gm. **Alternate Schedule:** 25-30 mg/kg BIW-TIW. **Max:** 1.5 gm. | ⊕D ❄v Increased risk of severe neurotoxic reactions with renal dysfunction. Avoid neurotoxic & nephrotoxic drugs. |

Upper Respiratory Tract Infection

CEPHALOSPORINS

| Cefaclor (Ceclor, Ceclor CD) | **Cap:** 250 mg, 500 mg; **Susp:** 125 mg/5 ml, 187 mg/5 ml, 250 mg/5 ml, 375 mg/5 ml; **Tab,ER:** (CD) 375 mg, 500 mg | **Adults: Cap/Susp:** 250 mg q8h. **Tab,ER:** 375 mg q12h. **Peds:** ≥1 mth: **Cap/Susp:** 20 mg/kg/d given q8h. **Max:**1 gm/d. | ⊕B ❄> |

| Cefadroxil (Duricef) | **Cap:** 500 mg; **Susp:** 250 mg/5 ml, 500 mg/5 ml; **Tab:** 1 gm | **Adults:** 1 gm qd or 500 mg bid x 10d. **Peds:** 15 mg/kg q12h or 30 mg/kg qd. | ⊕B ❄> R |

| Cefdinir (Omnicef) | **Cap:** 300 mg; **Susp:** 125 mg/5 ml | **Pharyngitis/Tonsillitis:** ≥13 yo: **Caps:** 300 mg q12h x 5-10d or 600 mg q24h x 10d. **6 mths-12 yo: Susp:** 7 mg/kg q12h x 5-10d or 14 mg/kg q24h x 10d. **Sinusitis:** ≥13 yo: **Caps:** 300 mg q12h or 600 mg q24h x 10d. **6 mths-12 yo: Susp:** 7 mg/kg q12h or 14 mg/kg q24h x 10d. | ⊕B ❄> R |

[14] INH associated with hepatitis. Avoid in acute hepatic diseases

NAME	FORM/STRENGTH	DOSAGE	COMMENTS
Cefditoren Pivoxil (Spectracef)	**Tab:** 200 mg	**≥12 yo: Pharyngitis/Tonsillitis:** 200 mg bid x 10d.	⊕B ✲> R
Cefixime (Suprax)	**Susp:** 100 mg/5 ml; **Tab:** 200 mg, 400 mg	**>12 yo or >50 kg: Tab/Susp:** 400 mg qd or 200 mg bid. **≤50 kg or >6 mths: Susp:** 8 mg/kg qd or 4 mg/kg bid.	⊕B ✲v R
Cefpodoxime Proxetil (Vantin)	**Susp:** 50 mg/5 ml, 100 mg/5 ml; **Tab:** 100 mg, 200 mg	**≥12 yo: Pharyngitis/Tonsillitis:** 100 mg q12h x 5-10d. **2 mths-11 yo:** 5 mg/kg q12h x 5-10d. **≥12 yo: Sinusitis:** 200 mg q12h x 10d. **2 mths-11 yo:** 5 mg/kg q12h x 10d.	⊕B ✲v R
Cefprozil (Cefzil)	**Susp:** 125 mg/5 ml, 250 mg/5 ml; **Tab:** 250 mg, 500 mg	**Adults & Peds ≥13 yo: Pharyngitis/Tonsillitis:** 500 mg q24h x 10d. **Sinusitis:** 250-500 mg q12h x 10d. **6 mths-12 yo: Pharyngitis/Tonsillitis:** 7.5 mg/kg q12h x 10d. **Sinusitis:** 7.5-15 mg/kg q12h x 10d. **Max:** Adult dose.	⊕B ✲v R
Ceftibuten (Cedax)	**Cap:** 400 mg; **Susp:** 90 mg/5 ml	**≥12 yo:** 400 mg qd x 10d. **≥6 mths:** 9 mg/kg qd x 10d. **Max:** 400 mg/d.	⊕B ✲> R
Cefuroxime Axetil (Ceftin)	**Susp:** 125 mg/5 ml, 250 mg/5 ml; **Tab:** 125 mg, 250 mg, 500 mg	**Adults & Peds ≥13 yo: Tab:** 250 mg bid x 10d. **3 mths-12 yo: Pharyngitis/Tonsillitis: Tab:** 125 mg bid x 10d. **Susp:** 10 mg/kg bid x 10d. **Max:** 500 mg/d. **Sinusitis: Tab:** 250 mg bid x 10d. **Susp:** 15 mg/kg bid x 10d. **Max:** 1 gm/d.	⊕B ✲v R Tabs & susp are not bioequivalent.
Cephalexin (Keflex)	**Cap:** 250 mg, 500 mg; **Susp:** 125 mg/5 ml, 250 mg/5 ml; **Tab:** 250 mg, 500 mg	**Adults: Usual:** 250 mg q6h. **Max:** 4 gm/d. **Streptococcal Pharyngitis:** 500 mg q12h. **Peds: >1 yo: Usual:** 25-50 mg/kg/d given q12h.	⊕B ✲>

Cephradine (Velosef)	**Cap:** 250 mg, 500 mg; **Susp:** 250 mg/5 ml	**Tonsillitis/Pharyngitis: Adults:** 250 mg q6h or 500 mg q12h. **Peds: >9 mths:** 25-50 mg/kg/d given q6h or q12h (up to adult dose).	⬤B ❄> R
Loracarbef (Lorabid)	**Cap:** 200 mg, 400 mg; **Susp:** 100 mg/5 ml, 200 mg/5 ml	**Adults & Peds ≥13 yo: Pharyngitis/Tonsillitis:** 200 mg q12h x 7d. **Sinusitis:** 400 mg q12h x 12d. **6 mths-12 yo: Pharyngitis/Tonsillitis:** 7.5 mg/kg q12h x 10d. **Sinusitis:** 15 mg/kg q12h x 10d.	⬤B ❄> R

KETOLIDES

Telithromycin (Ketek)	**Tab:** 400 mg	**Adults: Sinusitis:** 800 mg qd x 5d.	⬤C ❄>

MACROLIDES

Azithromycin (Zithromax)	**Susp:** 100 mg/5 ml, 200 mg/5 ml, 1 gm/pkt; **Tab:** 250 mg, 600 mg	**Pharyngitis/Tonsillitis: Adults:** 500 mg qd x 1d, then 250 mg qd on d2-5. **≥2 yo:** 12 mg/kg qd x 5d. **Acute Bacterial Sinusitis: Adults:** 500 mg qd x 3d. **≥6mo:** 10 mg/kg qd x 3d.	⬤B ❄>
Clarithromycin (Biaxin)	**Susp:** 125 mg/5 ml, 250 mg/5 ml; **Tab:** 250 mg, 500 mg; **Tab,ER:** 500 mg	**Adults: Pharyngitis/Tonsillitis: Susp/Tab:** 250 mg q12h x 10d. **Sinusitis: Susp/Tab:** 500 mg q12h x 14d. **Tab,ER:** 1 gm qd x 14d. **Peds: ≥6 mths: Pharyngitis/Tonsillitis/Sinusitis: Susp/Tab:** 7.5 mg/kg q12h x 10d.	⬤C ❄> R
Dirithromycin (Dynabac)	**Tab,Delay:** 250 mg	**Adults & Peds ≥12 yo:** 500 mg qd x 7-10d.	⬤C ❄>
Erythromycin Base	**Tab:** 250 mg	**Adults: Usual:** 250 mg q6h or 500 mg q12h. **Peds: Usual:** 30-50 mg/kg/d in divided doses. **Max:** 4 gm/d.	⬤B ❄>

NAME	FORM/STRENGTH	DOSAGE	COMMENTS
Erythromycin Ethylsuccinate (E.E.S., EryPed)	**Chewab:** (EryPed) 200 mg; **Sus:** (EryPed) 100 mg/2.5 ml, 200 mg/5ml, 5 ml, 400 mg/5 ml, (E.E.S.) 200 mg/5 ml, 400 mg/5 ml; **Tab:** (E.E.S.) 400mg	**Adults: Usual:** 1600 mg/d given q6h, q8h, or q12h. **Peds: Usual:** 30-50 mg/kg/d in divided doses q6h, q8h, or q12h. Double dose for more severe infections. **Max:** 4 gm/d.	©B ✽ >
Erythromycin (Ery-Tab, PCE)	**Tab,Enteric:** (Ery-Tab) 250 mg, 333 mg, 500 mg; **Tab,ER:** (PCE) 333 mg, 500 mg	**Adults: Usual:** 250 mg qid, 333 mg q8h, or 500 mg q12h. **Peds: Usual:** 30-50 mg/kg/d in divided doses. **Max:** 4 gm/d.	©B ✽ >
Erythromycin Stearate (Erythrocin)	**Tab:** 250 mg, 500 mg	**Adults: Usual:** 250 mg q6h or 500 mg q12h. **Peds: Usual:** 30-50 mg/kg/d in divided doses. **Max:** 4 gm/d.	©B ✽ >
PENICILLINS			
Amoxicillin (Amoxil, DispermMox, Trimox)	**Cap:** (Amoxil, Trimox) 250 mg, 500 mg; **Chewab:** (Amoxil) 200 mg, 400 mg; **Susp:** (Amoxil) 50 mg/ml, 125 mg/5 ml, 200 mg/5 ml, 250 mg/5 ml, 400 mg/5 ml, (Trimox) 125 mg/5 ml, 250 mg/5 ml; **Tab:** (Amoxil) 5 ml	**Adults & Peds >40 kg:** 500-875 mg q12h or 250-500 mg q8h, depending on severity; **>3 mths:** 25-45 mg/kg/d divided q12h or 20-40 mg/kg/d divided q8h, depending on severity; **≤3 mths: Usual/Max:** 15 mg/kg q12h.	©B ✽ >R

	500 mg, 875 mg; **Tab, Dispersible:** (DisperMox) 200 mg, 400 mg, 600 mg		
Amoxicillin/Clavulanate (Augmentin)	**Chewtab:** 125-31.25 mg, 200-28.5 mg, 250- 62.5 mg, 400-57 mg; **Susp:** (per 5 ml) 125- 31.25 mg, 200-28.5 mg, 250-62.5 mg, 400-57 mg; **Tab:** 250-125 mg, 500- 125 mg, 875-125 mg	Dose based on amoxicillin component. **Adults & Peds ≥40 kg: Tab:** 500-875 mg q12h or 250-500 mg q8h, depending on severity. May use 125 mg/5 ml or 250 mg/5 ml susp in place of 500 mg tab & 200 mg/5 ml susp or 400 mg/5 ml susp in place of 875 mg tab. **≥12 wks: Chewtab/Susp:** 25-45 mg/kg/d given q12h or 20-40 mg/kg/d given q8h, depending on severity. **<12 wks: Susp:** 15 mg/kg q12h (use 125 mg/5 ml susp).	⬤B ✿> H R 2-250 mg tabs are not equivalent to 1-500 mg tab. Only use 250 mg tab if peds ≥40 kg. Chewtab & tab not interchangeable.
Amoxicillin/Clavulanate (Augmentin XR)	**Tab,ER:** 1000 mg- 62.5 mg	**≥16 yo:** 2 tabs q12h x 10d.	⬤ B ✿>
Ampicillin (Principen)	**Cap:** 250 mg, 500 mg; **Susp:** 125 mg/5ml, 250 mg/5ml	**Adults & Peds: >20 kg:** 250 mg qid. **Peds: ≤20 kg:** 50 mg/kg/d given tid-qid.	⬤B ✿>
Ampicillin Sodium	**Inj:** 125 mg, 250 mg, 500 mg, 1 gm, 2 gm, 10 gm	**Adults & Peds: ≥40 kg:** 250-500 mg IM/IV q8h. **Peds: <40 kg:** 25-50 mg/kg q6-8h.	⬤B ✿>
Dicloxacillin Sodium (Dynapen)	**Cap:** 250 mg, 500 mg; **Susp:** 62.5 mg/5 ml	**Adults & Peds ≥40 kg: Mild-Moderate:** 125 mg q6h. **Severe:** 250 mg q6h. **Peds <40 kg: Mild-Moderate:** 3.125 mg/kg q6h. **Severe:** 6.25 mg/kg q6h.	⬤B ✿>

NAME	FORM/STRENGTH	DOSAGE	COMMENTS
Penicillin V Potassium (Penicillin VK, Veetids)	**Susp:** 125 mg/5 ml, 250 mg/5 ml; **Tab:** 250 mg, 500 mg	**Adults & Peds ≥12 yo: Streptococcal:** 125-500 mg q6h x 10d. **Fusospirochetosis:** (Oropharynx) 250-500 mg q6-8h. **Pneumococcal:** 250-500 mg q6h until afebrile x 2d.	◐B ❄>

QUINOLONES

NAME	FORM/STRENGTH	DOSAGE	COMMENTS
Gatifloxacin (Tequin)	**Inj:** 2 mg/ml; 10 mg/ml; **Tab:** 200 mg, 400 mg	**≥18 yo: Sinusitis:** 400 mg PO/IV qd x 10d.	◐C ❄> R
Levofloxacin (Levaquin)	**Inj:** 5 mg/ml, 25 mg/ml; **Tab:** 250 mg, 500 mg, 750 mg	**≥18 yo: Sinusitis:** 500 mg IV/PO qd x 10-14d.	◐C ❄v R
Moxifloxacin HCl (Avelox)	**Inj:** 400 mg/250 ml; **Tab:** 400 mg	**≥18 yo: Sinusitis:** 400 mg PO/IV qd x 10d.	◐C ❄v

TETRACYCLINES

NAME	FORM/STRENGTH	DOSAGE	COMMENTS
Demeclocycline (Declomycin)	**Tab:** 150 mg, 500 mg	**Adults:** 150 mg qid or 300 mg bid. **Peds: ≥8 yo:** 3-6 mg/lb/d given bid-qid.	◐N ❄v
Doxycycline Hyclate (Vibramycin, Vibra-Tabs)	**Cap:** 50 mg, 100 mg; **Tab:** 100 mg	**Adults:** 100 mg q12h on d1, then 100 mg qd or 50 mg q12h. **Severe:** 100 mg q12h. **Peds: >8 yo & ≤100 lbs:** 1 mg/lb bid on d1, then 1 mg/lb qd or 0.5 mg/lb bid. **Severe:** 2 mg/lb. **>100 lbs:** Adult dose.	◐D ❄v
Doxycycline Monohydrate (Monodox, Vibramycin)	**Cap:** (Monodox) 50 mg, 100 mg; **Susp:** (Vibramycin) 25 mg/5 ml	**Adults:** 100 mg q12h or 50 mg q6h on d1, then 100 mg qd or 50 mg q12h. **Peds: >8 yo & ≤100 lbs:** 1 mg/lb bid on d1, then 1 mg/lb qd or 0.5 mg/lb bid. **>100 lbs:** Adult dose.	◐D ❄v

Minocycline HCl (Dynacin, Minocin)	**Cap:** 50 mg, 75 mg, 100 mg; **Inj:** 100 mg	**Adults:** 200 mg PO/IV, then 100 mg q12h or 50 mg qid. **>8 yo:** 4 mg/kg PO/IV, then 2 mg/kg q12h.	◉D ❄v R
Tetracycline HCl (Sumycin)	**Cap:** 250 mg, 500 mg; **Susp:** 125 mg/5 ml	**Adults:** 250 mg qid or 500 mg bid. **Peds: >8 yo:** 25-50 mg/kg divided bid-qid.	◉D ❄v R

Urinary Tract Infection

CARBAPENEM

Ertapenem Sodium (Invanz)	**Inj:** 1 gm	**Adults:** 1 gm qd x 10-14d. May give IV up to 14d; IM up to 7d.	◉B ❄> R

CEPHALOSPORINS

Cefaclor (Ceclor, Ceclor CD)	**Cap:** 250 mg, 500 mg; **Susp:** 125 mg/5 ml, 187 mg/5 ml, 250 mg/5 ml, 375 mg/5 ml	**Adults:** 250 mg q8h. **Peds: ≥1 mth:** 20 mg/kg/d q8h.	◉B ❄>
Cefadroxil (Duricef)	**Cap:** 500 mg; **Susp:** 250 mg/5 ml, 500 mg/5 ml; **Tab:** 1 gm	**Adults: Uncomplicated Lower UTI:** 1-2 gm/d given qd-bid. **Other UTIs:** 1 gm bid. **Peds:** 15 mg/kg q12h.	◉B ❄> R
Cefepime HCl (Maxipime)	**Inj:** 500 mg, 1 gm, 2 gm	**Adults: Mild-Moderate:** 0.5-1 gm IM/IV q12h x 7-10d. **Severe:** 2 gm IV q12h x 10d. **Peds: 2 mths-16 yo:** ≤**40 kg:** 50 mg/kg IV q12h. **Max:** Do not exceed adult dose.	◉B ❄> R
Cefixime (Suprax)	**Susp:** 100 mg/5 ml; **Tab:** 200 mg, 400 mg	**>12 yo or >50 kg:** Tab/Susp: 400 mg qd or 200 mg bid. **≤50 kg or >6 mths:** Susp: 8 mg/kg qd or 4 mg/kg bid.	◉B ❄v R

NAME	FORM/STRENGTH	DOSAGE	COMMENTS
Cefpodoxime Proxetil (Vantin)	**Susp:** 50 mg/5 ml, 100 mg/5 ml; **Tab:** 100 mg, 200 mg	**≥12 yo:** 100 mg q12h x 7d.	▣B ❀v R
Ceftriaxone Sodium (Rocephin)	**Inj:** 1 gm/50 ml, 2 gm/50 ml, 250 mg, 500 mg, 1 gm, 2 gm, 10 gm	**IM/IV: Adults:** 1-2 gm qd (or in equally divided doses bid). **Max:** 4 gm/d.	▣B ❀>
Cefuroxime Axetil (Ceftin)	**Tab:** 125 mg, 250 mg, 500 mg	**Adults & Peds ≥13 yo:** 125-250 mg bid x 7-10d.	▣B ❀v R
Cefuroxime (Kefurox, Zinacef)	**Inj:** 750 mg, 1.5 gm, 7.5 gm	**IM/IV: Adults: Uncomplicated:** 750 mg q8h x 5-10d. **Peds: >3 mths:** 50-100 mg/kg/d given q6-8h. **Max:** 4.5 gm/d.	▣B ❀> R
Cephalexin (Keflex)	**Cap:** 250 mg, 500 mg; **Susp:** 125 mg/5 ml, 250 mg/5 ml; **Tab:** 250 mg, 500 mg	**Adults: Usual:** 250 mg q6h. **Max:** 4 gm/d. **Peds: Usual:** 25-50 mg/kg/d in divided doses.	▣B ❀>
Cephradine (Velosef)	**Cap:** 250 mg, 500 mg; **Susp:** 250 mg/5 ml	**Adults: Uncomplicated:** 500 mg q12h. **Serious (Prostatitis):** 500 mg q6h or 1 gm q12h. **Peds: >9 mths:** 25-50 mg/kg/d given q6h or q12h (up to adult dose).	▣B ❀> R

MONOBACTAMS

NAME	FORM/STRENGTH	DOSAGE	COMMENTS
Loracarbef (Lorabid)	**Cap:** 200 mg, 400 mg; **Susp:** 100 mg/5 ml, 200 mg/5 ml	**Adults & Peds: ≥13 yo: Cystitis:** 200 mg qd x 7d. **Pyelonephritis:** 400 mg q12h x 14d.	▣B ❀> R

Amoxicillin (Amoxil, DisperMox, Trimox)	**Cap:** (Amoxil, Trimox) 250 mg, 500 mg; **Chewtab:** (Amoxil) 200 mg, 400 mg; **Susp:** (Amoxil) 50 mg/ml, 125 mg/5 ml, 200 mg/5 ml, 250 mg/5 ml, 400 mg/5 ml, (Trimox) 125 mg/5 ml, 250 mg/5 ml; **Tab:** (Amoxil) 500 mg, 875 mg; **Tab, Dispersible:** (DisperMox) 200 mg, 400 mg, 600 mg	**Adults & Peds >40 kg:** 500-875 mg q12h or 250-500 mg q8h, depending on severity. **>3 mths:** 25-45 mg/kg/d divided q12h or 20-40 mg/kg/d divided q8h, depending on severity. **≤3 mths: Usual/Max:** 15 mg/kg q12h.	⓪B ❄️> R
Amoxicillin/Clavulanate (Augmentin)	**Chewtab:** 125-31.25 mg, 200-28.5 mg, 250-62.5 mg, 400-57 mg; **Susp:** (per 5 ml) 125-31.25 mg, 200-28.5 mg, 250-62.5 mg, 400-57 mg; **Tab:** 250-125 mg, 500-125 mg, 875-125 mg	Dose based on amoxicillin component. **Adults & Peds: ≥40 kg: Tab:** 500 mg q12h or 250 mg q8h. May use 125 mg/5 ml or 250 mg/5 ml susp in place of 500 mg tab & 200 mg/5 ml susp or 400 mg/5 ml susp in place of 875 mg tab. **≥12 wks: Chewtab/Susp:** 25 mg/kg/d given q12h or 20 mg/kg/d given q8h. **<12 wks: Susp:** 15 mg/kg q12h (use 125 mg/5 ml susp).	⓪B ❄️> H R 2-250 mg tabs are not equivalent to 1-500 mg tab. Only use 250 mg tab if peds ≥40 kg. Chewtab & tab not interchangeable.
Ampicillin (Principen)	**Cap:** 250 mg, 500 mg; **Susp:** 125 mg/5ml, 250 mg/5ml	**Genitourinary Tract: Adults & Peds: >20 kg:** 500 mg qid. **Peds: ≤20 kg:** 25 mg/kg qid.	⓪B ❄️>

NAME	FORM/STRENGTH	DOSAGE	COMMENTS
Carbenicillin Disodium (Geocillin)	**Tab:** 382 mg	**Adults:** *E.coli, Proteus, Enterobacter:* 1-2 tabs qid. *Pseudomonas, Enterococcus:* 2 tabs qid.	⬤B ❄️> R
QUINOLONES			
Ciprofloxacin (Cipro)	**Inj:** 10 mg/ml, 200 mg/ 100 ml, 400 mg/200 ml; **Susp:** 250 mg/5 ml, 500 mg/5 ml; **Tab:** 100 mg, 250 mg, 500 mg, 750 mg	**Adults: Mild-Moderate UTI:** 250 mg PO q12h or 200 mg IV q12h x 7-14d. **Severe-Complicated UTI:** 500 mg PO q12h or 400 mg IV q12h x 7-14d. **Peds 1-17yo: Complicated UTI/Pyelonephritis:** 10-20 mg/kg PO q12h or 6-10 mg/kg IV q8h x 10-21d. **Max:** 750 mg PO or 400 mg IV/dose.	⬤C ❄️v R (adults)
Ciprofloxacin (Cipro XR)	**Tab,ER:** 500 mg, 1000 mg	**Adults: ≥18 yrs: Uncomplicated UTI:** 500 mg qd x 3d. **Complicated UTI:** 1000 mg qd x 7-14d. **Acute Uncomplicated Pyelonephritis:** 1000 mg qd x 7-14d.	⬤C ❄️v R
Gatifloxacin (Tequin)	**Inj:** 2 mg/ml; 10 mg/ml; **Tab:** 200 mg, 400 mg	**≥18 yo: Complicated/Pyelonephritis:** 400 mg PO/IV qd x 7-10d. **Uncomplicated:** 400 mg PO/IV single dose or 200 mg PO/IV qd x 3d.	⬤C ❄️> R
Levofloxacin (Levaquin)	**Inj:** 5 mg/ml, 25 mg/ml; **Tab:** 250 mg, 500 mg, 750 mg	**≥18 yo: Complicated/Pyelonephritis:** 250 mg PO/IV qd x 10d. **Chronic Bacterial Prostatitis:** 500 mg PO/IV qd x 28d.	⬤C ❄️v R
Lomefloxacin (Maxaquin)	**Tab:** 400 mg	**≥18 yo: Complicated:** 400 mg qd x 14d.	⬤C ❄️v R
Norfloxacin (Noroxin)	**Tab:** 400 mg	**≥18 yo: Uncomplicated:** 400 mg q12h x 3d if due to *K. pneumoniae, E. coli,* or *P. mirabilis,* or x 7-10d if due to other organisms. **Complicated:** 400 mg q12h x 10-21d.	⬤C ❄️v R

Ofloxacin (Floxin)	**Tab:** 200 mg, 300 mg, 400 mg	≥18 yo: **Complicated:** 200 mg q12h x 10d.	⬤C ❋v **H R**

SULFONAMIDE

Sulfisoxazole (Gantrisin Pediatric)	**Susp:** 500 mg/5 ml	**Peds: >2 mths: Initial:** 1/2 of 24h dose. **Maint:** 150 mg/kg/d or 4 gm/m²/d in divided doses. **Max:** 6 gm/d.	⬤C ❋v Cl in pregnancy & nursing.

SULFONAMIDES AND COMBINATIONS

Sulfamethoxazole/ Trimethoprim (Bactrim, Bactrim DS, Septra, Septra DS, Sulfatrim Pediatric)	**Inj:** 80-16 mg/ml; **Susp:** 200-40 mg/5 ml; **Tab:** (SS) 400-80 mg; (DS) 800-160 mg	**PO: Adults:** 800 mg SMX & 160 mg TMP (1 DS tab, 2 SS tabs, or 20 ml) q12h x 10-14d. **Peds: ≥2 mths:** 4 mg/kg TMP & 20 mg/kg SMX q12h x 10d. **IV: Adults & Peds: Severe:** 8-10 mg/kg/d (based on TMP) given q6-12h up to 14d.	⬤C ❋v **R** Cl in pregnancy & nursing.

TETRACYCLINES

Doxycycline Hyclate (Vibramycin, Vibra-Tabs)	**Cap:** 50 mg, 100 mg; **Tab:** 100 mg	**Adults:** 100 mg q12h on d1, then 100 mg qd or 50 mg q12h. **Peds: >8 yo & ≤100 lbs:** 1 mg/lb bid on d1, then 1 mg/lb qd or 0.5 mg/lb bid. **>100 lbs:** Adult dose.	⬤D ❋v
Doxycycline Monohydrate (Monodox, Vibramycin)	**Cap:** (Monodox) 50 mg, 100 mg; **Susp:** (Vibramycin) 25 mg/5 ml	**Adults:** 100 mg q12h or 50 mg q6h on d1, then 100 mg qd or 50 mg q12h. **Peds: >8 yo & ≤100 lbs:** 1 mg/lb bid on d1, then 1 mg/lb qd or 0.5 mg/lb bid. **>100 lbs:** Adult dose.	⬤D ❋v
Minocycline HCl (Dynacin, Minocin)	**Cap:** 50 mg, 75 mg, 100 mg; **Inj:** 100 mg	**Adults:** 200 mg PO/IV, then 100 mg q12h or 50 mg qid. **>8 yo:** 4 mg/kg PO/IV, then 2 mg/kg q12h.	⬤D ❋v **R**

NAME	FORM/STRENGTH	DOSAGE	COMMENTS
Tetracycline HCl (Sumycin)	**Cap:** 250 mg, 500 mg; **Susp:** 125 mg/5 ml	**Adults:** 250 mg qid or 500 mg bid. **Peds: >8 yo:** 25-50 mg/kg divided bid-qid.	Ⓓ ❉ ∨ R
MISCELLANEOUS			
Cycloserine (Seromycin)	**Cap:** 250 mg	**Adults:** 500 mg-1 gm/d in divided doses.	Ⓒ❉∨
Fosfomycin Tromethamine (Monurol)	**Granules:** 3 gm/sachet	**Women: ≥18 yo:** One 3 gm single-dose sachet. Mix with 3-4 oz of water.	Ⓑ ❉∨
Methenamine Hippurate (Hiprex, Urex)	**Tab:** 1 gm	**Adults & Peds: >12 yo:** 1 gm bid. **6-12 yo:** 0.5-1 gm bid.	Ⓝ ❉∨
Methenamine Mandelate (Mandelamine)	**Susp:** 0.5 gm/5 ml; **Tab:** 0.5 gm, 1 gm	**Adults: Usual:** 1 gm tid pc & qhs (4 gm/d). **Peds: 6-12 yo:** 500 mg tid & qhs (2 gm/d). **<6 yo:** 250 mg/30 lbs qid.	Ⓒ❉<
Nalidixic Acid (NegGram)	**Susp:** 250 mg/5 ml; **Tab:** 250 mg, 500 mg	**Adults:** 1 gm qid x 1-2 wks. **Peds: 3 mths-12 yo:** 55 mg/kg/d given qid.	Ⓒ❉∨
Nitrofurantoin (Furadantin)	**Susp:** 25 mg/5 ml	**Adults:** 50-100 mg qid x 7d. **Peds: >1 mth:** 5-7 mg/kg/d given as qid x 7d.	Ⓑ ❉∨ R
Nitrofurantoin, Macrocrystals (Macrobid, Macrodantin)	**Cap:** (Macrobid) 100 mg, (Macrodantin) 25 mg, 50 mg, 100 mg	**Macrobid: Adults & Peds >12 yo:** 100 mg q12h x 7d. **Macrodantin: Adults:** 50-100 mg qid x 7d. **Peds: >1 mth:** 5-7 mg/kg/d given as qid x 7d.	Ⓑ ❉∨ R
Trimethoprim (Proloprim)	**Tab:** 100 mg, 200 mg	**Adults & Peds: >12 yo:** 100 mg bid or 200 mg qd x 10d.	Ⓒ❉> R

Miscellaneous Anti-Infectives

Iodoquinol (Yodoxin)	Tab: 210 mg, 650 mg	Intestinal Amebiasis: Adults: Usual: 630-650 mg tid pc x 20d. Peds: Usual: 10-13.3 mg/kg tid pc x 20d. Max: 1.95 gm/24h.	⊙N ❄>
Tinidazole (Tindamax)	Tab: 250 mg, 500 mg	Giardiasis: Adults: 2 gm single dose. >3 yo: 50 mg/kg single dose. Max: 2 gm/d. Amebiasis: Intestinal: Adults: 2 gm qd x 3d. >3 yo: 50 mg/kg qd x 3d. Max: 2 gm/d. Amebic Liver Abscess: Adults: 2 gm qd x 3-5d. >3 yo: 50 mg/kg qd x 3-5d. Max: 2 gm/d. May crush tabs in cherry syrup. Take with food.	⊙X (1st trimester) ⊙C (2nd/3rd trimester) ❄v R Avoid unnecessary use.

ANTINEOPLASTICS
Antineoplastics

Alemtuzumab (Campath)	Inj: 10 mg/ml	Adults: B-cell Chronic Lymphocytic Leukemia: Initial: 3 mg IV qd. When tolerated, increase to 10 mg/d. Maint: When 10 mg tolerated, increase to 30 mg/d TIW up to 12 wks.	⊙C ❄v Hematologic toxicity. Infusion reactions. Opportunistic infections.
Anastrozole (Arimidex)	Tab: 1 mg	Adults: Adjuvant/Advanced/Metastatic Breast Cancer: 1 mg qd.	⊙D ❄>
Asparaginase (Elspar)	Inj: 10,000 IU	Adults & Peds: Acute Lymphocytic Leukemia: 1000 IU/kg IV qd x 10d beginning day 22 of treatment period or 6000 IU/m² IM on days 4, 7, 10, 13, 16, 19, 22, 25, & 28.	⊙C ❄v Be prepared to treat anaphylaxis. [3]

[3] Give only under supervision of a physician experienced with antineoplastics.

NAME	FORM/STRENGTH	DOSAGE	COMMENTS
Bevacizumab (Avastin)	Inj: 100 mg, 400 mg	**Adults: Metastatic Colon/Rectum Carcinoma:** 5 mg/kg IV infusion over 90 mins once q14d until disease progression is detected. If 1st infusion is well tolerated, administer 2nd infusion over 60 mins. If 2nd infusion is well tolerated, administer subsequent doses over 30 mins.	◉C ❊v GI perforation. Wound dehiscence. Hemoptysis.
Bicalutamide (Casodex)	Tab: 50 mg	**Adults: Stage D$_2$ Metastatic Carcinoma of Prostate:** 50 mg qd. Intiate with LHRH analogue therapy.	◉X ❊> [3]
Bleomycin (Blenoxane)	Inj: 15 U, 30 U	**Adults: Squamous Cell Carcinoma/non-Hodgkin's Lymphomas/Testicular Carcinoma:** 0.25-0.5 U/kg IV/IM/SC qwk-BIW. **Hodgkin's Disease:** 0.25-0.5 U/kg IV/IM/SC qwk-BIW. After 50% response, 1 U/d or 5 U/wk IV/IM.	◉D ❊v Pulmonary fibrosis & severe idiosyncratic reaction. [3]
Bortezomib (Velcade)	Inj: 3.5 mg	**Adults: Initial:** 1.3 mg/m^2/dose IV bolus biw x 2 wks (days 1, 4, 8, and 11) followed by a 10-day rest period (days 12-21). At least 72 hrs should elapse between consecutive doses. **Grade 3 Non-Hematological/Grade 4 Hematological Toxicities (excluding neuropathy):** Withhold therapy until symptoms of toxicity resolve. Reinitiate at 25% reduced dose. **Peripheral Neuropathy: Grade 1 with pain or Grade 2 (interfering with function but not activities of daily living):** Reduce dose to 1 mg/m^2. **Grade 2 with pain or Grade 3 (interfering with activities of daily living):** Withhold dose until toxicity resolves. Reinitiate at 0.7 mg/m^2 qwk. **Grade 4 (permanent sensory loss interfering with function):** D/C therapy.	◉D ❊v

Drug	Form	Dosage	Notes
Busulfan (Myleran)	**Tab:** 2 mg	**Adults & Peds: CML:** 60 mcg/kg/d or 1.8 mg/m²/d.	●D ✿v R Bone marrow hypoplasia. [3]
Capecitabine (Xeloda)	**Tab:** 150 mg, 500 mg	**≥18 yo: Metastatic Breast Cancer/Colorectal Cancer:** 1250 mg/m² bid x 2 wks, then 1 wk rest period. Give as 3 wk cycles. Interrupt and/or reduce dose if toxicity occurs. Readjust according to adverse effects.	●D ✿v R Bleeding & death reported w/coumarin.
Carboplatin (Paraplatin)	**Inj:** 50 mg, 150 mg, 450 mg	**Adults: Advanced Ovarian Carcinoma: Single Agent:** 360 mg/m² IV on d1 q4wks. **Combination Therapy:** 300 mg/m² IV on d1 q4wks x 6 cycles. Adjust based on platelet & neutrophil count.	●D ✿v R Bone marrow suppression. Anaphylactoid reactions. [3]
Carmustine (BiCNU)	**Inj:** 100 mg	**Adults: Brain Tumors/Multiple Myeloma/Hodgkin's Disease/non-Hodgkin's Lymphomas:** 150-200 mg/m² IV q6wks as single dose or 75-100 mg/m² IV qd x 2d. Adjust based on leukocyte & platelet count.	●D ✿v Bone marrow & pulmonary toxicity. [3]
Carmustine Implant (Gliadel Wafer)	**Wafer:** 7.7 mg/wafer	**Adults: Newly-Diagnosed High Grade Malignant Glioma/Recurrent Gliobastoma Multiforme:** Place 8 wafers in resection cavity if size and shape allows; if not, place max number of wafers allowed.	●D ✿v
Cetuximab (Erbitux)	**Inj:** 100 mg	**Adults: Metastatic Colorectal Carcinoma: Initial:** 400 mg/m² IV infusion over 120 mins. **Maint:** 250 mg/m² IV infusion over 60 mins once weekly. **Max Infusion Rate:** 5 ml/min.	●C ✿v Infusion reactions.

[3] Give only under supervision of a physician experienced with antineoplastics.

NAME	FORM/STRENGTH	DOSAGE	COMMENTS
Chlorambucil (Leukeran)	Tab: 2 mg	**Adults: CLL/Malignant Lymphoma/Hodgkin's Disease:** **Usual:** 1.1-0.2mg/kg/d x 3-6 wks. **Lymphocytic Infiltration of Bone Marrow/Hypoplastic Bone Marrow:** **Max:** 0.1mg/kg/day.	Bone marrow suppression. Infertility. Carcinogenic. ⊙D ☼v
Cisplatin (Platinol-AQ)	Inj: 1 mg/ml	**Adults: Metastatic Testicular Tumors:** 20 mg/m²/d IV x 5d per cycle. **Metastatic Ovarian Tumors (w/cyclophosphamide):** 75-100 mg/m² IV per cycle once q4wks. **Advanced Bladder Cancer:** 50-70 mg/m² IV per cycle once q3-4wks. Pretreat hydration with fluid 8-12h before therapy.	Renal toxicity. Ototoxicity. Anaphylactoid reactions. 3 ⊙D ☼v
Cladribine (Leustatin)	Inj: 10 mg	**Adults: Hairy Cell Leukemia:** 0.09 mg/kg/d continuous infusion x 7d.	Acute nephrotoxicity. 3 ⊙D ☼v
Cyclophosphamide (Cytoxan)	Inj: 100 mg, 200 mg, 500 mg, 1 gm, 2 gm; Tab: 25 mg, 50 mg	**Adults & Peds: Malignant Lymphomas/Leukemias/Multiple Myeloma/Mycosis Fungoides/Neuroblastoma/Ovary Adenocarcinoma/Retinoblastoma/Breast Carcinoma: IV:** 40-50 mg/kg in divided doses over 2-5d, or 10-15 mg/kg q7-10d, or 3-5 mg/kg BIW. **PO:** 1-5 mg/kg/d.	⊙D ☼v
Dacarbazine (DTIC-Dome)	Inj: 200 mg	**Metastatic Malignant Melanoma:** 2-4.5 mg/kg/d IV pd x 10d, repeat q4wks; or 250 mg/m² IV pd x 5d, repeat q3wks. **Hodgkin's Disease:** 150 mg/m²/d IV pd x 5d, repeat q4wks; 375 mg/m² on d1, repeat q15d.	Hemopoietic depression. Hepatic necrosis. 3 ⊙C ☼v

Drug	Form	Dosage	Notes
Dactinomycin (Cosmegen)	**Inj:** 0.5 mg	**Adults & Peds >6-12 mths: Wilms' Tumor, Rhabdomyosarcoma, Ewing's Sarcoma:** 15 mcg/kg/d IV x 5d. **Metastatic Nonseminomatous Testicular Cancer:** 1000 mcg/m² in combo treatment. **Recurrent or Locoregional Malignancies:** 50 mcg/kg for lower extremity or pelvis, 35 mcg/kg for upper extremity. **Gestational Trophoblastic Neoplasia:** 12 mcg/kg IV qd x 5d.	▣D ❄v Extremely corrosive to soft tissue. [3]
Docetaxel (Taxotere)	**Inj:** 20 mg/0.5 ml	**Adults: Locally Advanced/Metastatic Breast Cancer:** 60-100 mg/m² IV q3wks. **Unresectable (in combo with cisplatin)/Locally Advanced/Metastatic Non-Small Cell Lung Cancer:** 75 mg/m² IV q3wks.	▣D ❄v H Treatment related mortality. Severe hypersensitivity, fluid retention. Neutropenia. [3]
Doxorubicin HCl (Adriamycin, Rubex)	**Inj:** (Adriamycin) 2 mg/ml, 10 mg, 20 mg, 50 mg; (Rubex) 50 mg	**Acute Lymphoblastic & Myeloblastic Leukemia/ Wilms' Tumor/Neuroblastoma/Soft Tissue & Bone Sarcomas/Breast, Ovarian, Bronchogenic, Bladder, Thyroid, & Gastric Carcinoma/Hodgkin's Disease/ Malignant Lymphoma: Monotherapy:** 60-75 mg/m² IV q21d. **Combination Therapy:** 40-60 mg/m² IV q21-28d	▣D ❄v H Local tissue necrosis. Myocardial toxicity. Myelosuppression. Acute myelogenous leukemia. [3]
Doxorubicin HCl Liposome (Doxil)	**Inj:** 2 mg/ml	**Adults: Ovarian Cancer:** 50 mg/m² IV at 1 mg/min. If no reaction, increase rate to complete infusion in 1h. Dose once q4wks for min of 4 courses. **AIDS-related Kaposi's Sarcoma:** 20 mg/m² IV once q3wks. Do not substitute with doxorubicin HCl on mg per mg basis.	▣D ❄v H Myelosuppression. Myocardial toxicity. Infusion related reactions. [3]

[3] Give only under supervision of a physician experienced with antineoplastics.

NAME	FORM/STRENGTH	DOSAGE	COMMENTS
Estradiol (Estrace, Gynodiol)	**Tab:** (Estrace) 0.5 mg, 1 mg, 2 mg; (Gynodiol) 0.5 mg, 1 mg, 1.5 mg, 2 mg	**Advanced Prostate Cancer:** 1-2 mg tid. **Metastatic Breast Cancer:** 10 mg tid for min of 3 mths.	▨X ✿v [4,10]
Estramustine (Emcyt)	**Cap:** 140 mg	**Adults: Metastatic/Progressive Prostate Carcinoma:** 14 mg/kg/d given tid-qid.	▨N ✿>
Estrogens, Conjugated (Premarin)	**Tab:** 0.3 mg, 0.45 mg, 0.625 mg, 0.9 mg, 1.25 mg, 2.5 mg	**Advanced Prostate Cancer:** 1.25-2.5 mg tid. **Metastatic Breast Cancer:** 10 mg tid for min of 3 mths.	▨X ✿> [4,28]
Etoposide (Etopophos, Toposar)	**Inj:** (Etopophos) 100 mg, (Toposar) 20 mg/ml	**Adults: Refractory Testicular Tumors:** 50-100 mg/m²/d IV on days 1-5 to 100 mg/m²/d IV on days 1, 3, 5. **Small Cell Lung Cancer:** 35 mg/m²/d IV x 4d to 50 mg/m²/d x 5d.	▨D ✿v R (Etopophos) Severe myelosuppression. [3]
Etoposide (VePesid)	**Cap:** 50 mg; **Inj:** 20 mg/ml	**Adults: Refractory Testicular Tumors: IV:** 50-100 mg/m²/d on days 1-5 to 100 mg/m²/d on days 1, 3, 5. **Small Cell Lung Cancer: IV:** 35 mg/m²/d x 4d to 50 mg/m²/d x 5d. **Cap:** 2 x IV dose & round to nearest 50 mg.	▨D ✿v R Severe myelosuppression. [3]
Fludarabine Phosphate (Fludara)	**Inj:** 50 mg	**Adults: B-cell Chronic Lymphocytic Leukemia:** 25 mg/m²/d IV over 30 min x 5d, repeat q28d.	▨D ✿v R Autoimmune hemolytic anemia. Severe bone marrow suppression. [3]

Fluorouracil (Adrucil)	Inj: 50 mg/ml	Adults: Palliative Management of Colon, Rectum, Breast, Stomach & Pancreatic Carcinomas: Initial: 12 mg/kg/d (up to 800 mg/d) x 4d, then 6 mg/kg on days 6, 8, 10 & 12. Maint: Either repeat initial dose q30d or after toxic signs subside, give 10-15 mg/kg/wk as a single dose (up to 1 gm/wk).	⬤D ❄v [3]
Flutamide (Eulexin)	Cap: 125 mg	Stage B_2-C Prostatic Carcinoma/Stage D_2 Metastatic Carcinoma: 250 mg tid at 8h intervals.	⬤D ❄> Hepatic injury.
Fulvestrant (Faslodex)	Inj: 50 mg/ml	Hormone Receptor Positive Metastatic Breast Cancer in Postmenopausal Women: Adults: 250 mg IM into buttock monthly. Give as either single 5 ml inj or 2 concurrent 2.5 ml inj.	⬤D ❄v
Gallium Nitrate (Ganite)	Inj: 500 mg	Adults: Cancer-related Hypercalcemia: 200 mg/m² IV daily x 5d. Mild hypercalcemia: 100 mg/m²/d x 5d. If calcium levels are within normal range in <5d, may d/c treatment. Daily infusion must be given over 24 hrs.	⬤C ❄v R Avoid concurrent use with nephrotoxic drugs.

[3] Give only under supervision of a physician experienced with antineoplastics.
[4] Contraindicated in pregnancy. Increased risk of endometrial carcinoma in postmenopausal women.
[10] Attempt to taper or d/c at 3-6 mth intervals.
[28] Not for CV disease prevention. The WHI reported increased risks of MI, stroke, invasive breast cancer, pulmonary emboli, & DVT in postmenopausal women. Prescribe at lowest effective doses for shortest duration.

NAME	FORM/STRENGTH	DOSAGE	COMMENTS
Gefitinib (Iressa)	Tab: 250 mg	**Adults:** 250 mg/d. **Poorly Tolerated Diarrhea/Skin Adverse Reactions:** Provide brief (up to 14 days) therapy interruption followed by reinstatement of 250 mg/d. **Concomitant Potent CYP3A4 Inducers (eg, rifampicin, phenytoin):** Consider increasing dose to 500 mg/d, in the absence of severe adverse reactions.	▣D ❄v R
Gemcitabine HCl (Gemzar)	Inj: 200 mg, 1 gm	**Adults: Non-Small Cell Lung Cancer:** 1 gm/m² IV on days 1, 8, 15 of each 28d cycle; or 1250 mg/m² IV on days 1 & 8 of each 21d cycle. **Pancreatic Cancer:** 1 gm/m² IV qwk, up to 7 wks. Adjust based on hematologic toxicity.	▣D ❄v
Gemtuzumab Ozogamicin (Mylotarg)	Inj: 5 mg	**Adults: CD33 Positive Acute Myeloid Leukemia (1st relapse): ≥60 yo:** 9 mg/m² IV, repeat after 14d.	▣D ❄v Severe myelosuppression. Hypersensitivity reactions. Hepatotoxicity. 3
Goserelin Acetate (Zoladex 3-Month)	Implant: 10.8 mg	**Adults: Stage B₂-C Prostate Cancer:** 3.6 mg depot SC 8 wks before radiotherapy, then 10.8 mg depot SC 28d later. **Advanced Prostate Cancer:** 10.8 mg SC q12wks in upper abdominal wall.	▣X ❄v
Goserelin Acetate (Zoladex)	Implant: 3.6 mg	**Adults: Stage B₂-C Prostate Cancer:** 3.6 mg depot SC 8 wks before radiotherapy, then 10.8 mg depot SC 28d later. **Advanced Prostate or Breast Cancer:** 3.6 mg SC in upper abdominal wall q28d.	▣X ❄v

Hydroxyurea (Hydrea)	Cap: 500 mg	**Adults: Solid Tumors: Intermittent:** 80 mg/kg as a single dose q3d. **Continuous:** 20-30 mg/kg qd. **Resistant CML:** 20-30 mg/kg qd.	▣D ❀v R
Ifosfamide (Ifex)	Inj: 1 gm, 3 gm	**Adults: Germ Cell Testicular Cancer:** 1.2 g/m^2/d IV x 5d. Repeat q3wks.	▣D ❀v Urotoxic effects. CNS toxicity. Myelo-suppression. [3]
Imatinib Mesylate (Gleevec)	Cap: 100 mg, 400 mg	**Adults: CML: Chronic Phase:** 400 mg/d, may increase to 600 mg qd. **Accelerated Phase/Blast Crisis:** 600 mg/d, may increase to 400 mg bid. **GIST:** 400 mg/d or 600 mg/d. **Peds: ≥3 yrs: CML: Ph+ Chronic Phase: Recurrent After Stem Cell Transplant Or Resistant To Interferon-α Therapy:** 260 mg/m^2/day given qd or split into 2 doses (am and pm). Take with food and plenty of water.	▣D ❀v H
Interferon alfa-2a (Roferon-A)	Inj: 3 MIU, 6 MIU, 9 MIU, 36 MIU	**≥18 yo: Hairy Cell Leukemia: Induction:** 3 MIU SC/IM qd x 16- 24 wks. **Maint:** 3 MIU SC/IM TIW. **Kaposi's Sarcoma: Induction:** 36 MIU SC/IM qd x 10-12 wks. **Maint:** 36 MIU SC/IM TIW. **CML: Initial:** 9 MIU qd SC/IM.	▣C ❀v [13]

[3] Give only under supervision of a physician experienced with antineoplastics.

[13] May cause or aggravate neuropsychiatric, autoimmune, ischemic, & infectious disorders.

NAME	FORM/STRENGTH	DOSAGE	COMMENTS
Interferon alfa-2b (Intron-A)	**Inj:** 10 MIU/0.2 ml, 3 MIU/0.2 ml, 5 MIU/ 0.2 ml, 10 MIU/ml, 6 MIU/ml, 3 MIU/ 0.5 ml, 5 MIU/0.5 ml, 3 MIU, 5 MIU, 10 MIU, 18 MIU, 25 MIU, 50 MIU	**Hairy Cell Leukemia:** 2 MIU/m² SC/IM TIW up to 6 mths. **Malignant Melanoma: Induction:** 20 MIU/m² IV x 5d/wk x 4 wks. **Maint:** 10 MIU/m² SC TIW x 48 wks. **Follicular Lymphoma:** 5 MIU SC TIW up to 18 mths. **Condylomata Acuminata:** 1 MIU into lesions TIW x 3 wks. **Kaposi's Sarcoma:** 30 MIU/m² SC/IM TIW.	◕C ❄v [13]
Irinotecan HCl (Camptosar)	**Inj:** 20 mg/ml	**Adults: Metastatic Carcinoma of Colon/Rectum:** 125 mg/m² wkly x 4 wks, then 2-wk rest; or 350 mg/m² q3wks.	◕D ❄v Myelosuppression. Early & late diarrhea. [3]
Leuprolide Acetate (Eligard)	**Inj:** 7.5 mg, 22.5 mg, 30 mg	**Advanced Prostate Cancer: Adults:** 7.5 mg SC monthly, 22.5 mg SC q3mths or 30 mg SC q4mths. Rotate injection sites.	◕X ❄>
Leuprolide Acetate (Lupron)	**Inj:** 1 mg/ml	**Advanced Prostate Cancer:** 1 mg SC qd. Rotate injection sites.	◕X ❄>
Leuprolide Acetate (Lupron Depot)	**Inj:** (Depot) 7.5mg, (3 month) 22.5mg, (4 month) 30mg	**Advanced Prostate Cancer:** 7.5 mg IM monthly, 22.5 mg IM q3mths, or 30 mg IM q4mths. Give as single dose & rotate injection sites.	◕X ❄>
Medroxyprogesterone Acetate (Depo-Provera)	**Inj:** 400 mg/ml	**Inoperable, Recurrent, Metastatic Endometrial or Renal Carcinoma: Initial:** 400-1000 mg IM qwk. **Maint:** 400 mg IM qmth.	◕N ❄>

Megestrol Acetate (Megace)	**Tab:** 20 mg, 40 mg	**Advanced Breast Carcinoma:** 40 mg qid. **Advanced Endometrial Carcinoma:** 40-320 mg qd in divided doses. Treat for min of 2 mths.	⬤D ❄v
Melphalan (Alkeran)	**Inj:** 50 mg	**Adults: Multiple Myeloma:** 16 mg/m² q2wks x 4 doses, then q4wks after recovery from toxicity.	⬤D ❄v R [3, 23]
Melphalan (Alkeran)	**Tab:** 2 mg	**Adults: Multiple Myeloma:** 6 mg qd x 2-3 wks, then 2 mg qd after WBC & platelets are rising. **Epithelial Ovary Carcinoma:** 0.2 mg/kg/d x 5d. May repeat q4-5wks.	⬤D ❄v [3, 23]
Mercaptopurine (Purinethol)	**Tab:** 50 mg	**Adults & Peds: ALL: Induction: Initial:** 2.5 mg/kg/d. Calculate to nearest multiple of 25 mg. **Titrate:** May increase to 5 mg/kg/d after 4 wks if needed. **Maint:** 1.5-2.5 mg/kg/d. Dose peds in pm.	⬤D ❄v H R [3]
Mesna (Mesnex)	**Inj:** 100 mg/ml; **Tab:** 400 mg	**Prophylaxis to Reduce Ifosfamide-induced Hemorrhagic Cystitis: Usual: IV:** IV bolus as 20% of ifosfamide dose given concurrently, and 4 and 8 hrs after each ifosfamide dose. **Max:** 60% of ifosfamide dose/d. **IV/PO:** IV bolus as 20% of ifosfamide dose given concurrently, then give tabs as 40% of ifosfamide dose 2 and 6 hrs after each ifosfamide dose. **Max:** 100% of ifosfamide dose/d.	⬤B ❄v [3]

[3] Give only under supervision of a physician experienced with antineoplastics.

[13] May cause or aggravate neuropsychiatric, autoimmune, ischemic, & infectious disorders.

[23] Chromosomal aberrations. Severe bone marrow suppression.

NAME	FORM/STRENGTH	DOSAGE	COMMENTS
Methotrexate Sodium	**Inj:** 20 mg, 25 mg/ml, 1 gm; **Tab:** 2.5 mg	**Choriocarcinoma/Trophoblastic Diseases: Adults: PO/IM:** 15-30 mg qd x 5d, rest ≥1 wk & repeat 3-5x. **Meningeal Leukemia: Intrathecal:** Dilute preservative free MTX to 1 mg/ml. Dose q2-5d. **<1 yo:** 6 mg. **1 yo:** 8 mg. **2 yo:** 10 mg. **≥3 yo:** 12 mg. **Burkette's Lymphoma: Stages I-II: PO:** 10-25 mg/d x 4-8d for several courses; separate by 7-10d rest period. **Lymphosarcomas: Stage III: PO:** 0.625-2.5 mg/kg/d. **Leukemia: Induction:** 3.3 mg/m² with prednisone qd. **Remission Maint:** 15 mg/m² PO/IM twice wkly or 2.5 mg/kg IV q14d. **Mycosis Fungoides:** 5-50 mg qwk. If poor response, give 15-37.5 mg twice wkly. **Osteosarcoma: Initial:** 12 g/m² IV, increase to 15 g/m² if peak levels of 1000 micromolar not reached at end of infusion.	⊞X ❄v [3, 19]
Mitotane (Lysodren)	**Tab:** 500 mg	**Adults: Adrenal Cortical Carcinoma:** 2-6 gm/d given tid-qid. **Titrate:** Increase to 9-10 mg/d.	⊞C ❄v Stop after shock or severe trauma. [3]
Mitoxantrone (Novantrone)	**Inj:** 2 mg/ml	**Adults: IV: ANLL: Induction:** 12 mg/m² qd on days 1-3. **Advanced Hormone-Refractory Prostate Cancer Pain:** 12-14 mg/m² q21d.	⊞D ❄v Bone marrow suppression. Myocardial toxicity. Secondary AML. [3]
Nilutamide (Nilandron)	**Tab:** 150 mg	**Adults: Stage D₂ Prostate Cancer:** 300 mg qd x 30d, then 150 mg qd. Begin on day of surgical castration.	⊞C ❄> Interstitial pneumonitis.

Drug	Form	Dosage	Notes
Oxaliplatin (Eloxatin)	Inj: 50 mg, 100 mg	**Adults: IV: Metastatic Colon/Rectum Carcinoma: Day 1:** 85 mg/m² w/ leucovorin (LV) 200 mg/m² over 120 min; followed with 5-FU 400 mg/m² bolus, then 5-FU 600 mg/m² as 22h infusion. **Day 2:** LV 200 mg/m² over 120 min; followed by 5-FU 400 mg/m² bolus, then 5-FU 600 mg/m² as 22h infusion. Repeat cycle q2wks.	●D ✿v Anaphylactic reactions reported.
Paclitaxel (Taxol)	Inj: 6 mg/ml	**Adults: IV: Ovary Carcinoma: Previously Untreated:** 135 mg/m²/d q3wks. **Treated:** 135-175 mg/m² over 3h q3wks. **Breast Cancer:** 175 mg/m² over 3h q3wks. **Non-Small Cell Lung Cancer:** 135 mg/m² over 24h q3wks. **Kaposi's Sarcoma:** 135 mg/m² over 3h q3wks.	●D ✿v Anaphylaxis & severe hypersensitivity reactions. [3]
Pemetrexed (Alimta)	Inj: 500 mg	**Adults: Malignant Pleural Mesothelioma:** 500 mg/m² IV over 10 mins on Day 1 of each 21-day cycle with cisplatin 75 mg/m² infused over 2h beginning 30 mins after pemetrexed.	●D ✿v R
Procarbazine (Matulane)	Cap: 50 mg	**Stage III & IV Hodgkin's Disease: Adults:** 2-4 mg/kg/d x 1st wk then increase to 4-6 mg/kg/d until max response. **Maint:** 1-2 mg/kg/d. **Peds:** 50 mg/m²/d x 1st wk then increase to 100 mg/m²/d until max repsonse. **Maint:** 50 mg/m²/d.	●D ✿v [3]

[3] Give only under supervision of a physician experienced with antineoplastics.

[19] Monitor for bone marrow, lung, liver & kidney toxicities. Serious toxic reactions.

NAME	FORM/STRENGTH	DOSAGE	COMMENTS
Rituximab (Rituxan)	**Inj:** 10 mg/ml	**Adults: Non-Hodgkin's Lymphoma:** 375 mg/m² IV qwk x 4 or 8 doses. **Retreatment:** 375 mg/m² IV qwk x 4 doses.	▣C ❋v Fatal infusion & mucocutaneous reactions. Tumor lysis syndrome.
Tamoxifen Citrate (Nolvadex)	**Tab:** 10 mg, 20 mg	**Adults: Breast Cancer Treatment:** 20 mg qd or qam & qpm. **Ductal Carcinoma in Situ or Reduction of Breast Cancer (High Risk):** 20 mg qd x 5 yrs.	▣D ❋v Uterine malignancies, stroke, & PE reported.
Toremifene (Fareston)	**Tab:** 60 mg	**Adults: Metastatic Breast Cancer:** 60 mg qd.	▣D ❋>
Trastuzumab (Herceptin)	**Inj:** 440 mg	**Adults: Metastatic Breast Cancer: LD:** 4 mg/kg IV over 90 min. **Maint:** 2 mg/kg IV over 30 min qwk.	▣B ❋v Cardiomyopathy. Hypersensitivity, infusion reactions. Pulmonary events.

CARDIOVASCULAR AGENTS
Angina
BETA BLOCKERS

NAME	FORM/STRENGTH	DOSAGE	COMMENTS
Atenolol (Tenormin)	**Inj:** 0.5 mg/ml; **Tab:** 25 mg, 50 mg, 100 mg	**Angina Pectoris: Initial:** 50 mg qd. **Titrate:** May increase to 100 mg qd after 1 wk. **Max:** 200 mg/d.	▣D ❋> R
Metoprolol Succinate (Toprol-XL)	**Tab,ER:** 25 mg, 50 mg, 100 mg, 200 mg	**Angina Pectoris: Initial:** 100 mg qd. **Titrate:** May increase qwk. **Max:** 400 mg/d.	▣C ❋>

Metoprolol Tartrate (Lopressor)	Tab: 50 mg, 100 mg	Angina Pectoris: Initial: 50 mg bid. Titrate: May increase qwk. Maint: 100-400 mg/d. Max: 400 mg/d.	◖C ❄>
Nadolol (Corgard)	Tab: 20 mg, 40 mg, 80 mg, 120 mg, 160 mg	Angina Pectoris: Initial: 40 mg qd. Titrate: Increase by 40-80 mg q3-7d. Usual: 40-80 mg qd. Max: 240 mg/d.	◖C ❄v R [17]
Propranolol HCl (Inderal, Inderal LA)	Cap,ER: 60 mg, 80 mg, 120 mg, 160 mg; Tab: 10 mg, 20 mg, 40 mg, 60 mg, 80 mg	Adults: Angina Pectoris: Inderal LA: Initial: 80 mg qd. Titrate: Increase q3-7d intervals. Usual: 160 mg qd. Max: 320 mg/d. Inderal: 80-320 mg/d given bid-qid.	◖C ❄>

CALCIUM CHANNEL BLOCKER (DIHYDROPYRIDINES)

Amlodipine Besylate (Norvasc)	Tab: 2.5 mg, 5 mg, 10 mg	Chronic Stable/Vasospastic Angina: 5-10 mg qd.	◖C ❄v H
Nicardipine (Cardene)	Cap: 20 mg, 30 mg	Chronic Stable Angina: Initial: 20 mg tid. Maint: 20-40 mg tid.	◖C ❄v H
Nifedipine (Procardia, Procardia XL)	Cap: 10 mg, 20 mg; Tab,ER: 30 mg, 60 mg, 90 mg	Vasospastic/Chronic Stable: Procardia XL: Initial: 30-60 mg qd. Titrate: Increase over 7-14d. Max: 120mg/d. Procardia: Initial: 10 mg tid. Titrate: Increase over 7-14d. Usual: 10-20 mg tid. Max: 180 mg/d.	◖C ❄v

CALCIUM CHANNEL BLOCKER (NON-DIHYDROPYRIDINES)

| Bepridil (Vascor) | Tab: 200 mg, 300 mg | Chronic Stable Angina: Initial: 200 mg qd. Titrate: Adjust after 10d based on response. Max: 400 mg qd. | ◖C ❄v |

[17] Abrupt cessation may induce arrhythmia or MI.

NAME	FORM/STRENGTH	DOSAGE	COMMENTS
Diltiazem HCl (Cardizem, Cardizem CD, Cardizem LA, Cartia XT, Dilacor XR, Diltia XT, Tiazac)	**Cap,ER:** (Cardizem CD) 120 mg, 180 mg, 240 mg, 300 mg, 360 mg, (Cartia XT) 120 mg, 180 mg, 240 mg, 300 mg, (Dilacor XR/Diltia XT) 120 mg, 180 mg, 240 mg, (Tiazac) 120 mg, 180 mg, 240 mg, 300 mg, 360 mg, 420 mg; **Tab:** (Cardizem) 30 mg, 60 mg, 90 mg, 120 mg; **Tab, ER:** (Cardizem LA) 120 mg, 180 mg, 240 mg, 300 mg, 360 mg, 420 mg	**Chronic Stable Angina: Cardizem CD/Cartia XT: Initial:** 120-180 mg qd. **Titrate:** Adjust at 1-2 wk intervals. **Max:** 480 mg/d. **Cardizem: Initial:** 30 mg qid. **Titrate:** Adjust at 1-2d intervals. **Usual:** 180-360 mg/d. **Cardizem LA: Initial:** 180 mg qd. **Titrate:** Adjust at 1-2 wk intervals. **Dilacor XR/Diltia XT: Initial:** 120 mg qd. **Titrate:** Adjust at 1-2 wk intervals. **Max:** 480 mg/d. **Tiazac: Initial:** 120-180 mg qd. **Titrate:** Adjust at 1-2 wk intervals. **Max:** 540 mg/d.	●C ✿v
Verapamil (Calan, Covera-HS)	**Tab:** 40 mg, 80 mg, 120 mg; **Tab,ER:** 180 mg, 240 mg	**Vasospastic/Unstable/Chronic Stable: Calan: Usual:** 80-120 mg tid. **Titrate:** Increase by qd or qwk intervals. **Covera-HS: Initial:** 180 mg qhs. **Titrate:** Increase to 240 qhs, then 360 mg qhs, then 480 mg qhs.	●C ✿v H (Calan)

CALCIUM CHANNEL BLOCKER/HMG COA REDUCTASE INHIBITOR

| Amlodipine Besylate/ Atorvastatin Calcium (Caduet) | **Tab:** 5-10 mg, 5-20 mg, 5-40 mg, 5-80 mg, 10-10 mg, 10-20 mg, 10-40 mg, 10-80 mg | Dosing is based on the appropriate combination of recommendations for the monotherapies. **Amlodipine: Adults:** 5-10 mg qd. **Atorvastatin:** See under Antilipidemic Agents for dosing. | ▣X ❁v H |

VASODILATORS

Isosorbide Dinitrate (Dilatrate-SR, Isordil, Isordil Titradose)	**Cap,ER:** (Dilatrate-SR) 40 mg; **Tab,SL:** (Isordil) 2.5 mg, 5 mg, 10 mg; **Tab:** (Isordil Titradose) 5 mg, 10 mg, 20 mg, 30 mg, 40 mg	**Prevention: Dilatrate-DR: Usual:** 40 mg bid. Separate doses by 6h. **Max:** 160 mg/d. Take at least 18h nitrate-free interval. **Isordil (Tritradose): Initial:** 5-20 mg bid-tid. **Maint:** 10-40 mg bid-tid. Take at least 14h nitrate-free interval. **Acute Episode/Prevention: Isordil:** 2.5-5 mg SL 15 min before expected episode or to abort acute episode after failure of SL NTG.	▣C ❁>
Isosorbide Mononitrate (Imdur, Ismo, Monoket)	**Tab:** (Monoket) 10 mg, 20 mg, (Ismo) 20 mg; **Tab,ER:** (Imdur) 30 mg, 60 mg, 120 mg	**Prevention/Treatment: Monoket:** 20 mg bid (space 7h apart). **Small Patients: Initial:** 5 mg bid. **Titrate:** Increase to 10 mg by 2nd or 3rd day. **Maint:** 20 mg bid. **Prevention: Ismo:** 20 mg bid, 1st dose on awakening then 7h later. **Imdur: Initial:** 30-60 mg qam. **Titrate:** Increase after several days to 120 mg/d.	▣B (Imdur, Monoket) ▣C (Ismo) ❁>
Nitroglycerin (Minitran, Nitrek, Nitro-Dur)	**Patch:** (mg/h) (Minitran) 0.1, 0.2, 0.4, 0.6; (Nitrek) 0.2, 0.4, 0.6; (Nitro-Dur) 0.1, 0.2, 0.4, 0.6, 0.8	**Prevention: Initial:** 0.2-0.4 mg/h for 12-14h. Remove for 10-12h.	▣C ❁>

NAME	FORM/STRENGTH	DOSAGE	COMMENTS
Nitroglycerin (Nitro-Bid, Nitrol)	**Oint:** 2% (15 mg/inch)	**Prevention: Initial:** 0.5 inch qam & 6h later. **Titrate:** May increase to 1 inch bid, then to 2 inches bid. Should have 10-12h nitrate-free period.	⬤C ❄>
Nitroglycerin (Nitro-Time)	**Cap,ER:** 2.5 mg, 6.5 mg, 9 mg; **Inj:** 5 mg/ml	**Cap,ER: Initial:** 2.5-6.5 mg tid-qid. **Titrate:** Guide by symptoms and/or side effects. Should have 10-12h nitrate-free period. **Inj: Initial:** 5 mcg/min IV. **Titrate:** Increase by 5 mcg/min q3-5min.	⬤C ❄>
Nitroglycerin (Nitrolingual Spray, Nitroquick, Nitrostat, Nitrotab)	**Spray,SL:** (Nitrolingual) 0.4 mg/spray; **Tab,SL:** 0.3 mg, 0.4 mg, 0.6 mg	**Treatment: Tab:** 1 tab SL q5min, up to 3 tabs/15 min. **Spray:** 1-2 sprays SL, up to 3 sprays/15 min. **Prophylaxis: Tab/Spray:** Take tab or spray 5-10 min before precipitating activity.	⬤C ❄>

Antiarrhythmics

ENDOGENOUS NUCLEOSIDE

Adenosine (Adenocard)	**Inj:** 6 mg/2 ml, 12 mg/4 ml	**Adults & Peds: ≥50 kg:** 6 mg rapid IV bolus over 1-2 sec. If not converted to NSR within 1-2 min, give 12 mg rapid IV bolus; may give 2nd 12 mg dose if needed. **Max:** 12 mg/dose. **Peds: <50kg:** 0.05-0.1 mg/kg rapid IV bolus. If not converted to NSR within 1-2 min, give additional bolus doses incrementally increasing amount by 0.05-0.1 mg/kg. Follow each bolus with a saline flush. Continue process until NSR or a max single dose of 0.3 mg/kg is used.	⬤C ❄>

Disopyramide Phosphate (Norpace, Norpace CR)	**Cap:** 100 mg, 150 mg; **Cap,ER:** 100 mg, 150 mg	**Adults: <50 kg: Cap:** 100 mg q6h. **Cap,ER:** 200 mg q12h. **≥50 kg: Cap:** 150 mg q6h. **Cap,ER:** 300 mg q12h. **Peds: <1 yo:** 10-30 mg/kg/d. **1-4 yo:** 10-20 mg/kg/d. **4-12 yo:** 10-15 mg/kg/d. **12-18 yo:** 6-15 mg/kg/d.	●C ✿v H R [5]
Moricizine HCl (Ethmozine)	**Tab:** 200 mg, 250 mg, 300 mg	**≥18 yo:** Usual: 600-900 mg/d given as q8h.	●B ✿v H R [5]
Procainamide HCl (Procanbid, Pronestyl, Pronestyl-SR)	**(Pronestyl) Cap:** 250 mg; **Tab:** 250 mg, 375 mg, 500 mg; **Tab,ER:** (SR) 500 mg; **(Procanbid) Tab,ER:** 500 mg, 1000 mg	**Adults: Cap/Tab: Initial:** Up to 50 mg/kg/d in divided doses q3h. May give q3h, q4h, or q6h; adjust by patient response. **Tab,ER: Initial:** Up to 50 mg/kg/d given q6h. Adjust by patient response. **Procanbid: Initial:** Up to 50 mg/kg/d given q12h. Adjust by patient response.	●C ✿v H R May cause positive ANA titer. [5]
Quinidine Sulfate (Quinidex Extentabs)	**Tab,ER:** 300 mg	**Adults: A-Fib/Flutter Conversion: Initial:** 300 mg q8-12h. **Titrate:** Increase cautiously if no result and levels within therapeutic range. **A-Fib/Flutter Relapse Reduction:** 300 mg q8-12h. **Titrate:** Increase cautiously if needed. **Ventricular Arrhythmia:** Dosing regimens not adequately studied. Monitor ECG for QTc prolongation.	●C ✿v

[5] Proarrhythmic properties/drug should only be used in life-threatening arrhythmias.

NAME	FORM/STRENGTH	DOSAGE	COMMENTS
GROUP IB			
Lidocaine HCl (Xylocaine)	**Inj:** 0.5%, 1%, 2%	**Adults: Initial:** 50-100 mg IV given 25-50 mg/min, may repeat after 5 min. **Max:** 200-300 mg/h. Following bolus, initiate with 1-4 mg min continuous infusion. **Maint:** Adjust according to cardiac rhythm & toxicity. **Peds:** 1 mg/kg bolus, then 30 mcg/kg/min.	B ❋>
Mexiletine HCl (Mexitil)	**Cap:** 150 mg, 200 mg, 250 mg	**Adults: Initial:** 200 mg q8h. **Titrate:** Increase by 50-100 mg q2-3d. **Max:** 1200 mg/d.	C ❋v H [5]
GROUP IC			
Flecainide Acetate (Tambocor)	**Tab:** 50 mg, 100 mg, 150 mg	**Adults: PSVT/PAF: Initial:** 50 mg q12h. **Titrate:** Increase by 50 mg bid q4d. **Max:** 300 mg/d. **Sustained VT: Initial:** 100 mg q12h. **Titrate:** Increase by 50 mg bid q4d. **Max:** 400 mg/d. **Peds: <6 mths:** 50 mg/m²/d given bid-tid. **>6 mths:** 100 mg/m²/d given bid-tid. **Max:** 200 mg/m²/d.	C ❋> R
Propafenone HCl (Rythmol, Rythmol SR)	**Cap,ER:** (SR) 225 mg, 325 mg, 425 mg; **Tab:** 150 mg, 225 mg, 300 mg	**Adults: Tab: Initial:** 150 mg q8h, may increase q3-4d to 225 mg q8h, then to 300 mg q8h. **Max:** 900 mg/d. **Cap,ER: Initial:** 225 mg q12h, may increase at min 5d intervals to 325 mg q12h, then to 425 mg q12h if needed.	C ❋v (Rythmol) ❋> (Rythmol SR) H [5]
GROUP II			
Acebutolol HCl (Sectral)	**Cap:** 200 mg, 400 mg	**Adults: Ventricular Arrhythmia: Initial:** 200 mg bid. **Maint:** Increase gradually to 600-1200 mg/d.	B ❋v R

Esmolol HCl (Brevibloc)	**Inj:** 250 mg/ml, 10 mg/ml	**Adults: SVT: Initial:** 500 mcg/kg/min x 1 min, then 50 mcg/kg/min x 4 min. **Maint:** 50-200 (avg 100) mcg/kg/min. **Intra-/Post-op Tachycardia: Initial: Rapid:** 80 mg IVP, then 150 mcg/kg/min infusion. **Gradual:** 500 mcg/kg/min x 1 min, then 50 mcg/kg/min x 4 min. If inadequate response within 5 min, repeat LD & give maint 100 mcg/kg/min.	◑C ❄>
Propranolol HCl (Inderal)	**Inj:** 1 mg/ml; **Tab:** 10 mg, 20 mg, 40 mg, 60 mg, 80 mg	**Adults: PO:** 10-30 mg tid-qid, given ac & qhs. **IV:** 1-3 mg IV at 1 mg/min.	◑C ❄>
GROUP III			
Amiodarone HCl (Cordarone, Pacerone)	**Inj:** 50 mg/ml; **Tab:** 200 mg, 400 mg	**Adults: PO: LD:** 800-1600 mg/d PO x 1-3 wks until response. Reduce to 600-800 mg/d x 1 mth. **Maint:** 400 mg/d. **IV: LD:** 150 mg over 1st 10 min (15 mg/min), then 360 mg over next 6h (1 mg/min), then 540 mg over remaining 18h (0.5 mg/min). **Maint:** 0.5 mg/min x 2-3 wks.	◑D ❄v
Bretylium Tosylate	**Inj:** 50 mg/ml	**Adults: Life-Threatening Ventricular Arrhythmias: Initial:** 5 mg/kg IV, increase to 10 mg/kg if needed. **Maint:** 5-10 mg/kg q6h. **Other Ventricular Arrhythmias: Initial:** 5-10 mg/kg IM/IV repeat at 1-2h if needed. **Maint:** 5-10 mg/kg IV q6h or 5-10 mg/kg IM q6-8h.	◑C ❄>

5 Proarrhythmic properties/drug should only be used in life-threatening arrhythmias.

NAME	FORM/STRENGTH	DOSAGE	COMMENTS
Dofetilide (Tikosyn)	Cap: 0.125 mg, 0.25 mg, 0.5 mg	≥18 yo: A-Fib/Flutter: Usual: 500 mcg bid, modify using algorithm based on ECG, heart rate & CrCl. Reevaluate q3mths based on QTc & renal function.	◉C ✿v R Should be inpatient at least 3d when initiate. Monitor ECG.
Sotalol HCl (Betapace, Betapace AF)	Tab: (Betapace) 80 mg, 120 mg, 160 mg, 240 mg; Cap: (Betapace AF) 80 mg, 120 mg, 160 mg	Adults: Betapace: Life-Threatening Ventricular Arrhythmia: Initial: 80 mg bid. Titrate: Increase q3d prn to 120-160 mg bid. Usual: 160-320 mg/d given bid-tid. Adults: Betapace AF: Normal Sinus Rhythm Maint in A-Fib/Flutter: Dose according to CrCl, refer to PI. Peds (Betapace, Betapace AF): ≥2 yo: Initial: 30 mg/m² tid. Titrate: Wait ≥36h between dose increases. Guide dose by response, HR & QTc. Max: 60 mg/m². <2 yo: See dosing chart in PI. Reduce dose or d/c if QTc >550 msec.	◉B ✿v R Should be inpatient at least 3d when initiate. Monitor ECG. 5
GROUP IV			
Verapamil HCl (Calan)	Tab: 40 mg, 80 mg, 120 mg	Adults: A-Fib (Digitalized): Usual: 240-320 mg/d given tid-qid. PSVT Prophylaxis (Non-Digitalized): 240-480 mg/d given tid-qid. Max: 480 mg/d.	◉C ✿v

Digoxin (Digitek, Lanoxicaps, Lanoxin, Lanoxin Pediatric)	Cap: (Lanoxicaps) 0.05 mg, 0.1 mg, 0.2 mg; Inj: (Lanoxin Pediatric) 0.1 mg/ml, (Lanoxin) 0.25 mg/ml; Sol: (Lanoxin Pediatric) 0.05 mg/ml; Tab: (Digitek, Lanoxin) 0.125 mg, 0.25 mg	**Adults: A-Fib:** Titrate to minimum effective dose for desired response.	⊛C ✿> R
Ibutilide Fumarate (Corvert)	Inj: 0.1 mg/ml	**≥18 yo: A-Fib/Flutter: 1st Infusion: ≥60 kg:** 1 mg over 10 min. **<60 kg:** 0.01 mg/kg over 10 min. **2nd Infusion:** Repeat equal strength infusion 10 min after 1st dose if arrhythmia still present.	⊛C ✿v [5]

Antilipidemic Agents
BILE ACID SEQUESTRANTS

Cholestyramine (Questran, Questran Light, Prevalite)	Powder: 4 gm/pkt or scoopful	**Adults: Initial:** 1 pkt or 1 scoopful qd or bid. **Maint:** 2-4 pkts or 2-4 scoopfuls/d given bid. **Max:** 6 pkts or 6 scoopfuls/d.	⊛C ✿> May decrease vitamin content in breast milk.
Colesevelam (WelChol)	Tab: 625 mg	**Adults: Initial:** 3 tabs bid or 6 tabs qd w/meal. May increase to 7 tabs/d.	⊛B ✿>

[5] Proarrhythmic properties/drug should only be used in life-threatening arrhythmias.

NAME	FORM/STRENGTH	DOSAGE	COMMENTS
Colestipol Hydrochloride (Colestid)	**Granules:** 5 gm/pkt or scoopful; **Tab:** 1 gm	**Adults: Initial:** 2 gm (tabs) or 5 gm (1 pkt or scoopful) qd-bid. **Titrate:** Increase by 2 gm qd or bid at 1-2 mth intervals. **Usual:** 2-16 gm/d (tab) or 1-6 pkts or scoopfuls qd or in divided doses.	◉N ❄>

CALCIUM CHANNEL BLOCKER/HMG COA REDUCTASE INHIBITOR

Amlodipine Besylate/Atorvastatin Calcium (Caduet)	**Tab:** 5-10 mg, 5-20 mg, 5-40 mg, 5-80 mg, 10-10 mg, 10-20 mg, 10-40 mg, 10-80 mg	Dosing is based on the appropriate combination of recommendations for the monotherapies. **Amlodipine:** See under Angina and Hypertension for dosing. **Atorvastatin: Adults: Hypercholesterolemia/Mixed Dyslipidemia: Initial:** 10-20 mg qd (or 40 mg qd for LDL-C reduction >45%). **Titrate:** Adjust dose at 2-4 wk intervals. **Usual:** 10-80 mg qd. **Homozygous Familial Hypercholesterolemia:** 10-80 mg qd. **10-17 yo (postmenarchal): Heterozygous Familial Hypercholesterolemia: Initial:** 10 mg/d. **Titrate:** Adjust dose at ≥4 wks intervals. **Max:** 20mg/d.	◉X ❄v H

CHOLESTEROL ABSORPTION INHIBITOR

Ezetimibe (Zetia)	**Tab:** 10 mg	**Adults:** 10 mg qd. May give with statin for incremental effect. Give either ≥2h before or ≥4h after bile acid sequestrant.	◉C ❄v

FIBRIC ACIDS

Clofibrate	**Cap:** 500 mg	**Adults:** 2 gm/d in divided doses.	◉C ❄v H R

Fenofibrate (Lofibra)	Cap: 67 mg, 134 mg, 200 mg	Adults: Hypercholesterolemia/Mixed Dyslipidemia: Initial: 200 mg qd. Hypertriglyceridemia: Initial: 67-200 mg/d. Max: 200 mg/d.	C ✴v H R
Fenofibrate (Tricor)	Tab: 54 mg, 160 mg	Adults: Hypercholesterolemia/Mixed Dyslipidemia: Initial: 160 mg qd. Hypertriglyceridemia: Initial: 54-160 mg/d. Max: 160 mg/d.	C ✴v H R
Gemfibrozil (Lopid)	Tab: 600 mg	Adults: 600 mg bid 30 min ac.	C ✴v H R

HMG COA REDUCTASE INHIBITOR/NICOTINIC ACID

| Lovastatin/Niacin (Advicor) | Tab: 20-500 mg, 20-750 mg, 20-1000mg | ≥18 yo: Initial: 20-500 mg qhs. Titrate: Increase by ≤500 mg of niacin q4wks. Max: 40-2000 mg. Adjust with cyclosporine or fibrates. May pretreat with ASA/NSAID to reduce flushing. | X ✴v H |

HMG COA REDUCTASE INHIBITORS

| Atorvastatin Calcium (Lipitor) | Tab: 10 mg, 20 mg, 40 mg, 80 mg | Adults: Hypercholesterolemia/Mixed Dyslipidemia: Initial: 10-20 mg qd (or 40 mg qd for LDL-C reduction >45%). Titrate: Adjust at 2-4 week intervals. Usual: 10-80 mg qd. Homozygous Familial Hypercholesterolemia: 10-80 mg qd. 10-17 yo (postmenarchal): Heterozygous Familial Hypercholesterolemia: Initial: 10 mg/d. Titrate: Adjust at ≥4 wk intervals. Max: 20 mg/d. | X ✴v |

NAME	FORM/STRENGTH	DOSAGE	COMMENTS
Fluvastatin Sodium (Lescol, Lescol XL)	**Cap:** 20 mg, 40 mg; **Tab,ER:** 80 mg	**Adults: Initial:** (LDL reduction <25%) 20 mg cap qpm. (LDL reduction ≥25%) 40 mg cap qpm or 80 mg XL tab qpm (or 40 mg bid). **Usual:** 20-80 mg/d. Caution with <40 mg/d. Take 2h after bile-acid resins qhs.	☼X ✽∞ H
Lovastatin (Altoprev-formerly known as Altocor)	**Tab,ER:** 10 mg, 20 mg, 40 mg, 60 mg	**Adults: Initial:** 20, 40, or 60 mg qhs. Use 10 mg/d if patient requires smaller reductions. May adjust q4wks or more. Adjust with cyclosporine, fibrates, niacin, amiodarone, verapamil.	☼X ✽∞ H R
Lovastatin (Mevacor)	**Tab:** 10 mg, 20 mg, 40 mg	**Adults: Initial:** 20 mg qd w/pm meal (10 mg/d if need LDL-C reduction <20%). **Usual:** 10-80 mg/d as pb-bid. **Peds: 10-17 yo: Heterozygous Familial Hypercholesterolemia: Initial:** 20 mg qd (10 mg qd if need LDL-C reduction <20%). **Titrate:** May adjust q4wks. **Max:** 40 mg/d. Adjust with cyclosporine, fibrates, niacin, amiodarone, verapamil.	☼X ✽∞ H R
Pravastatin Sodium (Pravachol)	**Tab:** 10 mg, 20 mg, 40 mg, 80 mg	**Adults: ≥18 yo: Initial:** 40 mg qd. **Titrate:** Increase to 80 mg qd. **Heterozygous Familial Hypercholesterolemia: 14-18 yo: Initial:** 40mg qd. **8-13 yo: Initial:** 20mg qd. Adjust with cyclosporine. Take resins 1h before or 4h after.	☼X ✽∞ H R
Rosuvastatin (Crestor)	**Tab:** 5 mg, 10 mg, 20 mg, 40 mg	**Adults: Hypercholesterolemia/Mixed Dyslipidemia: Initial:** 10 mg (or 5 mg qd for less aggressive LDL-C reductions, 20 mg qd with LDL-C > 190 mg/dL). **Titrate:** Adjust dose if needed at 2-4 week intervals. **Range:** 5-40 mg qd. **Homozygous Familial Hypercholesterolemia:** 20 mg qd. **Max:** 40 mg qd. Adjust with cyclosporine, gemfibrozil.	☼X ✽∞ H R

| Simvastatin (Zocor) | **Tab:** 5 mg, 10 mg, 20 mg, 40 mg, 80 mg | **Adults: Initial:** 20-40 mg qpm, 40 mg if at high risk for CHD events. **Usual:** 5-80 mg/d.
Homozygous Familial Hypercholesterolemia: 40 mg qpm or 80 mg/d given as 20 mg bid plus 40 mg qpm. Adjust with cyclosporine, fibrates, amiodarone, verapamil, or niacin. **10-17 yo (at least 1-yr postmenarchal): Heterozygous Familial Hypercholesterolemia: Initial:** 10 mg qpm. **Usual:** 10-40 mg/d. **Titrate:** Adjust at ≥4 wk intervals. **Max:** 40 mg/d. | ◙X ❄v **H R** |

NICOTINIC ACID

| Niacin (Niaspan) | **Tab,ER:** 500 mg, 750 mg, 1000 mg | **Adults: Initial:** 500 mg qhs. **Titrate:** Increase by 500 mg q4wks. **Maint:** 1-2 gm qhs. May pretreat with ASA/NSAID to reduce flushing. | ◙C ❄v **H** |

SALICYLATE/HMG-COA REDUCTASE INHIBITOR

| Aspirin/Pravastatin Sodium (Pravigard PAC) | **Tab:** 81-20 mg, 325-20 mg, 81-40 mg, 325-40 mg, 81-80 mg, 325-80 mg | **Adults: Usual:** 81 mg-40 mg or 325 mg-40 mg qd. May increase to 81 mg-80 mg or 325 mg-80 mg qd. | ◙X ❄v **H** |

Coagulation Modifiers

ALPHA₂-GLYCOPROTEIN

| Antithrombin III, Human (Thrombate III) | **Inj:** 500 IU, 1000 IU | **Adults: Antithrombin III Deficiency: LD:** IU required = (desired-baseline ATIII level x kg)/1.4. **Maint:** Give 60% LD q24h to maintain 80-120% plasma level. | ◙B ❄> |

NAME	FORM/STRENGTH	DOSAGE	COMMENTS
DIRECT THROMBIN INHIBITORS			
Argatroban	**Inj:** 100 mg/ml	**Thrombosis in HIT:** D/C heparin and obtain baseline aPTT. **Initial:** 2 mcg/kg/min IV. Check aPTT after 2h. **Titrate:** Increase until aPTT is 1.5-3x the initial baseline. **Max:** 10 mcg/kg/min. **HIT with PCI: Initial:** 350 mcg/kg bolus with 25 mcg/kg/min IV. Adjust based on ACT. Continue infusion dose once therapeutic ACT (300-400 sec) achieved.	●B ❄v H
Lepirudin (Refludan)	**Inj:** 50 mg	**Adults: HIT and Associated Thromboembolic Disease:** 0.4 mg/kg (up to 110 kg) slow IV bolus, then 0.15 mg/kg/h (up to 110 kg) continuous IV infusion x 2-10d or longer if needed. **Max:** 44 mg bolus and 16.5 mg/h max initial infusion.	●B ❄v R
GLYCOPROTEIN IIB/IIIA INHIBITORS			
Abciximab (ReoPro)	**Inj:** 2 mg/ml	**Adults: PCI:** 0.25 mg/kg IV bolus over 10-60 min before PCI, then 0.125 mcg/kg/min IV infusion (Max: 10 mcg/min) x 12h. **Unstable Angina (PCI within 24h):** 0.25 mg/kg IV bolus, then 10 mcg/min infusion x 18-24h, concluding 1h after PCI.	●C ❄>
Eptifibatide (Integrilin)	**Inj:** 2 mg/ml, 0.75 mg/ml	**Adults: Acute Coronary Syndrome:** 180 mcg/kg IV bolus, then 2 mcg/kg/min IV infusion up to 72h. **PCI:** 180 mcg/kg IV bolus b/f PCI, then 2 mcg/kg/min IV infusion x 20-24h post-PCI. Give 2nd 180 mcg/kg IV bolus 10 min after 1st bolus.	●B ❄> R

| Tirofiban HCl (Aggrastat) | Inj: 0.05 mg/ml, 0.25 mg/ml | **≥18 yo: Acute Coronary Syndrome: Initial:** 0.4 mcg/kg/min IV x 30 min. **Maint:** 0.1 mcg/kg/min IV. Continue through angiography & 12-24h after angioplasty/atherectomy. | ●B ❄v R Use with ASA & heparin unless CI. |

GLYCOSAMINOGLYCAN

| Heparin Sodium | Inj: 1000 U/ml, 2500 U/ml, 5000 U/ml, 7500 U/ml, 10,000 U/ml | **Based on 68 kg: LD:** 5000 U IV, then 10,000-20,000 U SC. **Maint:** 8000-10,000 U q8h or 15,000-20,000 U q12h. **Intermittent IV Injection: LD:** 10,000 U. **Maint:** 5000-10,000 U q4-6h. **IV Infusion: LD:** 5,000 U. **Maint:** 20,000-40,000 U/d. **Peds: Initial:** 50 U/kg IV. **Maint:** 100 U/kg IV q4h or 20,000 U/m²/d continuous IV. | ●C ❄^ |

LOW MOLECULAR WEIGHT HEPARINS

| Dalteparin Sodium (Fragmin) | Inj: 2500 U/0.2 ml, 5000 U/0.2 ml, 10,000 U/ml | **Adults: SC: Unstable Angina/Non-Q-Wave MI:** 120 U/kg, up to 10,000 U q12h with 75-165 mg/d ASA x 5-8d. **Hip Replacement Surgery: Initial:** 2500 U 2h pre-op, then 2500 U 4-8h post-op. **Maint:** 5000 U qd x 5-10d post-op (up to 14d). **Abdominal Surgery:** 2500 U 2h pre-op, then qd x 5-10d post-op. **Severely Restricted Mobility During Acute Illness:** 5000 U qd x 12-14 d. | ●B ❄> 6 |
| Danaparoid Sodium (Organan) | Inj: 750 U/0.6 ml | **Adults: DVT/PE Prevention with Hip Replacement Surgery:** 750 U SC bid; 1-4h pre-op, then not before 2h post-op. Continue x 7-10d (up to 14d). | ●B ❄> 6 |

6 Risk of paralysis by spinal/epidural hematoma with neuraxial anesthesia/lumbar puncture. Increased risk with concomitant anticoagulation, NSAIDs, or traumatic/repeated lumbar puncture.

NAME	FORM/STRENGTH	DOSAGE	COMMENTS
Enoxaparin (Lovenox)	Inj: 30 mg/0.3 ml, 40 mg/0.4 ml, 60 mg/0.6 ml, 80 mg/0.8 ml, 100 mg/ml, 120 mg/0.8 ml, 150 mg/ml	**Adults: SC: Hip/Knee Replacement Surgery:** 30 mg q12h 12-24h post-op x 7-10d (up to 14d), or 40 mg qd for hip surgery up to 3 wks. **Abdominal Surgery:** 40 mg 2h pre-op x 7-10d (up to 14d). **DVT/PE Treatment:** 1 mg/kg q12h with warfarin (goal INR 2-3) x 7d (up to 17d). **Unstable Angina/Non-Q-Wave MI:** 1 mg/kg q12h with 100-325 mg/d ASA x 5-8d (up to 12.5d). **Acute Illness:** 40mg qd x 6-11d (up to 14d).	●B ❄>[6]
Tinzaparin (Innohep)	Inj: 20,000 IU/ml	**Adults: DVT/PE Treatment:** 175 IU/kg SC qd for at least 6d & until anticoagulated with warfarin.	●B ❄>[6]

PHOSPHODIESTERASE/PLATELET AGGREGATION-ADHESION INHIBITORS

NAME	FORM/STRENGTH	DOSAGE	COMMENTS
Anagrelide HCl (Agrylin)	Cap: 0.5 mg, 1 mg	**≥16 yo: Thrombocythemia: Initial:** 0.5 mg qid or 1 mg bid x 1 wk. **Maint:** Adjust based on platelet count; may increase by 0.5 mg/d qwk. **Max:** 10 mg/d or 2.5 mg/dose.	●C ❄v H R
Aspirin (Bayer Aspirin, Ecotrin)	Chewtab: 81 mg; Tab: 81 mg, 325 mg; Tab,Enteric: 81 mg, 325 mg, 500 mg	**Adults: Stroke/TIA:** 50-325 mg qd. **Suspected AMI: Initial:** 160-162.5 mg qd as soon as suspect MI. **Maint:** 160-162.5 mg x 30d post-infarct. **Prevention or Recurrent MI:** 75-325 mg qd.	●N ❄> H R Avoid use during 3rd trimester.
Cilostazol (Pletal)	Tab: 50 mg, 100 mg	**Adults: Intermittent Claudication:** 100 mg bid, 1h before or 2h after breakfast & dinner. Dose 50 mg bid with certain drugs.	●C ❄v CI in CHF.

Clopidogrel Bisulfate (Plavix)	Tab: 75 mg	Adults: MI/Stroke/Peripheral Arterial Disease: 75 mg qd. Acute Coronary Syndrome: LD: 300 mg. Maint: 75 mg qd. Take with 75-325 mg ASA qd.	◑B ❄v
Dipyridamole (Persantine)	Tab: 25 mg, 50 mg, 75 mg	Adults: Prophylaxis to Thromboembolism after Cardiac Valve Replacement: 75-100 mg qid as an adjunct to warfarin.	◑B ❄>
Dipyridamole/ASA (Aggrenox)	Cap,ER: 200-25 mg	Adults: Risk Reduction of Stroke: 1 cap qam & qpm.	◑B (Dipyridamole) ◑D (ASA) ❄> H R
Ticlopidine HCl (Ticlid)	Tab: 250 mg	Adults: Stroke: 250 mg bid. Coronary Artery Stenting: 250 mg bid with ASA up to 30d after stent implant. Take with food.	◑B ❄v H R [15]

SPECIFIC FACTOR XA INHIBITOR

| Fondaparinux Sodium (Arixtra) | Inj: 2.5 mg/0.5 ml | Adults: Hip Fracture or Replacement Surgery/Knee Replacement Surgery: 2.5 mg SC qd, starting 6-8h post-op for 5-9d (up to 11d). Hip Fracture Surgery: Extended prophylaxis up to 24 additional days. | ◑B ❄> R [6] |

[6] Risk of paralysis by spinal/epidural hematoma with neuraxial anesthesia/lumbar puncture. Increased risk with concomitant anticoagulation, NSAIDs, or traumatic/repeated lumbar puncture.

[15] Neutropenia. Agranulocytosis. TTP. Aplastic anemia.

THROMBOLYTICS

NAME	FORM/STRENGTH	DOSAGE	COMMENTS
Alteplase (Activase)	**Inj:** 50 mg, 100 mg	**Acute MI: <67 kg:** 100 mg IV bolus, then 50 mg over 30 min, then 35 mg infused over the next 60 min. **≤67 kg:** 15 mg IV bolus, then 0.75 mg/kg over next 30 min up to 50 mg, and then 0.50 mg/kg over the next 60 min up to 35 mg. **Acute Ischemic Stroke:** 0.9 mg/kg up to 90 mg given over 60 min (10% of total dose given as initial bolus over 1 min). **PE:** 100 mg IV over 2h.	▣C ✱ ⟨≋⟩
Alteplase (Cathflo Activase)	**Inj:** 2 mg	**Obstructed Catheters: Adults & Peds: ≥2 yo:** 2 mg in 2 ml. **10 to <30 kg:** 110% of catheter internal lumen volume, not to exceed 2 mg in 2 ml. Repeat if function not restored after 120 min. **Max:** 2 mg/dose. Reconstitute to 1 mg/ml.	▣C ✱ ⟨≋⟩
Reteplase (Retavase)	**Inj:** 10.4 U	**Acute MI:** 10 U IV over 2 min, repeat in 30 min.	▣C ✱ ⟨≋⟩
Streptokinase (Streptase)	**Inj:** 250,000 IU, 750,000 IU, 1.5 MIU	**Acute MI:** 1.5 MIU IV within 60 min. **PE, DVT:** 250,000 IU over 30 min, then 100,000 IU/h x 24h (72h if DVT). **Thrombosis/Embolism:** 250,000 IU over 30 min, then 100,000 IU/h x 24-72h.	▣C ✱ ⟨≋⟩
Tenecteplase (TNKase)	**Inj:** 50 mg	**Acute MI: <60 kg:** 30 mg. **60 to <70 kg:** 35 mg. **70 to <80 kg:** 40 mg. **80 to <90 kg:** 45 mg. **≥90 kg:** 50 mg. Give IV over 5 sec. **Max:** 50 mg/dose.	▣C ✱ ⟨≋⟩
Urokinase (Abbokinase)	**Inj:** 250,000 IU	**Adults: PE: LD:** 4400 IU/kg IV at 90 ml/h over 10 min. **Maint:** 4400 IU/kg/h IV for 12h. Flush line after each cycle.	▣B ✱ ⟨≋⟩

| Urokinase (Abbokinase Open-Cath) | Inj: 5000 IU, 9000 IU | **Obstructed Catheters:** Amount of drug should equal the internal volume of the catheter, may repeat in resistant cases. Specialized administration. | ●B ❄> |

VITAMIN K-DEPENDENT COAGULATION FACTOR INHIBITOR

| Warfarin Sodium (Coumadin) | Inj: 5 mg; Tab: 1 mg, 2 mg, 2.5 mg, 3 mg, 4 mg, 5 mg, 6 mg, 7.5 mg, 10 mg | **≥18 yo:** Adjust dose based on PT/INR. Give IV as alternate to PO. **Initial:** 2-5 mg qd. **Usual:** 2-10 mg qd. **Venous Thromboembolism (including PE):** INR of 2-3. **A-Fib:** INR of 2-3. **Post-MI:** Initiate 2-4 wks post-infarct & maintain INR of 2.5-3.5. **Mechanical/Bioprosthetic Heart Valve:** INR of 2-3 x 12 wks after valve insertion, then INR of 2.5-3.5 long term. | ●X ❄> |

Heart Failure

ACE INHIBITORS

Captopril (Capoten)	Tab: 12.5 mg, 25 mg, 50 mg, 100 mg	**Initial:** 25 mg tid. **Usual:** 50-100 mg tid. **Max:** 450 mg/d.	●C (1st trimester) ●D (2nd/3rd trimester) ❄v R [7]
Enalapril Maleate (Vasotec)	Tab: 1.25 mg, 2.5 mg, 5 mg, 10 mg, 20 mg	**Initial:** 2.5 mg. **Usual:** 2.5-20 mg given bid. **Titrate:** Increase over few days or wks. **Max:** 40 mg/d.	●C (1st trimester) ●D (2nd/3rd trimester) ❄v R [7]
Lisinopril (Prinivil, Zestril)	Tab: 2.5 mg, 5 mg, 10 mg, 20 mg, 30 mg, 40 mg	**Initial:** 5 mg qd. **Usual: Prinivil:** 5-20 mg qd. **Zestril:** 5-40 mg qd.	●C (1st trimester) ●D (2nd/3rd trimester) ❄v R [7]

[7] Ace Inhibitors can cause injury & death to developing fetus in 2nd & 3rd trimesters.

NAME	FORM/STRENGTH	DOSAGE	COMMENTS
Quinapril HCl (Accupril)	**Tab:** 5 mg, 10 mg, 20 mg, 40 mg	**Initial:** 5 mg bid. **Titrate:** Increase at wkly intervals. **Usual:** 10-20 mg bid.	▣C (1st trimester) ▣D (2nd/3rd trimester) ❖v R [7]

ALDOSTERONE BLOCKER

NAME	FORM/STRENGTH	DOSAGE	COMMENTS
Eplerenone (Inspra)	**Tab:** 25 mg, 50 mg	**Adults: CHF Post-MI: Initial:** 25 mg qd. **Titrate:** To 50 mg qd within 4 wks. **Maint:** 50 mg qd. **Adjust dose based on K+ level:** See labeling.	▣B ❖v R

ALPHA/BETA BLOCKERS

NAME	FORM/STRENGTH	DOSAGE	COMMENTS
Carvedilol (Coreg)	**Tab:** 3.125 mg, 6.25 mg, 12.5 mg, 25 mg	**Mild-Severe HF: Initial:** 3.125 mg bid x 2 wks. **Titrate:** Double dose q2wks. **Max:** 50 mg bid if >85 kg. Reduce dose if HR <55 beats/min. Take w/ food.	▣C ❖v

ANGIOTENSIN II RECEPTOR ANTAGONISTS

NAME	FORM/STRENGTH	DOSAGE	COMMENTS
Valsartan (Diovan)	**Cap:** 40 mg, 80 mg, 160 mg, 320 mg	**Adults: Initial:** 40 mg bid. **Titrate:** Increase to 80 mg or 160 mg bid (use highest dose tolerated). **Max:** 320 mg/day in divided doses.	▣C (1st trimester) ▣D (2nd/3rd trimester) ❖v R [9]

BETA BLOCKERS

NAME	FORM/STRENGTH	DOSAGE	COMMENTS
Metoprolol Succinate (Toprol-XL)	**Tab,ER:** 25 mg, 50 mg, 100 mg, 200 mg	**Initial: Class II HF:** 25 mg qd x 2 wks. **Severe HF:** 12.5 mg qd x 2 wks. **Titrate:** Double dose q2wks as tolerated. **Max:** 200 mg/d.	▣C ❖>

CARBONIC ANHYDRASE INHIBITOR

Acetazolamide (Diamox)	Inj: 500 mg; Tab: 125 mg, 250 mg	CHF/Drug Induced Edema: Initial: 250-375 mg IV/PO qam (5 mg/kg). Maint: May give qod or qd x 2d, then skip 1d.	⊙C ❋v

DIURETICS (INDOLINE)

Indapamide (Lozol)	Tab: 1.25 mg, 2.5 mg	Initial: 2.5 mg qam. Titrate: After 1 wk, may increase to 5 mg qd.	⊙B ❋v

DIURETICS (LOOP)

Bumetanide (Bumex)	Inj: 0.25 mg/ml; Tab: 0.5 mg, 1 mg, 2 mg	≥18 yo: PO: Usual: 0.5-2 mg qd. Maint: Give qod or q3-4d. Max: 10 mg/d. IV/IM: Initial: 0.5-1 mg, may repeat q2-3h x 2-3 doses. Max: 10 mg/d.	⊙C ❋v [8]
Ethacrynate Sodium (Edecrin Sodium)	Inj: 50 mg	Usual: 50 mg, or 0.5-1.0 mg/kg as single dose. May give 2nd dose if necessary.	⊙B ❋v [8]
Ethacrynic Acid (Edecrin)	Tab: 25 mg, 50 mg	Adults: 50-200 mg qd. Peds: Initial: 25 mg qd. Titrate: Increase by 25 mg.	⊙B ❋v [8]

[7] Ace Inhibitors can cause injury & death to developing fetus in 2nd & 3rd trimesters.

[8] Excess amounts may lead to water & electrolyte depletion.

[9] Drugs acting directly on the renin-angiotensin system can cause fetal & neonatal morbidity & death, primarily during the 3rd trimester.

NAME	FORM/STRENGTH	DOSAGE	COMMENTS
Furosemide (Furocot, Lasix)	**Inj:** 10 mg; **Sol:** 10 mg/ml, 40 mg/5 ml; **Tab:** 20 mg, 40 mg, 80 mg	**Adults: PO: Usual:** 20-80 mg as single dose, may repeat or increase by 20-40 mg after 6-8h. **Max:** 600 mg/d. **IV/IM:** 20-40 mg. May repeat or increase by 20 mg after 2h. **Peds: Usual: PO:** 2 mg/kg as single dose, may increase by 1-2 mg/kg after 6-8h. **Max:** 6 mg/kg. **IV/IM:** 1 mg/kg single dose. May increase by 1 mg/kg after 2h. **Max:** 6 mg/kg.	⊞C ❄> [8]
Torsemide (Demadex)	**Inj:** 10 mg/ml; **Tab:** 5 mg, 10 mg, 20 mg, 100 mg	**Initial:** 10-20 mg PO/IV qd. **Titrate:** Double dose until desired diuretic response. **Max:** 200 mg as single dose.	⊞B ❄>

DIURETICS (POTASSIUM SPARING)

NAME	FORM/STRENGTH	DOSAGE	COMMENTS
Amiloride HCl (Midamor)	**Tab:** 5 mg	**Initial:** 5 mg qd. **Titrate:** Increase to 10 mg/d. If hyperkalemia persists, may increase to 15 mg/d then to 20 mg/d. **Maint:** May give on an intermittent basis.	⊞B ❄v
Spironolactone (Aldactone)	**Tab:** 25 mg, 50 mg, 100 mg	**Initial:** 100 mg/d in single or divided doses. **Maint:** 25-200 mg/d.	⊞C ❄v [16]
Triamterene (Dyrenium)	**Cap:** 50 mg, 100 mg	**Initial:** 100 mg bid. **Max:** 300 mg/d.	⊞C ❄v

DIURETICS (POTASSIUM SPARING/THIAZIDE)

NAME	FORM/STRENGTH	DOSAGE	COMMENTS
Amiloride/HCTZ (Moduretic)	**Tab:** 5-50 mg	**Initial:** 1 tab qd. **Maint:** May be given on intermittent basis. **Max:** 2 tabs qd.	⊞B ❄v

Spironolactone/HCTZ (Aldactazide)	**Tab:** 25-25 mg, 50-50 mg	**Usual:** 100 mg/d per component qd or in divided doses. **Maint:** 25-200 mg/d per component.	⊙C ✿v Not for initial therapy. 16
Triamterene/HCTZ (Dyazide, Maxzide)	**Cap:** (Dyazide) 37.5-25 mg; **Tab:** (Maxzide) 37.5-25 mg, 75-50 mg	**Adults: Usual:** (37.5-25 mg cap/tab) 1-2 caps or tabs qd. (75-50 mg tab) 1 tab qd.	⊙C ✿v

DIURETICS (QUINAZOLINE)

Metolazone (Zaroxolyn)	**Tab:** 2.5 mg, 5 mg, 10 mg	**Adults:** 5-20 mg qd.	⊙B ✿v Rapid and slow formulations are not equivalent.

DIURETICS (THIAZIDE)

Chlorothiazide (Diuril)	**Inj:** 0.5 gm; **Susp:** 250 mg/5 ml; **Tab:** 250 mg, 500 mg	**Adults: PO/IV:** 0.5-1 gm qd-bid. May give qod or 3-5d per wk. **Peds: PO: Usual:** 10-20 mg/kg/d given qd-bid. **Max:** ≤2 yo: 375 mg/d. **2-12 yo:** 1 gm/d. **<6 mths:** 15 mg/kg bid.	⊙C ✿v
Chlorthalidone (Thalitone)	**Tab:** 15 mg	**Initial:** 30-60 mg qd or 60 mg qod, up to 90-120 mg qd. **Maint:** May be lower than initial; adjust to response.	⊙B ✿v
Methyclothiazide (Enduron)	**Tab:** 2.5 mg, 5 mg	**Usual:** 2.5-10 mg qd. **Max:** 10 mg/dose.	⊙B ✿v
Polythiazide (Renese)	**Tab:** 1 mg, 2 mg	**Adults:** 1-4 mg qd.	⊙N ✿v

8 Excess amounts may lead to water & electrolyte depletion.
16 Tumorigenic in chronic toxicity studies. Avoid unnecessary use.

NAME	FORM/STRENGTH	DOSAGE	COMMENTS

INOTROPIC AGENTS

NAME	FORM/STRENGTH	DOSAGE	COMMENTS
Digoxin (Digitek, Lanoxicaps, Lanoxin, Lanoxin Pediatric)	**Cap:** (Lanoxicaps) 0.05 mg, 0.1 mg. **Inj:** (Lanoxin Pediatric) 0.1 mg/mL, (Lanoxin) 0.25 mg/mL. **Sol:** (Lanoxin Pediatric) 0.05 mg/mL. **Tab:** (Digitek, Lanoxin) 0.125 mg, 0.25 mg	**HF: Adults: Rapid Digitalization: LD:** (Cap/Inj) 0.4-0.6 mg PO/IV or (Tab) 0.5-0.75 mg PO, may give additional (Cap/Inj) 0.1-0.3 mg or (Tab) 0.125-0.375 mg at 6-8h intervals until clinical effect. **Maint:** (Tab) 0.125-0.5 mg qd. **Peds: Sol/Ped Inj: Digitalizing Dose:** **Premature Infants:** 20-30 mcg/kg PO or 15-25 mcg/kg IV. **Full-Term Infants:** 25-35 mcg/kg PO or 20-30 mcg/kg IV. **1-24 months:** 35-60 mcg/kg PO or 30-50 mcg/kg IV. **2-5 yo:** 30-40 mcg/kg PO or 25-35 mcg/kg IV. **5-10 yo:** 20-35 mcg/kg PO or 15-30 mcg/kg IV. **>10 yo:** 10-15 mcg/kg PO or 8-12 mcg/kg IV. **Maint: Premature Infants:** 20-30% of digitalizing dose. **Full-Term Infants to < 10 yo:** 25-35% of digitalizing dose. **Cap: Digitalizing Dose: 2-5 yo:** 25-35 mcg/kg. **5-10 yo:** 15-30 mcg/kg. **>10 yo:** 8-12 mcg/kg. **Maint: ≥2 yo:** 25-35% of digitalizing dose. **Tab:** 10-15 mcg/kg. **Maint: 2-5 yo:** 10-15 mcg/kg. **5-10 yo:** 7-10 mcg/kg. **>10 yo:** 3-5 mcg/kg.	⊙C ✹ ☼ R

MISCELLANEOUS

NAME	FORM/STRENGTH	DOSAGE	COMMENTS
Milrinone Lactate (Primacor)	**Inj:** 1 mg/mL; 200 mcg/mL in D5W	**LD:** 50 mcg/kg IV over 10 min. **Maint:** Standard is 0.77 mcg/kg/d IV. **Titrate:** Adjust to desired response. **Max:** 1.13 mcg/kg/d. Not shown to be safe & effective >48h.	⊙C ✹ ☼ R

Hypertension

ACE INHIBITORS

Benazepril HCl (Lotensin)	**Tab:** 5 mg, 10 mg, 20 mg, 40 mg	**Initial:** 10 mg qd; 5 mg qd if on diuretic. **Maint:** 20-40 mg/d as qd-bid. **Max:** 80 mg/d.	◉C (1st trimester) ◉D (2nd/3rd trimester) ✿> R [7]
Captopril (Capoten)	**Tab:** 12.5 mg, 25 mg, 50 mg, 100 mg	**Initial:** 25 mg bid-tid. **Titrate:** Increase to 50 mg bid-tid after 1-2 wks. **Usual:** 25-150 mg bid-tid. **Max:** 450 mg/d.	◉C (1st trimester) ◉D (2nd/3rd trimester) ✿v R [7]
Enalapril Maleate (Vasotec)	**Tab:** 1.25 mg, 2.5 mg, 5 mg, 10 mg, 20 mg	**Adults: Initial:** 5 mg qd, 2.5 mg if on diuretic. **Usual:** 10-40 mg/d as qd-bid. **Peds: 1 mth-16 yo: Initial:** 0.08 mg/kg (up to 5 mg) qd. **Max:** 0.58 mg/kg/dose (or 40 mg/dose).	◉C (1st trimester) ◉D (2nd/3rd trimester) ✿v R [7]
Enalaprilat (Vasotec IV)	**Inj:** 1.25 mg/ml	**Usual:** 1.25 mg over 5 min q6h. **Max:** 20 mg/d. **Concomitant Diuretic: Initial:** 0.625 mg over 5 min, may repeat after 1h. **Maint:** 1.25 mg q6h. **PO/IV Conversion:** 5 mg/d PO for 1.25 mg IV q6h and 2.5 mg/d PO or 0.625 mg q6h IV.	◉C (1st trimester) ◉D (2nd/3rd trimester) ✿v R [7]
Fosinopril Sodium (Monopril)	**Tab:** 10 mg, 20 mg, 40 mg	**Initial:** 10 mg qd. **Usual:** 20-40 mg qd. **Max:** 80 mg/d.	◉C (1st trimester) ◉D (2nd/3rd trimester) ✿v [7]
Lisinopril (Prinivil, Zestril)	**Tab:** 2.5 mg, 5 mg, 10 mg, 20 mg, 30 mg, 40 mg	**Initial:** 10 mg qd, 5 mg qd if on diuretic. **Usual:** 20-40 mg qd. **Max:** 80 mg/d.	◉C (1st trimester) ◉D (2nd/3rd trimester) ✿v R [7]

[7] Ace Inhibitors can cause injury & death to developing fetus in 2nd & 3rd trimesters.

JOINT NATIONAL COMMITTEE (JNC) VII
ALGORITHM FOR HYPERTENSION

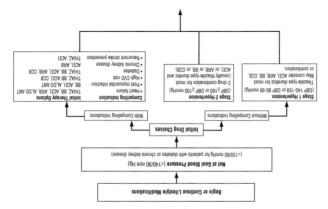

Begin or Continue Lifestyle Modifications

↓

Not at Goal Blood Pressure (<140/90 mm Hg)
(<130/80 mmHg for patients with diabetes or chronic kidney disease)

↓

Initial Drug Choices

With Compelling Indications ← → Without Compelling Indications

With Compelling Indications

Compelling Indication	Initial Therapy Options
• Heart failure	THIAZ, BB, ACEI, ARB, ALDO ANT
• Post myocardial infarction	BB, ACEI, ALDO ANT
• High CVD risk	THIAZ, BB, ACEI, CCB
• Diabetes	THIAZ, BB, ACEI, ARB, CCB
• Chronic kidney disease	ACEI, ARB
• Recurrent stroke prevention	THIAZ, ACEI

Stage 2 Hypertension
(SBP ≥160 or DBP ≥100 mmHg)
2-drug combination for most
(usually thiazide-type diuretic and
ACEI, or ARB, or BB, or CCB)

Stage 1 Hypertension
(SBP 140-159 or DBP 90-99 mmHg)
Thiazide-type diuretic for most.
May consider ACEI, ARB, BB, CCB,
or combination.

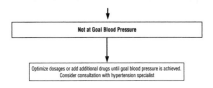

Not at Goal Blood Pressure

Optimize dosages or add additional drugs until goal blood pressure is achieved.
Consider consultation with hypertension specialist

Key:
THIAZ = thiazide diuretic
ACEI = angiotensin converting enzyme inhibitor
ARB = angiotension receptor blocker
BB = beta blocker
CCB = calcium channel blocker
ALDO ANT = aldosterone antagonist

NAME	FORM/STRENGTH	DOSAGE	COMMENTS
Moexipril HCl (Univasc)	**Tab:** 7.5 mg, 15 mg	**Initial:** 7.5 mg qd, 3.75 mg if on diuretic. **Usual:** 7.5-30 mg/d as qd-bid. **Max:** 60 mg/d.	⊙C (1st trimester) ⊙D (2nd/3rd trimester) ❋v R [7]
Perindopril Erbumine (Aceon)	**Tab:** 2 mg, 4 mg, 8 mg	**Initial:** 4 mg qd, 2-4 mg/d if on diuretic. **Usual:** 4-8 mg/d as qd-bid. **Max:** 16 mg qd.	⊙C (1st trimester) ⊙D (2nd/3rd trimester) ❋v R [7]

[7] Ace Inhibitors can cause injury & death to developing fetus in 2nd & 3rd trimesters.

123 KEY: ⊙ PREGNANCY RATING; ❋ BREASTFEEDING SAFETY; H HEPATIC ADJUSTMENT; R RENAL ADJUSTMENT

NAME	FORM/STRENGTH	DOSAGE	COMMENTS
Quinapril HCl (Accupril)	**Tab:** 5 mg, 10 mg, 20 mg, 40 mg	**Initial:** 10-20 mg qd; 5 mg qd if on diuretic. **Usual:** 20-80 mg/d given qd-bid.	●C (1st trimester) ●D (2nd/3rd trimester) ❋v R [7]
Ramipril (Altace)	**Tab:** 1.25 mg, 2.5 mg, 5 mg, 10 mg	**Initial:** 2.5 mg qd, 1.25 mg if an diuretic. **Usual:** 2.5-20 mg/d given as qd-bid.	●C (1st trimester) ●D (2nd/3rd trimester) ❋v H R [7]
Trandolapril (Mavik)	**Tab:** 1 mg, 2 mg, 4 mg	**Initial:** 1 mg qd in non-black patients; 2 mg qd in black patients; 0.5 mg if on diuretic. **Titrate:** Adjust at 1 wk intervals. **Usual:** 2-4 mg qd. **Max:** 8 mg/d.	●C (1st trimester) ●D (2nd/3rd trimester) ❋v H R [7]

ACE INHIBITORS/CALCIUM CHANNEL BLOCKERS

NAME	FORM/STRENGTH	DOSAGE	COMMENTS
Benazepril/Amlodipine (Lotrel)	**Cap:** 10-2.5 mg, 10-5 mg, 20-5 mg, 20-10 mg	**Usual:** If not controlled on monotherapy, or unacceptable edema with amlodipine, then 2.5-10 mg amlodipine & 10-80 mg benazepril per day.	●C (1st trimester) ●D (2nd/3rd trimester) ❋vH R [7,24]
Trandolapril/Verapamil HCl (Tarka)	**Tab:** 2-180 mg, 1-240 mg, 2-240 mg, 4-240 mg	**Replacement Therapy:** 1 tab qd with food.	●C (1st trimester) ●D (2nd/3rd trimester) ❋v H R [7]

ACE INHIBITORS/THIAZIDES

NAME	FORM/STRENGTH	DOSAGE	COMMENTS
Benazepril/HCTZ (Lotensin HCT)	**Tab:** 5-6.25 mg, 10-12.5 mg, 20-12.5 mg, 20-25 mg	**Initial (if not controlled on benazepril monotherapy):** 10-12.5 mg tab or 20-12.5 mg tab. **Titrate:** May increase after 2-3 wks. **Initial (if controlled on 25 mg HCTZ/d with hypokalemia):** 5-6.25 mg tab. **Replacement Therapy:** Substitute combination for titrated components.	●C (1st trimester) ●D (2nd/3rd trimester) ❋> R [7,24]

Captopril/HCTZ (Capozide)	**Tab:** 25-15 mg, 25-25 mg, 50-15 mg, 50-25 mg	**Initial:** 25-15 mg tab qd. **Titrate:** Adjust dose at 6-wk intervals. **Max:** 150 mg captopril/50 mg HCTZ per day. **Replacement Therapy:** Substitute combination for titrated components.	◧C (1st trimester) ◧D (2nd/3rd trimester) ❀v R [7]
Enalapril/HCTZ (Vaseretic)	**Tab:** 5-12.5 mg, 10-25 mg	**Initial (if not controlled on enalapril/HCTZ monotherapy):** 5-12.5 mg tab or 10-25 mg tab qd. **Titrate:** May increase after 2-3 wks. **Max:** 20 mg enalapril/50 mg HCTZ per day. **Replacement Therapy:** Substitute combination for titrated components.	◧C (1st trimester) ◧D (2nd/3rd trimester) ❀v R [7,24]
Lisinopril/HCTZ (Prinzide, Zestoretic)	**Tab:** 10-12.5 mg, 20-12.5 mg, 20-25 mg	**Initial (if not controlled with lisinopril/HCTZ monotherapy):** 10-12.5 mg tab or 20-12.5 mg tab daily. **Titrate:** May increase after 2-3 wks. **Initial (if controlled on 25 mg HCTZ/d with hypokalemia):** 10-12.5 mg tab. **Replacement Therapy:** Substitute combination for titrated components.	◧C (1st trimester) ◧D (2nd/3rd trimester) ❀v R [7,24]
Moexipril/HCTZ (Uniretic)	**Tab:** 7.5-12.5 mg, 15-12.5 mg, 15-25 mg	**Initial (if not controlled on moexipril/HCTZ monotherapy):** Switch to 7.5-12.5 mg tab, 15-12.5 mg tab, or 15-25 mg tab qd. **Titrate:** May increase after 2-3 wks. **Initial (if controlled on 25 mg HCTZ/d with hypokalemia):** 3.75-6.25 mg (1/2 of 7.5-12.5 mg tab). **Replacement Therapy:** Substitute combination for titrated components.	◧C (1st trimester) ◧D (2nd/3rd trimester) ❀v Avoid if CrCl ≤40 ml/min. [7]

[7] ACE Inhibitors can cause injury & death to developing fetus in 2nd & 3rd trimesters.
[24] Avoid if CrCl ≤30 ml/min.

NAME	FORM/STRENGTH	DOSAGE	COMMENTS
Quinapril/HCTZ (Accuretic)	Tab: 10-12.5 mg, 20-12.5 mg, 20-25 mg	**Initial (if not controlled on quinapril monotherapy):** 10-12.5 mg or 20-12.5 mg tab qd. **Titrate:** May increase after 2-3 wks. **Initial (if controlled on 25 mg HCTZ/d with hypokalemia):** 10-12.5 mg or 20-12.5 mg tab qd.	▣C (1st trimester) ▣D (2nd/3rd trimester) ✿v [7,24]

ALDOSTERONE BLOCKER

NAME	FORM/STRENGTH	DOSAGE	COMMENTS
Eplerenone (Inspra)	Tab: 25 mg, 50 mg	**Adults: Initial:** 50 mg qd. May increase to 50 mg bid if inadequate effect. **With Weak CYP450 3A4 Inhibitors: Initial:** 25 mg qd.	▣B ✿v R

ALPHA ADRENERGIC BLOCKERS

NAME	FORM/STRENGTH	DOSAGE	COMMENTS
Clonidine HCl (Catapres, Catapres-TTS)	Tab: 0.1 mg, 0.2 mg, 0.3 mg; Patch: (TTS) 0.1 mg/24h, 0.2 mg/24h, 0.3 mg/24h	**Patch: Initial:** 0.1 mg/24h patch wkly. **Titrate:** May increase after 1-2 wks. **Max:** 0.6 mg/24h. **Tab: Initial:** 0.1 mg bid. **Titrate:** May increase by 0.1 mg wkly. **Usual:** 0.2-0.6 mg/d. **Max:** 2.4 mg/d.	▣C ✿> R
Doxazosin Mesylate (Cardura)	Tab: 1 mg, 2 mg, 4 mg, 8 mg	**Initial:** 1 mg qd. Titrate: May double the dose q1-2wks. **Max:** 8 mg/d.	▣C ✿>
Guanadrel Sulfate (Hylorel)	Tab: 10 mg	**Initial:** 5 mg bid. **Titrate:** Increase by qwk-qmth. **Usual:** 20-75 mg/d given bid. **Max:** 400 mg/d.	▣B ✿v R
Guanfacine HCl (Tenex)	Tab: 1 mg, 2 mg	**Initial:** 1 mg qhs, may increase to 2 mg qhs after 3-4 wks. **Max:** 3 mg/d.	▣B ✿>
Methyldopa (Aldomet)	Tab: 125 mg, 250 mg, 500 mg	**Initial:** 250 mg bid-tid x 48h. **Titrate:** Adjust to desired response q2d. **Maint:** 500 mg-2 gm/d given bid-qid. **Max:** 3 gm/d. **Peds: Initial:** 10 mg/kg/d given bid-qid. **Max:** 65 mg/kg/d or 3 g/d.	▣B ✿> R

Methyldopate HCl	**Inj:** 50 mg/ml	**Usual:** 250-500 mg infused over 30-60 min q6h. **Max:** 1 gm q6h. **Peds:** 20-40 mg/kg/d IV given q6h. **Max:** 65 mg/kg/d or 3 g/d.	◐C ✽> R
Prazosin HCl (Minipress)	**Tab:** 1 mg, 2 mg, 5 mg	**Initial:** 1 mg bid-tid. **Usual:** 6-15 mg/d in divided doses. **Max:** 40 mg/d.	◐C ✽> Syncope with 1st dose.
Reserpine	**Tab:** 0.1 mg, 0.25 mg	**Initial:** 0.5 mg qd x 1-2 wks. **Maint:** 0.1-0.25 mg qd.	◐C ✽v
Terazosin HCl (Hytrin)	**Cap:** 1 mg, 2 mg, 5 mg, 10 mg	**Initial:** 1 mg qhs. **Titrate:** Increase stepwise as needed. **Usual:** 10 mg qd. May increase to 20 mg/day after 4-6 wks. **Max:** 20 mg/d. If d/c for several days, restart at initial dose.	◐C ✽> Syncope with 1st dose.

ALPHA ADRENERGIC BLOCKERS/THIAZIDES

Methyldopa/HCTZ (Aldoril)	**Tab:** 250-15 mg, 250-25 mg, 500-30 mg	**Initial:** 250-15 mg tab bid-tid, 250-25 mg tab bid, or 500-30 mg bid. **Max:** 50 mg HCTZ/d or 3 gm methyldopa/d.	◐C ✽v Not for initial therapy.

ALPHA/BETA BLOCKERS

Carvedilol (Coreg)	**Tab:** 3.125 mg, 6.25 mg, 12.5 mg, 25 mg	**Initial:** 6.25 mg bid x 7-14d. **Titrate:** Double dose q7-14d as tolerated. **Max:** 50 mg/d. Take with food.	◐C ✽v
Labetalol HCl (Normodyne)	**Inj:** 5 mg/ml; **Tab:** 100 mg, 200 mg, 300 mg	**PO: Initial:** 100 mg bid. **Titrate:** Increase by 100 mg bid q2-3d. **Maint:** 200-400 mg bid. **Max:** 2400 mg/d. **IV: Initial:** 20 mg over 2 min, then may give 40-80 mg q10min until desired response. **Max:** 300 mg.	◐C ✽>

7 ACE Inhibitors can cause injury & death to developing fetus in 2nd & 3rd trimesters.

24 Avoid if CrCl ≤30 mL/min.

NAME	FORM/STRENGTH	DOSAGE	COMMENTS
ANGIOTENSIN II RECEPTOR ANTAGONISTS			
Candesartan Cilexetil (Atacand)	Tab: 4 mg, 8 mg, 16 mg, 32 mg	Initial: 16 mg qd. Usual: 8-32 mg/d, given qd-bid.	C (1st trimester) D (2nd/3rd trimester) ✿ ❤ R 9
Eprosartan Mesylate (Teveten)	Tab: 400 mg, 600 mg	Initial: 600 mg qd. Usual: 400-800 mg/d, given qd-bid.	C (1st trimester) D (2nd/3rd trimester) ✿ ❤ 9
Irbesartan (Avapro)	Tab: 75 mg, 150 mg, 300 mg	6-12 yo: Initial: 75 mg qd. Titrate: May increase to 150 mg qd. ≥13 yo: Initial: 150 mg qd. Titrate: May increase to 300 mg qd.	C (1st trimester) D (2nd/3rd trimester) ✿ ❤ R 9
Losartan Potassium (Cozaar)	Tab: 25 mg, 50 mg, 100 mg	HTN: Initial: 50 mg qd. Usual: 25-100 mg given qd-bid. HTN with LVH: Initial: 50 mg qd. Add HCTZ 12.5 mg qd and/or increase losartan to 100 mg qd, followed by an increase in HCTZ to 25 mg qd based on BP response.	C (1st trimester) D (2nd/3rd trimester) ✿ ❤ H 9
Olmesartan Medoxomil (Benicar)	Tab: 5 mg, 20 mg, 40 mg	**Adults: Monotherapy Without Volume Depletion:** Initial: 20 mg qd. Titrate: May increase to 40 mg qd after 2 wks if needed. May add diuretic if BP not controlled. Intravascular Volume Depletion (eg, with diuretics, impaired renal function): Lower initial dose; monitor closely.	C (1st trimester) D (2nd/3rd trimester) ✿ ❤ 9
Telmisartan (Micardis)	Tab: 20 mg, 40 mg, 80 mg	Initial: 40 mg qd. Usual: 20-80 mg qd.	C (1st trimester) D (2nd/3rd trimester) ✿ ❤ 9

Valsartan (Diovan)	**Cap:** 40 mg, 80 mg, 160 mg, 320 mg	**Initial:** 80 or 160 mg qd. **Titrate:** Increase to 320 mg qd or add diuretic (greater effect than increasing dose >80 mg).	⊕C (1st trimester) ⊕D (2nd/3rd trimester)❈v H R[9]

ANGIOTENSIN II RECEPTOR ANTAGONISTS/THIAZIDES

Candesartan/HCTZ (Atacand HCT)	**Tab:** 16-12.5 mg, 32-12.5 mg	**Initial:** If not controlled on 25 mg HCTZ/d or controlled but serum K⁺ decreased, 16-12.5 mg tab qd. If not controlled on 32 mg candesartan/d, 32-12.5 mg qd; may increase to 32-25 mg qd.	⊕C (1st trimester) ⊕D (2nd/3rd trimester)❈v H R [9, 24]
Eprosartan Mesylate/HCTZ (Teveten HCT)	**Tab:** 600-12.5 mg, 600-25 mg	**Adults: Usual (Not Volume Depleted):** 600-12.5 mg qd. May increase to 600-25 mg qd if needed.	⊕C (1st trimester) ⊕D (2nd/3rd trimester)❈v H R [9]
Irbesartan/HCTZ (Avalide)	**Tab:** 150-12.5 mg, 300-12.5 mg	**Usual:** If not controlled on monotherapy, give 150-12.5 mg or 300-12.5 mg tab qd. **Max:** 2 tabs of 150-12.5 mg qd.	⊕C (1st trimester) ⊕D (2nd/3rd trimester)❈v R [9, 24]
Losartan/HCTZ (Hyzaar)	**Tab:** 50-12.5 mg, 100-25 mg	**Initial:** If not controlled on losartan, HCTZ alone, or 25 mg HCTZ/d, or controlled on 25 mg HCTZ/d but serum K⁺ decreased, 50-12.5 mg tab qd. **Max:** 2 tabs of 50-12.5 mg qd or 1 tab of 100-25 mg qd.	⊕C (1st trimester) ⊕D (2nd/3rd trimester)❈vH R [9, 24]

[9] Drugs acting directly on the renin-angiotensin system can cause fetal & neonatal morbidity & death, primarily during the 3rd trimester.
[24] Avoid if CrCl ≤30 ml/min.

NAME	FORM/STRENGTH	DOSAGE	COMMENTS
Olmesartan Medoxomil/ HCTZ (Benicar HCT)	Tab: (Olmesartan-HCTZ) 20-12.5 mg, 40-25 mg	Adults: Initial: If not controlled on olmesartan, add HCT 12.5 mg qd. May titrate to 25 mg qd after 2-4 wks. If not controlled on HCTZ, add olmesartan 20 mg qd. May titrate to 40 mg after 2-4 wks. Intravascular Volume Depletion (eg, with diuretics, impaired renal function): Lower initial dose; monitor closely.	C (1st trimester) D (2nd/3rd trimester) ❖ R 9
Telmisartan/HCTZ (Micardis HCT)	Tab: 40-12.5 mg, 80-12.5 mg	Initial: If not controlled on 80 mg telmisartan, or 25 mg HCTZ/d, or controlled on 25 mg HCTZ/d but serum K+ decreased, 80-12.5 mg tab qd. Max: 160 mg telmisartan-25 mg HCTZ/d.	C (1st trimester) D (2nd/3rd trimester) ❖ H R 9, 24
Valsartan/HCTZ (Diovan HCT)	Tab: 80-12.5 mg, 160-12.5 mg, 160-25 mg	Initial: If not controlled on valsartan on 25 mg HCTZ/d, or controlled on 25 mg HCTZ/d but serum K+ decreased, 80-12.5 mg tab or 160-12.5 mg tab qd. Max: 160 mg valsartan-25 mg HCT2/d.	C (1st trimester) D (2nd/3rd trimester) ❖ R 9, 24
BETA BLOCKERS			
Acebutolol HCl (Sectral)	Cap: 200 mg, 400 mg	Initial: 400 mg/d given qd-bid. Usual: 200-800 mg/d. Max: 1200 mg/d.	B ❖ R
Atenolol (Tenormin)	Tab: 25 mg, 50 mg, 100 mg	Initial: 50 mg qd. Titrate: May increase after 1-2 wks. Max: 100 mg qd.	D ❖ R
Betaxolol HCl (Kerlone)	Tab: 10 mg, 20 mg	Initial: 10 mg qd. Titrate: May increase to 20 mg qd after 7-14d. Max (usual): 20 mg/d.	C ❖ R
Bisoprolol Fumarate (Zebeta)	Tab: 5 mg, 10 mg	Initial: 2.5-5 mg qd. Max: 20 mg/d.	C ❖ H R
Carteolol HCl (Cartrol)	Tab: 2.5 mg, 5 mg	Initial: 2.5 mg qd. Maint: 2.5-5 mg qd. Max: 10 mg/d.	C ❖ R

Drug	Form/Strength	Dosage	
Esmolol HCl (Brevibloc)	**Inj:** 250 mg/ml, 10 mg/ml	**Adults: Intra-/Post-op HTN: Initial: Rapid:** 80 mg IVP, then 150 mcg/kg/min infusion. **Gradual:** 500 mcg/kg/min x 1 min, then 50 mcg/kg/min x 4 min. If inadequate response within 5 min, repeat LD & give maint 100 mcg/kg/min.	●C ❋>
Metoprolol Succinate (Toprol-XL)	**Tab,ER:** 25 mg, 50 mg, 100 mg, 200 mg	**Usual:** 50-100 mg qd. **Titrate:** Increase wkly. **Max:** 400 mg qd.	●C ❋>
Metoprolol Tartrate (Lopressor)	**Tab:** 50 mg, 100 mg	**Initial:** 50 mg bid or 100 mg qd. **Titrate:** Increase qwk. **Usual:** 100-450 mg/d. **Max:** 450 mg/d.	●C ❋> 17
Nadolol (Corgard)	**Tab:** 20 mg, 40 mg, 80 mg, 120 mg, 160 mg	**Initial:** 40 mg qd. **Titrate:** Increase by 40-80 mg. **Max:** 320 mg/d.	●C ❋v R 17
Penbutolol Sulfate (Levatol)	**Tab:** 20 mg	**Initial/Maint:** 20 mg qd.	●C ❋>
Pindolol	**Tab:** 5 mg, 10 mg	**Initial:** 5 mg bid. **Titrate:** Increase q3-4wks by 10 mg/d. **Max:** 60 mg/d.	●B ❋v 18
Propranolol HCl (Inderal, Inderal LA)	**Cap,ER:** 60 mg, 80 mg, 120 mg, 160 mg; **Tab:** 10 mg, 20 mg, 40 mg, 60 mg, 80 mg	**Adults: Tab: Initial:** 40 mg bid. **Maint:** 120-240 mg qd. **Cap,ER: Initial:** 80 mg qd. **Maint:** 120-160 mg qd.	●C ❋>
Timolol Maleate (Blocadren)	**Tab:** 5 mg, 10 mg, 20 mg	**Initial:** 10 mg bid. **Maint:** 20-40 mg/d. **Max:** 60 mg/d.	●C ❋v 18

9 Drugs acting directly on the renin-angiotensin system can cause fetal & neonatal morbidity & death, primarily during the 3rd trimester.

17 Abrupt cessation may induce arrhythmia or MI.

18 Abrupt cessation may exacerbate angina.

24 Avoid if CrCl ≤30 ml/min.

NAME	FORM/STRENGTH	DOSAGE	COMMENTS
BETA BLOCKERS/THIAZIDES			
Atenolol/Chlorthalidone (Tenoretic)	**Tab:** 50-25 mg, 100-25 mg	**Initial:** 50-25 mg tab qd. **Titrate:** May increase to 100-25 mg tab qd.	◉D ❋ < R
Bisoprolol/HCT2 (Ziac)	**Tab:** 2.5-6.25 mg, 5-6.25 mg, 10-6.25 mg	**Initial:** 2.5-6.25 mg tab qd. **Titrate:** Increase q14d up to 20 mg bisoprolol-12.5 mg HCTZ/d.	◉C ❋^ H R
Nadolol/ Bendroflumethiazide (Corzide)	**Tab:** 40-5 mg, 80-5 mg	**Initial:** 40-5 mg tab qd. **Max:** 80-5 mg tab qd.	◉C ❋^ R
Propranolol/HCTZ (Inderide, Inderide LA)	**Tab:** 40-25 mg, 80-25 mg; **Cap,ER:** 80-50 mg, 120-50 mg, 160-50 mg	**Initial:** 80-160 mg propranolol/d; 25-50 mg HCTZ/d. **Max:** (propranolol-HCTZ) 160-50mg/d. Do not substitute mg-for-mg of Cap,ER for Tab plus HCT2.	◉C ❋^
Timolol Maleate/HCT2 (Timolide)	**Tab:** 10-25 mg	**Initial/Maint:** 1 tab bid or 2 tabs qd.	◉C ❋^
CALCIUM CHANNEL BLOCKER/HMG COA REDUCTASE INHIBITOR			
Amlodipine Besylate/ Atorvastatin Calcium (Caduet)	**Tab:** 5-10 mg, 5-20 mg, 5-40 mg, 5-80 mg, 10-10 mg, 10-20 mg, 10-40 mg, 10-80 mg	Dosing is based on the appropriate combination of recommendations for the monotherapies. **Amlodipine: Adults: Initial:** 5 mg qd. Titrate over 7-14d. **Max:** 10 mg qd. **Peds ≥10 yrs (postmenarchal):** 2.5-5 mg qd. **Atorvastatin:** See under Antilipidemic Agents for dosing.	◉ X ❋^ H

Amlodipine Besylate (Norvasc)	**Tab:** 2.5 mg, 5 mg, 10 mg	**Adults: Initial:** 5 mg qd. **Max:** 10 mg qd. **Peds: 6-17yo:** 2.5-5 mg qd.	⊙C ❄v H
Felodipine (Plendil)	**Tab,ER:** 2.5 mg, 5 mg, 10 mg	**Initial:** 5 mg qd. **Maint:** 2.5-10 mg qd.	⊙C ❄v H
Isradipine (DynaCirc, DynaCirc CR)	**Cap:** 2.5 mg, 5 mg; **Tab,ER:** (CR) 5 mg, 10 mg	**Initial: Cap:** 2.5 mg bid. **Tab,ER:** 5 mg qd. **Titrate:** Increase by 5 mg/d q2-4wks. **Max:** 20 mg/d.	⊙C ❄v
Nicardipine (Cardene, Cardene SR)	**Cap:** 20 mg, 30 mg; **Inj:** 2.5 mg/ml; **Cap,ER:** (SR) 30 mg, 45 mg, 60 mg	**IV: Initial:** 50 ml/h (5 mg/h). **Titrate:** May increase by 25 ml/h (2.5 mg/h) q5-15min. **Max:** 150 ml/h (15 mg/h). **Equ. IV/PO Cardene Dose:** 20 mg q8h= 0.5 mg/h, 30 mg q8h=1.2 mg/h, 40 mg q8h=2.2 mg/h. **PO: Cap: Initial:** 20 mg tid. **Usual:** 20-40 mg tid. **Cap,ER: Initial:** 30 mg bid. **Usual:** 30-60 mg bid.	⊙C ❄v H
Nifedipine (Adalat CC, Procardia XL)	**Tab,ER:** 30 mg, 60 mg, 90 mg	**Initial: XL:** 30-60 mg qd. **CC:** 30 mg qd. **Titrate:** Increase over 7-14d. **Max: XL:** 120 mg/d. **CC:** 90 mg/d.	⊙C ❄v (CC) ❄v (XL)
Nisoldipine (Sular)	**Tab,ER:** 10 mg, 20 mg, 30 mg, 40 mg	**Initial:** 20 mg qd. **Titrate:** Increase by 10 mg qwk or longer interval. **Maint:** 20-40 mg qd. **Max:** 60 mg/d. Avoid high fat meals & grapefruit pre- and post-dosing.	⊙C ❄v H

NAME	FORM/STRENGTH	DOSAGE	COMMENTS
CALCIUM CHANNEL BLOCKERS (NON-DIHYDROPYRIDINES)			
Diltiazem HCl (Cardizem, Cardizem CD, Cardizem LA, Cardizem SR, Cartia XT, Dilacor XR, Diltia XT, Tiazac)	**Cap,ER:** (Cardizem CD) 120 mg, 180 mg, 240 mg, 300 mg, 360 mg, (Cardizem SR) 60 mg, 90 mg, 120 mg, (Cartia XT) 120 mg, 180 mg, 240 mg, 300 mg, (Dilacor XR/Diltia XT) 120 mg, 180 mg, 240 mg, (Tiazac) 120 mg, 180 mg, 240 mg, 300 mg, 360 mg, 420 mg; **Tab,ER:** (Cardizem LA) 120 mg, 180 mg, 240 mg, 300 mg, 360 mg, 420 mg	**Cardizem CD/Cartia XT: Initial:** 180-240 mg qd. **Titrate:** Adjust at 2 wk intervals. **Max:** 480 mg/d. **Cardizem SR: Initial:** 60-120 mg qd. **Titrate:** Adjust at 2 wk intervals. **Usual:** 240-360 mg/d. **Dilacor XR/Diltia XT: Initial:** 180-240 mg qd. **Max:** 540 mg/d. **Tiazac: Initial:** 120-240 mg qd. **Max:** 540 mg/d. **Cardizem LA: Initial:** 180-240 mg qd. Adjust at 2 week intervals. **Max:** 540 mg qd.	●C ❄v
Verapamil (Calan, Calan SR, Covera-HS, Isoptin SR, Verelan, Verelan PM)	**Cap,ER:** (Verelan) 120 mg, 180 mg, 240 mg, 360 mg, (Verelan PM) 100 mg, 200 mg, 300 mg; **Tab:** (Calan) 40 mg, 80 mg, 120 mg; **Tab,ER:** (Calan SR, Isoptin SR) 120 mg, 180 mg, 240 mg, (Covera-HS) 180 mg, 240 mg	**Calan: Initial:** 80 mg tid. **Usual:** 360-480 mg/d. **Calan SR/Isoptin SR: Initial:** 180 mg qam. **Titrate:** Increase to 240 mg qam, then 180 mg bid; or 240 mg + 120 mg qpm, then 240 mg q12h. **Covera-HS: Initial:** 180 mg qhs. **Titrate:** Increase to 240 mg qhs, then 360 mg qhs, then 480 mg qhs. **Verelan: Usual:** 240 mg qam. **Titrate:** Increase by 120 mg qam. **Max:** 480 mg qam. **Verelan PM: Initial:** 200 mg qhs. **Titrate:** Increase to 300 mg qhs, then 400 mg qhs.	●C ❄v H (Calan, Verelan) R (Verelan)

DIURETIC (LOOP)

Furosemide (Furocot, Lasix)	**Sol:** 10 mg/ml, 40 mg/5 ml; **Tab:** 20 mg, 40 mg, 80 mg	**Initial:** 40 mg bid. **Maint:** Adjust according to response.	C ❄>[8]
Torsemide (Demadex)	**Inj:** 10 mg/ml; **Tab:** 5 mg, 10 mg, 20 mg, 100 mg	**Initial:** 5 mg PO/IV qd. **Maint:** May increase to 10 mg PO/IV qd after 4-6 wks.	B ❄>

DIURETICS (INDOLINE)

Indapamide (Lozol)	**Tab:** 1.25 mg, 2.5 mg	**Initial:** 1.25 mg qam. **Titrate:** After 4 wks, increase to 2.5 mg qd; after another 4 wks increase to 5 mg qd.	B ❄v

DIURETICS (POTASSIUM SPARING)

Amiloride HCl (Midamor)	**Tab:** 5 mg	**Initial:** 5 mg qd. **Titrate:** Increase to 10 mg/day. If hyperkalemia persists, may increase to 15 mg/day then to 20 mg/day **Maint:** May be on an intermittent basis.	B ❄v
Spironolactone (Aldactone)	**Tab:** 25 mg, 50 mg, 100 mg	**Initial:** 50-100 mg/d as single or divided doses. **Maint:** After 2 wks, adjust by response.	C ❄v [16]
Triamterene (Dyrenium)	**Cap:** 50 mg, 100 mg	**Initial:** 100 mg bid. **Max:** 300 mg/d.	C ❄v

DIURETICS (POTASSIUM SPARING/THIAZIDE)

Amiloride/HCTZ (Moduretic)	**Tab:** 5-50 mg	**Initial:** 1 tab qd. **Maint:** May be given on intermittent basis. **Max:** 2 tabs qd.	B ❄v

[8] Excess amounts may lead to water & electrolyte depletion.

[16] Tumorigenic in chronic toxicity studies. Avoid unnecessary use.

NAME	FORM/STRENGTH	DOSAGE	COMMENTS
Spironolactone/HCTZ (Aldactazide)	Tab: 25-25 mg, 50-50 mg	Adults: 50-100 mg/d per component qd or in divided doses.	●C ❄v Not for initial therapy. 16
Triamterene/HCTZ (Dyazide, Maxzide)	Cap: (Dyazide) 37.5-25 mg; Tab: (Maxzide) 37.5-25 mg, 75-50 mg	Adults: Usual: (37.5-25 mg cap/tab) 1-2 caps or tabs qd. (75-50 mg tab) 1 tab qd.	●C ❄v

DIURETICS (QUINAZOLINE)

NAME	FORM/STRENGTH	DOSAGE	COMMENTS
Metolazone (Mykrox, Zaroxolyn)	Tab: (Mykrox) 0.5 mg, (Zaroxolyn) 2.5 mg, 5 mg, 10 mg	Mykrox: Initial: 0.5 mg qam. Titrate/Max: 1 mg qam. Zaroxolyn: 2.5-5 mg qd.	●B ❄v Rapid and slow formulations are not equivalent.

DIURETICS (THIAZIDE)

NAME	FORM/STRENGTH	DOSAGE	COMMENTS
Chlorothiazide (Diuril)	Susp: 250 mg/5 ml; Tab: 250 mg, 500 mg	Adults: Initial: 0.5-1 gm qd or in divided doses. Max: 2 gm/d. Peds: Usual: 10-20 mg/kg/d given qd-bid. Max: ≤2 yo: 375 mg/d. 2-12 yo: 1 gm/d. <6 mths: 15 mg/kg bid.	●C ❄v
Chlorthalidone (Thalitone)	Tab: 15 mg	Initial: 15 mg qd. Titrate: Increase to 30 mg qd, then 45-50 mg qd.	●B ❄v
Hydrochlorothiazide (HydroDiuril, Microzide)	Tab: (HydroDiuril) 25 mg, 50 mg; Cap: (Microzide) 12.5 mg	Adults: Microzide: Initial: 12.5 qd. Max: 50 mg/d. HydroDiuril: Initial: 25 mg qd. Titrate: May increase to 50 mg/d. Peds: Usual: 1-2 mg/kg/d given qd-bid. Max: ≤2 yo: 37.5 mg/d. 2-12 yo: 100 mg/d.	●B ❄v
Methyclothiazide (Enduron)	Tab: 2.5 mg, 5 mg	Adults: 2.5-5 mg qd.	●B ❄v
Polythiazide (Renese)	Tab: 1 mg, 2 mg	Adults: 2-4 mg qd.	●N ❄v

Trichlormethiazide (Naqua)	Tab: 4 mg	Adults: 2-4 mg qd.	⊕B ❄v

VASODILATORS (PERIPHERAL)

Hydralazine	Inj: 20 mg/ml; Tab: 10 mg, 25 mg, 50 mg, 100 mg	PO: Initial: 10 mg qid x 2-4d. Titrate: Increase to 25 mg qid x 3-5d, then 50 mg qid. Max: 300 mg/d. IM/IV: 20-40 mg, repeat as necessary.	⊕C ❄>
Minoxidil (Loniten)	Tab: 2.5 mg, 10 mg	>12 yo: Initial: 5 mg qd. Maint: 10-40 mg qd. Max: 100 mg/d. <12 yo: Initial: 0.2 mg/kg qd. Maint: 0.25-1 mg/kg/d. Max: 50 mg/d.	⊕C ❄v Pericardial effusion. Exacerbates angina.

Miscellaneous

Epoprostenol (Flolan)	Inj: 0.5 mg, 1.5 mg	PPH: Continuous Chronic Infusion: Initial: 2 ng/kg/min, decrease if not tolerated. Titrate: Increase by 2 ng/kg/min q15min or longer until dose-limiting effects seen.	⊕B ❄>
Isoxsuprine (Vasodilan)	Tab: 10 mg, 20 mg	PVD/Cerebrovascular Insufficiency/Raynaud's Disease: 10-20 mg tid-qid.	⊕C ❄v For PVD & cerebrovascular symptoms.
Papaverine (Papacon)	Cap,ER: 150 mg	Cerebral/Peripheral Ischemia: 1 cap q12h, may increase to 1 cap q8h or 2 caps q12h.	⊕N ❄>

Tumorigenic in chronic toxicity studies. Avoid unnecessary use.

NAME	FORM/STRENGTH	DOSAGE	COMMENTS

DERMATOLOGY
Acne Preparations
ANTI-INFECTIVES

NAME	FORM/STRENGTH	DOSAGE	COMMENTS
Clindamycin (Cleocin T)	Gel, Lot, Sol, Swab: 1%	**Adults & Peds: ≥12 yo:** Apply to affected area bid.	●B ❋v
Erythromycin (A/T/S)	Gel: 2%; Sol: 2%	**Adults: Gel:** Apply to affected area qd-bid. **Sol:** Apply to affected area bid.	Gel: ●B ❋v Sol: ●C ❋>
Erythromycin (Emgel)	Gel: 2%	**Adults:** Apply to affected area qd-bid.	●B ❋v
Erythromycin (Erycette)	Swab: 2%	**Adults:** Apply to affected area bid (qam & qpm).	●B ❋>
Erythromycin (Akne-Mycin)	Oint: 2%	**Adults:** Apply to affected area bid (qam & qpm).	●N ❋>
Sodium Sulfacetamide (Klaron)	Lot: 10%	**Adults & Peds: ≥12 yo:** Apply bid.	●C ❋>
Sodium Sulfacetamide/ Sulfur (Rosula)	Cleanser, Gel: 10%-5%	**Adults & Peds: ≥12 yo:** (Gel) Apply thin film qd-tid. (Cleanser) Wash for 10-20 sec qd-bid.	●C ❋>
Sodium Sulfacetamide/ Sulfur (Sulfacet-R)	Lot: 10%-5%	**Adults & Peds: ≥12 yo:** Apply qd-tid.	●C ❋>
Tetracycline HCl (Sumycin)	Cap: 250 mg, 500 mg; Susp: 125 mg/5 ml	**Severe Acne: Adults & Peds >8 yo:** 1 gm/d in divided doses. **Maint:** After improvement, 125-500 mg/d.	●D ❋v R

DICARBOXYLIC ACID

NAME	FORM/STRENGTH	DOSAGE	COMMENTS
Azelaic Acid (Azelex)	Cre: 20%	**≥12 yo:** Apply to affected area bid (qam & qpm).	●B ❋>

Azelaic Acid (Finacea)	**Gel:** 15%	**Adults:** Wash and dry skin. Apply to affected area bid (qam & qpm) x up to 12 wks.	◙B ❄>

ESTROGEN/PROGESTIN COMBINATION

Ethinyl Estradiol/Norethindrone (Estrostep)	**Tab:** (Phase 1) 35 mcg-1 mg; (Phase 2) 30 mcg-1 mg; (Phase 3) 20 mcg-1 mg	**Women: ≥15 yo:** 1 tab qd. See PI for initiation instructions.	◙X ❄v
Ethinyl Estradiol/Norgestimate (Ortho Tri-Cyclen)	**Tab:** (Phase 1) 35 mcg-0.18 mg; (Phase 2) 35 mcg-0.215 mg; (Phase 3) 35 mcg-0.25 mg	**Women: ≥15 yo:** 1 tab qd. Start 1st Sunday after menses begin or 1st day of menses.	◙X ❄v

KERATOLYTIC/ANTI-INFECTIVES

Benzoyl Peroxide/ Clindamycin (BenzaClin)	**Gel:** 5%-1%	**≥12 yo:** Apply to affected area bid.	◙C ❄v
Benzoyl Peroxide/ Erythromycin (Benzamycin)	**Gel:** 5%- 3%	**≥12 yo:** Apply to affected area bid (qam & qpm).	◙C ❄>

KERATOLYTICS

Benzoyl Peroxide (Benzac AC, Benzac AC Wash, Brevoxyl)	**(Benzac) Gel, Sol: (Wash):** 2.5%, 5%, 10%; **(Brevoxyl) Gel, Lot: (Cleanser/Wash):** 4%, 8%	**Benzac AC Wash: Adults:** Wash area qd-bid; rinse & dry. **Benzac AC: Adults:** Apply to clean area qd-bid. **Brevoxyl: ≥12 yo: Lot:** Wash area qd x 1st wk, then bid as tolerated. **Gel:** Apply to clean area qd-bid.	◙C ❄>

NAME	FORM/STRENGTH	DOSAGE	COMMENTS
Benzoyl Peroxide/ Clindamycin (Duac)	**Gel:** 5%-1%	≥**12 yo:** Apply qpm.	◐C ❄v

RETINOID-LIKE AGENTS

NAME	FORM/STRENGTH	DOSAGE	COMMENTS
Adapalene (Differin)	**Cre, Gel, Sol:** 0.1%	≥**12 yo:** Apply to affected area qhs. Avoid eyes, lips and mucous membranes.	◐C ❄>

RETINOIDS

NAME	FORM/STRENGTH	DOSAGE	COMMENTS
Isotretinoin (Accutane)	**Cap:** 10 mg, 20 mg, 40 mg	**Adults & Peds: ≥12 yo: Initial:** 0.5-1 mg/kg/day given bid x 15-20 wks w/food. Repeat if needed after 2 mths off of drug.	◐X ❄v Fetal abnormalities reported. Max 1 mth/Rx.
Tazarotene (Tazorac)	**Cre:** 0.1%; **Gel:** 0.1%	≥**12 yo:** Apply to affected area qpm.	◐X ❄>
Tretinoin (Avita)	**Cre:** 0.025%; **Gel:** 0.025%	**Adults:** Apply to affected area qpm.	◐C ❄>
Tretinoin (Retin-A, Retin-A Micro)	**Cre:** 0.025%, 0.05%, 0.1%; **Gel:** 0.01%, 0.025%, (Micro) 0.04%, 0.1%; **Sol:** 0.05%	**Retin-A: Adults:** Apply to affected area qhs. **Retin-A Micro:** ≥**12 yo:** Apply to affected area qhs.	◐C ❄>

Anti-Infective Agents

ANTIBACTERIALS

NAME	FORM/STRENGTH	DOSAGE	COMMENTS
Bacitracin (Baciguent)	**Oint:** 500 U/gm	**Adults & Peds:** Apply small amount qd-tid.	◐N ❄>
Gentamicin (Garamycin)	**Cre, Oint:** 0.1%	**Adults & Peds >1 yo:** Apply to lesions tid-qid.	◐N ❄>

Metronidazole (MetroCream, MetroGel, MetroLotion, Noritate)	Cre: (Noritate) 1%; Cre, Gel, Lot: 0.75%	**Adults: Rosacea: MetroCream, MetroGel, MetroLotion:** Apply to affected areas qam & qpm. **Noritate:** Apply to affected areas qd.	⊞B ❄v
Mupirocin (Bactroban, Bactroban Nasal)	Cre, Oint: 2%; Oint, Nas: 2%	**S. aureus/S. pyogenes: Adults & Peds ≥2 mths: Oint:** Apply tid. **≥3 mths: Cre:** Apply tid x 10d. **Nasal Colonization with MRSA: ≥12 yrs:** Apply nasal oint 1/2 tube per nostril bid x 5d.	⊞B ❄v
Neomycin	Oint: 3.5 mg/gm	**Adults & Peds:** Apply small amount qd-tid.	⊞N ❄>
Polymyxin B Sulfate/ Bacitracin Zinc (Polysporin)	Oint: 10,000 U-500 U; Powder: 10,000 U-500 U	**Adults & Peds: Prevent Infection in Minor Cuts, Scrapes, & Burns:** Apply to affected area qd-tid.	⊞N ❄>
Polymyxin B Sulfate/ Bacitracin Zinc/Neomycin (Neosporin)	Oint: 5,000 U-400 U-3.5 mg/gm	**Adults & Peds: Prevent Infection in Minor Cuts, Scrapes, & Burns:** Apply to affected area qd-tid.	⊞N ❄>
Sodium Sulfacetamide (Ovace)	Lot: 10%	**Adults & Peds: ≥12 yo:** Massage into wet skin, rinse thoroughly, & pat dry. **Seborrheic Dermatitis/Dandruff:** Wash affected area bid (qam & qpm) x 8-10d. To prevent recurrence, apply qwk or BIW, or every other wk. **Cutaneous Bacterial Infection:** Wash affected area qd x 8-10d.	⊞C ❄>
Sodium Sulfacetamide/ Sulfur (Plexion, Sulfacet-R)	Lot: 10%-5%	**Adults & Peds: ≥12 yo: Acne/Rosacea/Seborrheic Dermatitis:** Apply qd-tid.	⊞C ❄> Cl in kidney disease.
Sodium Sulfacetamide/ Sulfur (Rosula)	Cleanser, Gel: 10%-5%	**Adults & Peds: ≥12 yo: Seborrheic Dermatitis** (Gel) Apply thin film qd-tid. (Cleanser) Wash for 10-20 seconds qd-bid.	⊞C ❄>

ANTIFUNGALS

NAME	FORM/STRENGTH	DOSAGE	COMMENTS
Butenafine (Mentax)	Cre: 1%	**≥12 yo: Interdigital Tinea Pedis:** Apply bid x 7d or qd x 4 wks. **Tinea Corporis/Tinea Cruris/Tinea Versicolor:** Apply qd x 2 wks.	▣B ✿ ▷<
Ciclopirox (Loprox)	Cre, Gel, Lot: 0.77%; Shampoo: 1%	**Shampoo: Seborrheic Dermatitis: Adults:** Apply about 5 ml (up to 10 ml for long hair) to wet scalp. Lather and rinse off after 3 minutes. Repeat 2x/wk x 4 wks, at least 3d apart. **Cream/Gel/Lotion: Tinea Pedis/Tinea Cruris/Tinea Corporis/Cutaneous Candidiasis/Tinea Versicolor: ≥10 yo:** Apply qam & qpm x 4 wks. Avoid gel or shampoo in peds <16 yo.	▣B ✿ ▷<
Clioquinol/Hydrocortisone (Ala-Quin)	Cre: 3%-0.5%	**Adults & Peds:** Apply tid-qid.	▣N ✿ ▷<
Clotrimazole (Lotrimin)	Cre, Lot, Sol: 1%	**Adults & Peds: Candidiasis/Tinea Versicolor:** Apply qam & qpm.	▣B ✿ ▷<
Econazole (Spectazole)	Cre: 1%	**Adults & Peds: Tinea Cruris/Tinea Corporis/Tinea Pedis:** Apply qd x 4 wks. **Candidiasis:** Apply qam & qpm x 2 wks. **Tinea Versicolor:** Apply qd x 2 wks.	▣C ✿ ▷<
Ketoconazole (Nizoral, Nizoral A-D)	Sham: (A-D) 1%, (Nizoral) 2%	**Tinea Versicolor (2%): Adults:** Apply to damp skin of affected area, lather & rinse off after 5 min. **Dandruff (1%): >12 yo:** Apply to wet hair q3-4d up to 8 wks if needed.	▣C ✿ ▷<

Ketoconazole (Nizoral)	Cre: 2%	**Adults: Tinea Cruris/Tinea Corporis/Tinea Versicolor/ Cutaneous Candidiasis:** Apply qd x 2 wks. **Tinea Pedis:** Apply qd x 6 wks. **Seborrheic Dermatitis:** Apply bid x 4 wks.	⬤C ❄v
Miconazole (Monistat-Derm)	Cre: 2%	**Adults: Tinea Cruris/Tinea Corporis/Cutaneous Candidiasis:** Apply qam & qpm x 2 wks. **Tinea Pedis:** Apply qam & qpm x 4 wks. **Tinea Versicolor:** Apply qd x 2 wks.	⬤N ❄>
Naftifine (Naftin)	Cre, Gel: 1%	**Adults: Tinea Pedis/Tinea Cruris/Tinea Corporis:** (Cream) Apply qd. (Gel) Apply gel qam & qpm.	⬤B ❄>
Nystatin (Nystop)	Powder: 100,000 U/gm	**Adults & Peds:** Candida Species: Apply to lesions bid-tid.	⬤N ❄>
Oxiconazole (Oxistat)	Cre, Lot: 1%	**Adults: Tinea Cruris/Tinea Corporis (cre/lot):** Apply qd-bid x 2 wks. **Tinea Pedis (cre/lot):** Apply qd-bid x 4 wks. **Tinea Versicolor (cre):** Apply qd x 2 wks. **Peds: ≥12 yo: Cream:** Same as adult dose.	⬤B ❄>
Sertaconazole Nitrate (Ertaczo)	Cre: 2%	**Adults & Peds ≥12 yo: Interdigital Tinea Pedis:** Apply bid x 4 wks. Reevaluate if no improvement after 2 wks.	⬤C ❄>
Sulconazole (Exelderm)	Cre, Sol: 1%	**Adults: Tinea Corporis/Tinea Cruris/Tinea Versicolor:** Apply to affected area qd-bid x 3 wks. **Tinea Pedis:** Apply to affected area bid x 4 wks.	⬤C ❄>
Terbinafine (Lamisil AT)	Cre: 1%	**≥12 yo: Tinea Pedis:** Apply to area bid x 1 wk (interdigital) or x 2 wks (bottom/sides of foot). **Tinea Cruris/Tinea Corporis:** Apply to area qd x 1 wk. Wash & dry area before applying.	⬤N ❄>

NAME	FORM/STRENGTH	DOSAGE	COMMENTS
Tolnaftate (Tinactin)	Cre, Pow, Spray, Sol: 1%	**Adults & Peds: Tinea Pedis/Tinea Cruris/Tinea Corporis/Tinea Versicolor:** Apply bid x 2-3 wks, up to 4-6 wks.	⦿N ❄>

ANTIVIRALS

NAME	FORM/STRENGTH	DOSAGE	COMMENTS
Acyclovir (Zovirax)	Cre, Oint: 5%	**Adults: Herpes Genitalis/Herpes Labialis: Oint:** Apply q3h, 6x/d x 7d. Initiate with 1st sign/symptom. **Adults & Peds ≥12 yo: Herpes Labialis: Cre:** Apply 5x/d x 4d	⦿B ❄>
Imiquimod (Aldara)	Cre: 5%	**Adults: Actinic Keratosis:** Apply 2x/wk qhs to area on face/scalp (but not both concurrently). Wash off after 8 h. **Max:** 16 wks of therapy. **Adults & Peds: ≥12 yo: Genital/Perianal Warts (Condyloma Acuminata):** Apply 3x/wk qhs. Wash off after 6-10h. Use until warts clear. **Max:** 16 wks of therapy. Do not occlude treatment area.	⦿C ❄>
Penciclovir (Denavir)	Cre: 1%	**Adults: Recurrent Herpes Labialis (Cold Sores):** Apply q2h w/a x 4d. Start with earliest sign or symptom.	⦿B ❄v
Podofilox (Condylox)	Sol, Gel: 0.5%	**Adults: External Genital Warts (Condyloma Acuminata) (Gel/Sol), Perianal Warts (Gel):** Apply q12h x 3d, then withhold x 4d. May repeat up to 4 treatment cycles. **Max:** 0.5 gm/d or 0.5 ml/d & <10 cm² of wart tissue.	⦿C ❄v
Podophyllin (Podocon-25)	Liq: 25%	**Adults: Removal of Soft Genital Warts (Condylomata Acuminata): Initial:** Apply to intact lesion; remove after 30-45 min for 1st time use. **Usual:** Apply to lesion; remove when achieve desired result (1-4 hrs). Remove with alcohol or soap & water.	⦿N ❄v CI in pregnancy. Apply by physician.

OTHER AGENTS

Gentian Violet	Sol: 2%	Adults: Apply bid.	◉N ✿>

Anti-Infective Combinations
ANTIBIOTIC/ANTI-INFLAMMATORY AGENTS

Neomycin/Polymyxin B/ Hydrocortisone (Cortisporin)	Cre: 3.5 mg-10,000 U-0.5%	Adults: Apply to affected area bid-qid up to 7d.	◉C ✿>
Neomycin/Polymyxin B/ Bacitracin/Hydrocortisone (Cortisporin)	Oint: 3.5 mg-5,000 U-400 U-1%	Adults: Apply to affected area bid-qid up to 7d.	◉C ✿>
Nystatin/Triamcinolone (Mycolog II)	Cre, Oint: 10,000 U-0.1%	Adults & Peds: Apply to affected area bid.	◉C ✿>

Antipruritics/Anti-Inflammatory Agents
HISTAMINE RECEPTOR BLOCKER & COMBINATIONS

Calamine/Pramoxine HCl (Caladryl)	Cre, Lot: 8%-1%	≥2 yo: Apply tid-qid.	◉N ✿>
Diphenhydramine/Zinc Acetate (Benadryl)	Cre: 2%-0.1%; Gel: 2%-0.1%, 2%-1%	≥2 yo: Cre: Apply 1% tid-qid. ≥6 yo: Gel: Apply 1% tid-qid. ≥12 yo: Cre/Gel: Apply 2% tid-qid.	◉N ✿>
Doxepin (Zonalon)	Cre: 5%	Adults: Apply a thin film qid up to 8d.	◉B ✿v
Pramoxine HCl/ Zinc Acetate (Caladryl Clear)	Lot: 1%-0.1%	≥2 yo: Apply tid-qid.	◉N ✿>

TOPICAL CORTICOSTEROIDS — RELATIVE POTENCY AND DOSAGE

DRUG	DOSAGE FORM (S)	STRENGTH (%)	POTENCY	FREQUENCY
Alclometasone Dipropionate (Aclovate)	Cre, Oint	0.05	Low	bid/tid
Amcinonide (Cyclocort)	Cre, Lot, Oint	0.1	High	bid/tid
Augmented Betamethasone Dipropionate	Gel, Oint	0.05	Very High	bid/pb
Diprolene, Diprolene AF	Cre, Lot	0.05	High	bid/pb
Betamethasone Dipropionate (Maxivate, Alphatrex)	Cre, Lot, Oint	0.05	High	bid/pb (Alpha), qid-bid (Maxi)
Betamethasone Valerate (Betatrex, Beta-Val)	Cre, Lot, Oint	0.1	Medium	bid/pb
Betamethasone Valerate (Luxiq)	Foam	0.12	Medium	bid
Clobetasol Propionate (Cormax, Olux, Temovate)	Cre, Foam, Gel, Oint, Sol	0.05	Very High	bid
Clocortolone Pivalate (Cloderm)	Cre	0.1	Low	tid
Desonide (DesOwen, Tridesilon)	Cre, Lot, Oint	0.05	Low	bid/tid
Desoximetasone (Topicort)	Cre	0.05	Medium	bid
	Gel	0.05	High	bid
	Cre, Oint	0.25	High	bid

Diflorasone Diacetate (Maxiflor, Psorcon)	Cre, Oint (Maxiflor)	0.05	High	qd/tid
	Cre, Oint (Psorcon)	0.05	Very High	qd/qid
Fluocinolone Acetonide (Capex, Derma-Smoothe/FS, Synalar)	Cre, Oint	0.025	Medium	bid/qid
	Oil	0.01	Medium	qd/tid
	Shampoo (Capex)	0.01	Medium	qd
	Sol	0.01	Medium	bid/qid
Fluocinonide (Lidex, Lidex-E)	Cre, Gel, Oint, Sol	0.05	High	bid/qid
Flurandrenolide (Cordran)	Cre, Oint	0.025	Medium	bid/tid
	Cre, Lot, Oint	0.05	Medium	bid/qid
	Tape	4 mcg/cm^2	Medium	qd/bid
Fluticasone Propionate (Cutivate)	Cre	0.05	Medium	qd/bid
	Oint	0.005	Medium	bid
Halcinonide (Halog, Halog-E)	Cre, Oint, Sol	0.1	High	qd/tid
Halobetasol Propionate (Ultravate)	Cre, Oint	0.05	Very High	qd/bid
Hydrocortisone (Ala-Scalp HP, Ala-Cort, Cortaid, Hydrocort, Hytone, Nutracort, Texacort, Cetacort)	Cre, Oint	0.5	Low	tid/qid
	Cre, Lot, Oint, Sol	1	Low	tid/qid
	Lot	2	Low	tid/qid
	Cre, Lot, Oint, Sol	2.5	Low	bid/qid
Hydrocortisone Butyrate (Locoid)	Cre, Oint, Sol	0.1	Medium	bid/tid
Hydrocortisone Probutate (Pandel)	Cre	0.1	Medium	qd/bid
Hydrocortisone Valerate (Westcort)	Cre, Oint	0.2	Medium	bid/tid

DRUG	DOSAGE FORM (S)	STRENGTH (%)	POTENCY	FREQUENCY
Mometasone Furoate (Elocon)	Cre, Lot, Oint	0.1	Medium	qd
Prednicarbate (Dermatop E)	Cre, Oint	0.1	Medium	bid
Triamcinolone Acetonide (Aristocort A, Kenalog, Triacet)	Cre, Lot, Oint	0.025	Medium	bid/qid
	Cre, Lot, Oint	0.1	Medium	bid/tid
	Cre, Oint	0.5	High	bid/tid
	Spr	0.147 mg/gm	Medium	tid/qid

NAME	FORM/STRENGTH	DOSAGE	COMMENTS
TOPICAL CORTICOSTEROIDS/LOCAL ANESTHETIC AGENTS			
Lidocaine HCl/ Hydrocortisone Acetate (AnaMantle HC)	**Cre:** 3%-0.5%	**Adults: Hemorrhoids/Anal Fissures/Pruritus Ani:** Apply rectally bid.	⊞B ❊>
Pramoxine HCl/ Hydrocortisone Acetate (Analpram-HC, ProctoFoam-HC)	**Aer:** 1%-1%; **Cre:** 1%-1%, 2.5%-1%; **Lot:** 2.5%-1%	**Adults & Peds: Anal Dermatoses:** Apply to affected area tid-qid. Use applicator for anal administration with ProctoFoam-HC.	⊡C ❊>
MISCELLANEOUS			
Pimecrolimus (Elidel)	**Cre:** 1%	**Moderate-Severe Atopic Dermatitis:** ≥2 yrs: Apply bid. D/C upon resolution.	⊡C ❊v
Tacrolimus (Protopic)	**Oint:** 0.03%, 0.1%	**Moderate-Severe Atopic Dermatitis: Adults:** ≥16 yo: Apply bid. **Peds:** 2-15 yo: Apply 0.03% ointment bid. Continue x 1 wk after symptoms clear.	⊡C ❊v

Psoriasis

ANTIMETABOLITES

| Methotrexate | **Inj:** 20 mg, 1 gm, 25 mg/ml; **Tab:** 2.5 mg, 5 mg, 7.5 mg, 10 mg,15 mg | **Adults: Usual:** 10-25 mg/wk PO/IV/IM until adequate response achieved or use 2.5 mg q12h x 3 doses. **Titrate:** May increase gradually. **Max:** 30 mg/wk. | ●X ❀v [19] |

COAL TAR AGENTS

| Coal Tar (Tegrin) | **Cre:** 5%; **Sham:** 7% | **Adults:** Apply shampoo 2x/wk. Apply cream qd-qid. | ●N ❀> |

IMMUNOSUPPRESSIVES

Alefacept (Amevive)	**Inj:** (IV) 7.5 mg, (IM) 15 mg	**Adults:** 7.5 mg IV bolus or 15 mg IM once wkly x 12 wks. May retreat x 12 wks if >12 wk interval since 1st course. Adjust dose, D/C, and/or retreat, based on CD4+ T-lymphocyte counts.	●B ❀v
Cyclosporine (Neoral)	**Cap:** 25 mg, 100 mg; **Sol:** 100 mg/ml	**Adults: Initial:** 1.25 mg/kg bid x 4 wks. **Maint:** If no improvement, increase q2wks by 0.5 mg/kg/d. **Max:** 4.0 mg/kg/d.	●C ❀v Infection. Neoplasia. Nephrotoxicity. Malignancy risk w/certain psoriasis therapies.
Efalizumab (Raptiva)	**Inj:** 125 mg	**Adults ≥18 yo: Initial:** 0.7 mg/kg SQ single dose. **Maint:** 1 mg/kg SQ once weekly. **Max:** 200 mg/dose.	●C ❀v

[19] Monitor for bone marrow, lung, liver & kidney toxicities. Serious toxic reactions.

NAME	FORM/STRENGTH	DOSAGE	COMMENTS
PSORALENS			
Methoxsalen (8-MOP)	**Cap:** 10 mg	**Adults: Initial:** <30 kg: 10 mg. 30-50 kg: 20 mg. 51-65 kg: 30 mg. 66-80 kg: 40 mg. 81-90 kg: 50 mg. 91-115 kg: 60 mg. >115 kg: 70 mg. Take 2h before UVA exposure with food or milk. **Titrate:** May increase by 10 mg after 15th treatment under certain conditions. **Max:** Do not treat more often than qod.	●C ✿ V 20
Methoxsalen (Oxsoralen-Ultra)	**Cap:** 10 mg	**Adults: Initial:** <30 kg: 10 mg. 30-50 kg: 20 mg. 51-65 kg: 30 mg. 66-80 kg: 40 mg. 81-90 kg: 50 mg. 91-115 kg: 60 mg. >115 kg: 70 mg. Take 1.5-2h before UVA exposure with a low fat meal or milk. **Titrate:** May increase by 10 mg after 15th treatment under certain conditions. **Max:** Do not treat more often than qod.	●C ✿ V 21
RETINOIDS			
Acitretin (Soriatane)	**Cap:** 10 mg, 25 mg	**Adults:** 25-50 mg qd with food. Individualize dose based on intersubject variation in pharmacokinetics, clinical efficacy, & incidence of side effects. Terminate therapy when lesions resolve. May retreat relapses.	●X ✿ V CI in pregnancy & up to 3 yrs after stop med. Females should avoid ethanol. Hepatotoxicity, Pancreatitis, Pseudotumor cerebri.
Tazarotene (Tazorac)	**Cre:** 0.05%, 0.1%; **Gel:** 0.05%, 0.1%	**Adults & Peds: ≥12 yo:** Apply to lesions qpm. Apply gel to no more than 20% of BSA.	●X ✿ V

Calcipotriene (Dovonex)	**Cre, Oint, Sol:** 0.005%	**Adults: Sol:** Apply only to lesions on scalp bid up to 8 wks, rub in gently & completely. **Oint:** Apply to affected area qd-bid. **Cre:** Apply to affected area bid up to 8 wks.	●C ❄>

Miscellaneous

ALPHA-REDUCTASE INHIBITORS

Finasteride (Propecia)	**Tab:** 1 mg	**Androgenetic Alopecia:** 1 mg qd.	●X ❄v

ORNITHINE DECARBOXYLASE INHIBITOR

Eflornithine (Vaniqa)	**Cre:** 13.9%	**Facial Hair Reduction: Adults & Peds ≥12 yo:** Apply bid; at least 8h between doses. May wash off after 4h.	●C ❄>

PROTOPORPHYRIN PRECURSOR

Aminolevulinic Acid (Levulan Kerastick)	**Sol:** 20%	**Non-Hyperkeratotic Actinic Keratoses (Head/Scalp) Adults:** Apply to target lesion. After 14-18h, expose area to BLU-U blue light photodynamic illumination. May repeat after 8 wks if not completely resolved.	●C ❄>

PSORALENS

Methoxsalen (8-MOP)	**Cap:** 10 mg	**Vitiligo: Adults:** 20 mg 2-4 hrs before UV exposure with food or milk.	●C ❄> [20]

[20] Risk of ocular damage, aging skin, & skin cancer. Do not interchange with Oxsoralen-Ultra without re-titration.

[21] Risk of ocular damage, aging skin, & skin cancer. Do not interchange with regular Oxsoralen or 8-Mop. Determine minimum phototoxic dose & phototoxic peak time.

NAME	FORM/STRENGTH	DOSAGE	COMMENTS
Methoxsalen (Oxsoralen)	**Lot:** 1%	**Vitiligo: Adults & Peds ≥12 yo:** Apply to small well defined lesions before UVA exposure. Determine treatment intervals by erythema response; generally 1 wk or less often.	◑C ✿>

RETINOID COMBINATION

NAME	FORM/STRENGTH	DOSAGE	COMMENTS
Fluocinolone/Hydroquinone/ Tretinoin (Tri-Luma)	**Cre:** 0.01%-4%-0.05%	**Moderate to Severe Melasma of the Face: Adults:** Wash face and neck with mild cleanser. Apply thin film to hyperpigmented areas including 0.5 inch of normal skin surrounding lesion, at least 30 min before hs.	◑C ✿>
Mequinol/Tretinoin (Solage)	**Sol:** 2%-0.01%	**Solar Lentigines: Adults:** Apply to solar lentigines qam and qpm, at least 8h apart.	◑X ✿v

RETINOIDS

NAME	FORM/STRENGTH	DOSAGE	COMMENTS
Tazarotene (Avage)	**Cre:** 0.1%	**Facial Wrinkles/Hyperpigmentation or Hypopigmentation/Lentigines: ≥17 yo:** Cleanse and dry skin. Apply a pea-sized (1/4 inch or 5 mm diameter) amount to face (including eyelids, if desired) qhs.	◑X ✿>
Tretinoin (Renova)	**Cre:** 0.02%, 0.05%	**Wrinkles/Hyperpigmentation/Facial Skin Roughness: 0.05%: 18-50 yo:** Apply qpm. **Max:** 48 wks. **Wrinkles: 0.02%: 18-71 yo:** Apply qpm. **Max:** 52 wks.	◑C ✿> (0.05%) ✿v (0.02%)

VASODILATORS (PERIPHERAL)

NAME	FORM/STRENGTH	DOSAGE	COMMENTS
Minoxidil (Rogaine)	**Sol:** 5%	**Men:** Apply 1 ml bid to scalp.	◑N ✿>
Minoxidil (Rogaine)	**Sol:** 2%	**Women:** Apply 1 ml bid to scalp.	◑N ✿>

ANTIHISTAMINES

DRUG	RX/OTC	FORM/STRENGTH	DOSAGE	COMMENTS
Azelastine (Astelin)	RX	**Spray:** 137 mcg/spray	**Seasonal Allergic Rhinitis:** ≥12 yo: 2 sprays per nostril bid. **5-11 yo:** 1 spray per nostril bid. **Vasomotor Rhinitis:** ≥12 yo: 2 sprays per nostril bid	⊚C ❋>
Carbinoxamine Maleate (Palgic)	RX	**Sol:** 4 mg/5 ml; **Tab:** 4 mg	**Adults & Peds:** ≥6 yo: Usual: 4 mg prn. **Max:** 24 mg/day given q6-8h; **1-6 yo:** Usual: 2 mg prn. May increase to 0.2-0.4 mg/kg/day given q6-8h.	⊚C ❋v
Cetirizine HCl (Zyrtec)	RX	**Chewtab:** 5mg, 10 mg; **Syr:** 1 mg/ml; **Tab:** 5 mg, 10 mg	**Seasonal or Perennial Allergic Rhinitis/ Urticaria: Adults & Peds** ≥6 yo: 5-10 mg qd. **2-5 yo:** 2.5 mg qd. **Max:** 5 mg/d. **Perennial Allergic Rhinitis/Urticaria: 6 mo-23 mo:** 2.5 mg qd. **12 mo-23 mo:** May increase to max 5 mg/d.	⊚B ❋v H R
Chlorpheniramine Maleate (Chlor-Trimeton)	OTC	**Syr:** 2 mg/5 ml; **Tab:** 4 mg; **Tab,ER:** 8 mg, 12 mg	**Adults & Peds** ≥12 yo: Syr/Tab: 4 mg q4-6h. **Tab,ER:** 8 mg q8-12h or 12 mg q12h. **Max:** 24 mg/d. **6-11 yo:** Syr/Tab: 2 mg q4-6h. **Max:** 12 mg/d.	⊚N ❋>

NAME	RX/OTC	FORM/STRENGTH	DOSAGE	COMMENTS
Clemastine Fumarate (Tavist)	OTC (Tab 1.34 mg); RX (Tab 2.68 mg, Syr 0.5 mg/5 ml)	**Syr:** 0.5 mg/5 ml; **Tab:** 1.34 mg, 2.68 mg	**Adults & Peds ≥12 yo: Tab:** 1.34 mg bid or 2.68 mg qd. **Max:** 8.04 mg/d. **Syr:** 1-2 mg bid. **Max:** 6 mg/d. **6-12 yo: Syr:** 0.5-1 mg bid. **Max:** 3 mg/d.	■B ❄v
Cyproheptadine HCl	RX	**Syr:** 2 mg/5 ml; **Tab:** 4 mg	**Adults: Initial:** 4 mg tid. **Usual:** 4-20 mg/d. **Max:** 0.5 mg/kg/d. **7-14 yo:** 4 mg bid-tid. **Max:** 16 mg/d. **2-6 yo:** 2 mg bid-tid. **Max:** 12 mg/d.	■B ❄v
Desloratadine (Clarinex, Clarinex Reditabs)	RX	**ODT:** (Reditab) 5 mg; **Tab:** 5 mg	**Adults & Peds ≥12 yo:** 5 mg qd.	■C ❄v H R
Diphenhydramine HCl (Benadryl)	OTC (PO); RX (Inj); OTC/RX (50 mg cap)	**Cap:** 25 mg, 50 mg; **Chewtab:** 12.5 mg; **Inj:** 50 mg/ml; **Syr:** 12.5 mg/5 ml; **Tab:** 25 mg, 50 mg	**Adults: PO:** 25-50 mg q4-6h. **Max:** 300 mg/d **Inj:** 10-50 mg IV or up to 100 mg deep IM. **Max:** 400 mg/d. **6-11 yo: PO:** 12.5-25 mg q4-6h. **Max:** 150 mg/d. **Peds: Inj:** 5 mg/kg/d or 150 mg/m²/d IV/IM in 4 divided doses. **Max:** 300 mg/d.	■B ❄v
Fexofenadine HCl (Allegra)	RX	**Tab:** 30 mg, 60 mg, 180 mg	**Seasonal Allergic Rhinitis: Adults & Peds ≥12 yo:** 60 mg bid or 180 mg qd. **6-11 yo:** 30 mg bid. **Chronic Idiopathic Urticaria: Adults & Peds ≥12 yo:** 60 mg bid. **6-11 yo:** 30 mg bid.	■C ❄> R
Hydroxyzine HCl	RX	**Syr:** 10 mg/5 ml; **Tab:** 10 mg, 25 mg, 50 mg, 100 mg	**Adults:** 25 mg tid-qid. **≥6 yo:** 50-100 mg/d in divided doses. **<6 yo:** 50 mg/d in divided doses.	■N ❄v

Drug	RX	Form	Dosage	Rating
Hydroxyzine Pamoate (Vistaril)	RX	**Cap:** 25 mg; 50 mg, 100 mg; **Sus:** 25 mg/5 ml	**Adults:** 25 mg tid-qid. **≥6 yo:** 50-100 mg/d in divided doses. **<6 yo:** 50 mg/d in divided doses.	◙N ❄v
Loratadine (Claritin, Claritin Reditabs)	OTC/RX	**ODT:** (Reditab) 10 mg; **Syr:** 1 mg/ml; **Tab:** 10 mg	**Adults & Peds ≥6 yo:** ODT/Syr/Tab: 10 mg qd. **2-5 yo:** Syr: 5 mg qd.	◙B ❄> H R
Promethazine HCl (Phenergan)	RX	**Inj:** 25 mg/ml, 50 mg/ml; **Sup:** 12.5 mg, 25 mg, 50 mg; **Syr:** 6.25 mg/5 ml; **Tab:** 12.5 mg, 25 mg, 50 mg	**Adults:** 25 mg PO/PR qhs or 12.5 mg ac & qhs; 25 mg IM/IV and repeat in 2h if needed. **≥2 yo:** 25 mg or 0.5 mg/lb PO/PR qhs or 6.25-12.5 mg tid; up to 12.5 mg IM/IV.	◙C ❄v

COUGH & COLD COMBINATIONS

DRUG	RX/OTC	ANTIHISTAMINE	DECONGESTANT	COUGH SUPPRESSANT	OTHER CONTENT	DOSE
Actifed Cold & Sinus Caplets	OTC	Chlorpheniramine Maleate, 2 mg	Pseudoephedrine HCl, 30 mg		Acetaminophen, 500 mg	≥12 yo: 2 q6h.
Allegra-D Tablet	RX	Fexofenadine HCl, 60 mg	Pseudoephedrine HCl, 120 mg			≥12 yo: 1 bid.
Bromfed Capsule	RX	Brompheniramine Maleate, 12 mg	Pseudoephedrine HCl, 120 mg			≥12 yo: 1 q12h.
Cheracol with Codeine Syrup	CV			Codeine Phosphate, 10 mg/5 ml	Guaifenesin, 100 mg/5 ml	≥12 yo: 2 tsp q4h. 6 to <12 yo: 1 tsp q4h.

DRUG	RX/OTC	ANTIHISTAMINE	DECONGESTANT	COUGH SUPPRESSANT	OTHER CONTENT	DOSE
Claritin-D 12 Hour Tablet	OTC/RX	Loratadine, 5 mg	Pseudoephedrine Sulfate, 120 mg			≥12 yo: 1 q12h.
Claritin-D 24 Hour Tablet	OTC/RX	Loratadine, 10 mg	Pseudoephedrine Sulfate, 240 mg			≥12 yo: 1 qd.
Comtrex Maximum Strength Nightime Cold & Cough Caplet	OTC	Chlorpheniramine Maleate, 2 mg	Pseudoephedrine HCl, 30 mg	Dextromethorphan HBr, 15 mg	Acetaminophen, 500 mg	≥12 yo: 2 q6h.
Contac Severe Cold & Flu Maximum Strength Caplet	OTC	Chlorpheniramine Maleate, 2 mg	Pseudoephedrine HCl, 30 mg	Dextromethorphan HBr, 15 mg	Acetaminophen, 500 mg	≥12 yo: 2 q6h.
Coricidin HBP Cough/Cold Tablet	OTC	Chlorpheniramine Maleate, 4 mg		Dextromethorphan HBr, 30 mg		≥12 yo: 1 q6h.
Deconsal II Tablet	RX		Phenylephrine HCl, 20 mg		Guaifenesin, 375 mg	≥12 yo: 1-2 q12h. 6 to <12 yo: 1 qd
Delsym Suspension	OTC			Dextromethorphan Polistirex, 30 mg/5 ml		≥12 yo: 2 tsp. 6 to <12 yo: 1 tsp. 2 to <6 yo: 1/2 tsp. May repeat q12h.
Dimetapp Cold & Allergy Elixir	OTC	Brompheniramine Maleate, 1 mg/5 ml	Pseudoephedrine HCl, 15 mg/5 ml			≥12 yo: 4 tsp. 6 to <12 yo: 2 tsp. May repeat q4h. Max: 4 doses/24h.

Drixoral Cold & Allergy Tablet	OTC	Dexbrompheniramine Maleate, 6 mg	Pseudoephedrine Sulfate, 120 mg			≥12 yo: 1 q12h.
Entex PSE Tablet	RX		Pseudoephedrine HCl, 120 mg		Guaifenesin, 600 mg	≥12 yo: 1 q12h. 6 to <12 yo: 1/2 q12h.
Humibid DM Capsule	RX			Dextromethorphan HBr, 50 mg	Guaifenesin, 400 mg; Potassium Guaiacolsulfonate; 200 mg	>12 yo: 1 q12h. 6-12 yo: 1 qd.
Humibid LA Tablet	RX				Guaifenesin, 600 mg; Potassium Guaiacolsulfonate, 300 mg	>12 yo: 1 q12h.
Hycodan Syrup	CIII			Hydrocodone Bitartrate, 5 mg/5 ml	Homatropine MBr, 1.5 mg/5 ml	>12 yo: 1 tsp q4-6h. 6-12 yo: 1/2 tsp q4-6h.
Nucofed Pediatric Expectorant Syrup	CV		Pseudoephedrine HCl, 30 mg/5 ml	Codeine Phosphate, 10 mg/5 ml	Guaifenesin, 100 mg/5 ml	≥12 yo: 2 tsp q6h. 6 to <12 yo: 1 tsp q6h. 2 to <6 yo: 1/2 tsp q6h.

DRUG	RX/OTC	ANTIHISTAMINE	DECONGESTANT	COUGH SUPPRESSANT	OTHER CONTENT	DOSE
Robitussin DM Syrup	OTC			Dextromethorphan HBr, 10 mg/5 ml	Guaifenesin, 100 mg/5 ml	≥12 yo: 2 tsp q4h. 6 to <12 yo: 1 tsp q4h. 2 to <6 yo: 1/2 tsp q4h.
Robitussin PE Syrup	OTC		Pseudoephedrine HCl, 30 mg/5 ml		Guaifenesin, 100 mg/5 ml	≥12 yo: 2 tsp q4h 6 to <12 yo: 1 tsp q4h. 2 to <6 yo: 1/2 tsp q4h.
Rondec Syrup	RX	Brompheniramine Maleate, 4 mg/5 ml	Pseudoephedrine HCl, 45 mg/5 ml			≥6 yo: 5 ml qid. 2-6 yo: 2.5 ml qid.
Rondec-DM Syrup	RX	Brompheniramine Maleate, 4 mg/5 ml	Pseudoephedrine HCl, 45 mg/5 ml	Dextromethorphan HBr, 15 mg/5 ml		>6 yo: 5 ml qid. 2-6 yo: 2.5 ml qid.
Rynatan Tablet	RX	Chlorpheniramine Tannate, 9 mg	Phenylephrine Tannate, 25 mg			≥12 yo: 1-2 q12h.
Semprex-D Capsule	RX	Acrivastine, 8 mg	Pseudoephedrine HCl, 60 mg			≥12 yo: 1 q4-6h, qid.
Sudafed Sinus & Cold Liquid Caps	OTC		Pseudoephedrine HCl, 30 mg		Acetaminophen, 325 mg	≥12 yo: 2 q4-6h. Max: 8/24h.

TheraFlu Cold & Sore Throat Nighttime Liquid	OTC	Chlorpheniramine Maleate, 4 mg	Pseudoephedrine HCl, 60 mg		Acetaminophen, 650 mg — ≥12 yo: 1 pkt q4-6h. Max: 4 pkts/24h.
Triaminic Cold & Cough Liquid	OTC	Chlorpheniramine Maleate, 1 mg/5 ml	Pseudoephedrine HCl, 15 mg/5 ml	Dextromethorphan HBr, 5 mg/5 ml	6 to <12 yo: 2 tsp q4-6h. Max: 4 doses/24h.
Triaminic Cold & Cough Softchews	OTC	Chlorpheniramine Maleate, 1 mg	Pseudoephedrine HCl, 15 mg	Dextromethorphan HBr, 5 mg	6 to <12 yo: 2 tabs q4-6h. Max: 4 doses/24h.
Triaminic Flu, Cough & Fever Liquid	OTC	Chlorpheniramine Maleate, 1 mg/5 ml	Pseudoephedrine HCl, 15 mg/5 ml	Dextromethorphan HBr, 7.5 mg/5 ml	Acetaminophen, 160 mg/5 ml — 6 to <12 yo: 2 tsp q6h. Max: 4 doses/24h.
Triaminic Night Time Cough & Cold Liquid	OTC	Chlorpheniramine Maleate, 1 mg/5 ml	Pseudoephedrine HCl, 15 mg/5 ml	Dextromethorphan HBr, 7.5 mg/5 ml	6 to <12 yo: 2 tsp q6h. Max: 4 doses/24h.
Triaminic Cough & Sore Throat Softchews	OTC		Pseudoephedrine HCl 15 mg	Dextromethorphan HBr, 5 mg	Acetaminophen, 160 mg — 6 to <12 yo: 2 tabs. 2 to <6 yo: 1 tab. May repeat q4-6h. Max: 4 doses/24h.

DRUG	RX/OTC	ANTIHISTAMINE	DECONGESTANT	COUGH SUPPRESSANT	OTHER CONTENT	DOSE
Tussi-12 Suspension	RX	Chlorpheniramine Tannate, 4 mg/5 ml		Carbetapentane Tannate, 30 mg/5 ml		>6 yo: 5-10 ml q12h. 2-6 yo: 2.5-5 ml q12h.
Tussionex Pennkinetic Suspension	CIII	Chlorpheniramine Polistirex, 8 mg/5 ml		Hydrocodone Polistirex, 10 mg/5 ml		>12 yo: 1 tsp q12h. 6-12 yo: 1/2 tsp q12h.
Tussi-Organidin DM NR Liquid	RX			Dextromethorphan HBr, 10 mg/5 ml	Guaifenesin, 100 mg/5 ml	≥12 yo: 2 tsp. 6 to <12 yo: 1 tsp. 2 to <6 yo: 1/2 tsp. 6 mth to <2 yo: 1/8-1/4 tsp. May repeat q4h.
Tussi-Organidin NR Liquid	CV			Codeine Phosphate, 10 mg/5 ml	Guaifenesin, 100 mg/5 ml	≥12 yo: 2 tsp q4h. 6 to < 12 yo: 1 tsp q4h. 2 to <6 yo: 1 mg/kg/d of codeine in 4 divided doses.
Tylenol Cold Day Caplet	OTC		Pseudoephedrine HCl, 30 mg	Dextromethorphan HBr, 15 mg	Acetaminophen, 325 mg	≥12 yo: 2 q6h.
Zyrtec-D Tablet	RX	Cetirizine HCl, 5 mg	Pseudoephedrine HCl, 120 mg			≥12 yo: 1 bid.

NAME	FORM/STRENGTH	DOSAGE	COMMENTS

Anticholinergics

Ipratropium Bromide (Atrovent)	**Spray:** 0.03% (21 mcg/spray), 0.06% (42 mcg/spray)	**Rhinorrhea w/Common Cold: Adults & Peds:** ≥12 yo: 2 sprays 0.06% per nostril tid-qid. **5-11 yo:** 2 sprays 0.06% per nostril tid. **Allergic/Nonallergic Perennial Rhinitis: Adults & Peds:** ≥6 yo: 2 sprays 0.03% per nostril bid-tid.	●B ❄>

Corticosteroids

Beclomethasone (Beconase, Beconase AQ, Vancenase, Vancenase AQ Double Strength)	**Spray:** 42 mcg/spray, (Double Strength) 84 mcg/spray	**Allergic/Nonallergic (Vasomotor) Rhinitis: Beconase AQ:** ≥6 yo: 1-2 sprays per nostril bid. **Vancenase AQ DS:** ≥6 yo: 1-2 sprays per nostril qd. **Beconase:** ≥12 yo: 1 spray per nostril bid-qid. **6-12 yo:** 1 spray per nostril tid. **Vancenase:** ≥12 yo: 1 spray per nostril bid-qid. **6-12 yo:** 1 spray per nostril tid.	●C ❄v
Budesonide (Rhinocort, Rhinocort Aqua)	**Aerosol:** (Rhinocort) 32 mcg/inh; **Spray:** (Rhinocort Aqua) 32 mcg/spray	**Seasonal/Perennial Rhinitis: Rhinocort Aqua:** ≥6 yo: **Initial:** 1 spray per nostril qd. **Max:** ≥12 yo: 8 sprays/d. **6-12 yo:** 4 sprays/d. **Rhinocort:** ≥6 yo: 2 sprays per nostril qam & qpm or 4 sprays per nostril qam. **Max:** 8 sprays/d.	●C ❄>
Flunisolide (Nasalide, Nasarel)	**Spray:** 29 mcg/spray	**Seasonal/Perennial Rhinitis: Adults: Initial:** 2 sprays per nostril bid. **Titrate:** Increase to 2 sprays per nostril tid. **Max:** 16 sprays/day. **6-14 yo:** 1 spray per nostril tid or 2 sprays per nostril bid. **Max:** 8 sprays/day.	●C ❄>

NAME	FORM/STRENGTH	DOSAGE	COMMENTS
Fluticasone (Flonase)	**Spray:** 50 mcg/spray	**Seasonal and Perennial Allergic/Nonallergic Rhinitis: Adults: Initial:** 2 sprays per nostril qd or 1 spray per nostril bid. **Maint:** 1 spray per nostril qd. **≥4 yo: Initial:** 1-2 sprays per nostril qd. **Maint:** 1 spray per nostril qd. **Max:** 2 sprays per nostril/d. **Seasonal Allergic Rhinitis: ≥12 yo:** May also dose as 2 sprays per nostril qd prn.	◑C ❄>
Mometasone (Nasonex)	**Spray:** 50 mcg/spray	**Allergic Seasonal/Perennial Rhinitis: ≥12 yo: Treatment/Prophylaxis:** 2 sprays per nostril qd. **2-11 yo: Treatment:** 1 spray per nostril qd.	◑C ❄>
Triamcinolone (Nasacort AQ, Tri-Nasal Spray)	**Spray:** (Nasacort AQ) 55 mcg/spray; (Tri-Nasal) 50 mcg/spray	**Allergic/Nonallergic Rhinitis: Nasacort AQ: ≥12 yo: Initial/Max:** 2 sprays per nostril qd. **Maint:** 1 spray per nostril qd. **6-12 yo: Initial:** 1 spray per nostril qd. **Max:** 4 sprays/d. **Tri-Nasal Spray:** 2 sprays per nostril qd. **Max:** 8 sprays/d.	◑C ❄>

Decongestant Agents

NAME	FORM/STRENGTH	DOSAGE	COMMENTS
Oxymetazoline (Afrin, Neo-Synephrine, Vicks Sinex 12-Hour)	**Drops:** 0.05%; **Spray:** 0.05%	**Nasal Congestion: ≥6 yo: Usual:** 2-3 gtts/sprays q10-12h. **Max:** 2 doses/24h.	◑N ❄>
Phenylephrine (Vicks Sinex)	**Spray:** 0.5%	**Nasal Congestion: ≥12 yo:** 2-3 sprays per nostril q4h prn.	◑N ❄>

Anesthetics

Proparacaine (Alcaine, Ocu-Caine, Ophthetic, Parcaine)	**Sol:** 0.5%	**Adults: Foreign Bodies/Sutures:** 1-2 gtts pre-op. **Deep Ophthalmic Anesthesia:** 1 gtt q5-10min x 5-7 doses.	◉C ❊>
Tetracaine (Pontocaine, Tetcaine)	**Sol:** 0.5%	**Adults: Foreign Bodies/Sutures:** 1-2 gtts before operating/suture removal. **Tonometry:** 1-2 gtts before measurement. **Cataract Extraction:** 1 gtts q5-10min x 5-7 doses.	◉N ❊>

Antibiotic Agents

Bacitracin	**Oint:** 500 U/gm	**Adults:** Apply 1/4 inch qd-tid.	◉N ❊>
Bacitracin Zinc/Neomycin Sulfate/Polymyxin B Sulfate (Neosporin)	**Oint:** 400 U-3.5 mg-10,000 U/gm	**Adults:** Apply q3-4h x 7-10d.	◉C ❊>
Bacitracin Zinc/Polymyxin B Sulfate (Polysporin)	**Oint:** 500 U-10,000 U/gm	**Adults:** Apply q3-4h x 7-10d.	◉C ❊>
Chloramphenicol (Chloroptic, Ocu-Chlor)	**(Chloroptic) Oint:** 1%; **Sol:** 0.5%; **(Ocu-Chlor) Oint:** 1%	**Adults: Oint:** 1/2 inch q3h x 48h, then increase frequency. Treat x 7d; continue x 48h after normal. **Max:** 3 wks. **Sol:** 1-2 gtts 4-6x/d x 72h. May increase interval after 48h. Continue x 48h after normal.	◉C ❊v Bone marrow hypoplasia including aplastic anemia & death.

NAME	FORM/STRENGTH	DOSAGE	COMMENTS
Ciprofloxacin HCl (Ciloxan)	Oint, Sol: 0.3%	**Bacterial Conjunctivitis: Sol: Adults & Peds:** ≥1 yo: 1-2 gtts q2h w/a x 2d, then 1-2 gtts q4h w/a x 5d. **Oint: Adults & Peds:** ≥**2 yo:** 1/2 in tid x 2d, then bid x 5d. **Corneal Ulcers: Sol: Adults & Peds:** ≥**2 yo:** 2 gtts q15 min x 6h, then 2 gtts q30min on d1, then 2 gtts q1h on d2, then 2 gtts q4h on d3-14.	●C ✿>
Erythromycin (Romycin)	Oint: 5 mg/gm	**Adults & Peds:** Apply 1 cm up to 6x/d. **Neonatal Gonococcal/Chlamydia Ophthalmia Prophylaxis:** 1 cm in lower conjunctival sac.	●B ✿>
Gatifloxacin (Zymar)	Sol: 0.3%	**Adults & Peds:** ≥1 yo: 1 gtt q2h w/a, up to 8x/d for 2d; then 1 gtt up to qid w/a for 5d.	●C ✿>
Gentamicin Sulfate (Garamycin, Genoptic, Gentak, Ocu-mycin)	Oint, Sol: 0.3%	**Adults & Peds:** Usual: 1/2 inch bid-tid or 1-2 gtts q4h. **Severe Infection:** 2 gtts q1h.	●C ✿>
Gramicidin/Neomycin Sulfate/Polymyxin B Sulfate (AK-Spore, Neocidin, Neosporin)	Sol: 0.025 mg-1.75 mg-10,000 U/ml	**Adults:** Usual: 1-2 gtts q4h x 7-10d. **Severe Infection:** 2 gtts q1h.	●C ✿>
Levofloxacin (Quixin)	Sol: 0.5%	**Adults & Peds:** ≥1 yo: Conjunctivitis: Day 1-2: 1-2 gtts q2h w/a up to 8x/d. **Day 3-7:** 1-2 gtts q4h w/a up to qid.	●C ✿>
Moxifloxacin HCl (Vigamox)	Sol: 0.5%	**Adults & Peds:** 1 gtt tid x 7d.	●C ✿>
Norfloxacin (Chibroxin)	Sol: 0.3%	**Adults & Peds:** ≥1 yo: Usual: 1-2 gtts qid up to 7d. **Severe Infection:** 1-2 gtts q2h w/a on d1, then qid up to 7d.	●C ✿v

Ofloxacin (Ocuflox)	Sol: 0.3%	**Adults & Peds: ≥1 yo: Bacterial Conjunctivitis:** 1-2 gtts q2-4h x 2d, then 1-2 gtts qid x 5d. **Bacterial Corneal Ulcer:** 1-2 gtts q30min w/a & 1-2 gtts 4-6h after retiring x 2d, then 1-2 gtts q1h w/a x 5-7d, then 1-2 gtts qid x 2d.	●C ❊v
Oxytetracycline/Polymyxin B Sulfate (Terak, Terramycin with Polymyxin B Sulfate)	Oint: 5 mg-10,000 U/gm	**Adults:** Apply 1/2 inch bid-qid.	●N ❊>
Polymyxin B Sulfate/ Trimethoprim Sulfate (Polytrim)	Sol: 10,000 U-1 mg/ml	**Adults & Peds: ≥2 mth:** Usual: 1 gtt q3h x 7-10d. **Max:** 6 doses/d.	●C ❊>
Sulfacetamide Sodium (AK-Sulf, Bleph-10, Ocu-Sul, Sodium Sulamyd)	Oint: 10%; Sol: 10%, 15%, 30%	**Adults: Initial:** Apply 1/2 inch qid & qhs or 1-2 gtts q2-3h w/a x 7-10d. **Maint:** Increase dose interval as condition responds. **Trachoma:** 2 gtts q2h with systemic administration.	●C ❊v
Tobramycin (Tobrasol, Tobrex, Tomycine)	Oint: 0.3%; Sol: 0.3%	**Adults: Usual:** 1/2 inch bid-tid or 1-2 gtts q4h. **Severe Infection:** 1/2 inch q3-4h or 2 gtts q1h until improvement.	●B ❊v

Antibiotic/Corticosteroid Combinations

Bacitracin Zinc/ Hydrocortisone/Neomycin Sulfate/Polymyxin B Sulfate (Cortisporin)	Oint: 400 U-1%- 3.5 mg-10,000 U/gm	**Adults:** Apply q3-4h, depending on severity.	●C ❊v

NAME	FORM/STRENGTH	DOSAGE	COMMENTS
Dexamethasone Sodium Phosphate/Neomycin Sulfate (NeoDecadron)	**Sol:** 1 mg-3.5 mg/ml	**Adults: Initial:** 1-2 gtts q1h (day) & q2h (night). **Maint:** If good response, decrease to 1 gtt q4h, then to tid-qid.	◐C ✳v
Dexamethasone/Neomycin Sulfate/Polymyxin B Sulfate (AK-Trol, Maxitrol, Poly-Dex)	**Oint, Susp:** 1 mg-3.5 mg-10,000 U/gm or ml	**Adults: Oint:** Apply up to tid-qid or use susp hs. **Susp:** 1-2 gtts 4-6x/d. Severe Infection: 1-2 gtts q1h; taper to 4-6x/d.	◐C ✳>
Dexamethasone/Tobramycin (TobraDex)	**Oint:** 0.1%-0.3%; **Susp:** 0.1%-0.3%	**Adults & Peds:** ≥2 yo: **Oint:** Apply 1/2 inch up to tid-qid. **Susp:** 1-2 gtts q2h x 24-48h, then 1-2 gtts q4-6h thereafter.	◐C ✳>
Fluorometholone/ Sulfacetamide Sodium (FML-S Liquifilm)	**Susp:** 0.1%-10%	**Adults:** 1 gtt qid.	◐C ✳v
Gentamicin Sulfate/ Prednisolone Acetate (Pred-G)	**Oint:** 0.3%-0.6%; **Susp:** 0.3%-1%	**Adults: Usual:** Apply 1/2 inch qd-tid or 1 gtt bid-qid. May give drops q1h x 1st 24-48h.	◐C ✳v
Neomycin Sulfate/Polymyxin B Sulfate/Hydrocortisone (Cortisporin)	**Susp:** 1%-3.5 mg-10,000 U/ml	**Adults:** 1-2 gtts q3-4h, depending on severity.	◐C ✳v
Neomycin Sulfate/Polymyxin B Sulfate/Prednisolone Acetate (Poly Pred)	**Susp:** 0.35%-10,000 U-0.5%/ml	**Adults:** 1-2 gtts q3-4h. **Acute Infection:** 1-2 gtts q30min. Reduce dose as infection resolves.	◐N ✳>

| Prednisolone Acetate/Sulfacetamide Sodium (AK-Cide, Blephamide, Metimyd, Ocu-Lone C) | Oint, Susp: (Blephamide) 0.2%-10%, (Metimyd) 0.5%-10%; Oint: (AK-Cide, Ocu-Lone C) 0.5%-10% | Adults & Peds: ≥6 yo: Initial: Apply 1/2 inch 3-4x/d & 1-2x/qpm or instill 2 gtts q4h & qhs. Reduce dose when condition improves. | ⊞C ✿v |
| Prednisolone Sodium Phosphate/Sulfacetamide Sodium (Vasocidin) | Sol: 0.25%-10% | Adults & Peds: ≥6 yo: 2 gtts q4h. | ⊞C ✿v |

Corticosteroids

Dexamethasone (Maxidex)	Susp: 0.1%	Adults: 1-2 gtts q4-6h. Severe Disease: 1-2 gtts q1h, & taper to discontinuation.	⊞C ✿v
Dexamethasone Sodium Phosphate (Decadron, Ocu-Dex)	Oint: 0.05%; Sol: 0.1%	Adults: Initial: Apply oint tid-qid or instill 1-2 gtts q1h w/a & q2h during night. With improvement, apply oint qd-bid or instill 1 gtt 3-6x/d. Ear: 3-4 gtts bid-tid with gradual dose reduction.	⊞C ✿v
Fluorometholone Acetate (Eflone, Flarex)	Susp: 0.1%	Adults: 1-2 gtts qid. May increase to 2 gtts q2h during 1st 24-48h.	⊞C ✿v
Fluorometholone (Fluor-Op, FML)	Oint: 0.1%; Susp: 0.1%, 0.25%	≥2 yo: 1 gtt bid-qid or 1/2 inch oint qd-tid x 24-48h.	⊞C ✿v
Loteprednol Etabonate (Alrex, Lotemax)	Susp: (Alrex) 0.2%, (Lotemax) 0.5%	Adults: Lotemax: 1-2 gtts qid, may increase to 1 gtt q1h during 1st wk. Post-Op: 1-2 gtts qid starting 24h post-op. Continue x 2 wks. Alrex: Adults: 1 gtt qid.	⊞C ✿v
Medrysone (HMS)	Susp: 1%	Adults & Peds: ≥3 yo: 1 gtt up to q4h.	⊞C ✿>

NAME	FORM/STRENGTH	DOSAGE	COMMENTS
Prednisolone Acetate (Econopred Plus, Ocu-Pred A, Pred Forte, Pred Mild)	Susp: 0.12%, 0.125%, 1%	**Adults:** 1-2 gtts bid-qid. May increase frequency during 1st 24-48h.	◐C ❄v
Prednisolone Sodium Phosphate (AK Pred, Inflamase)	Sol: (Inflamase) 0.125%, 1%, (AK-Pred) 1%	**Adults:** 1-2 gtts q1h w/a & q2h at night. With improvement, 1 gtt q4h, then 1 gtt tid-qid.	◐C ❄>
Rimexolone (Vexol)	Susp: 1%	**Adults: Post-op:** 1-2 gtts qid starting 24h post-op, x 2 wks. **Anterior Uveitis:** 1-2 gtts q1h w/a x 1wk, then 1 gtt q2h x 1wk, then taper until resolved.	◐C ❄v

Fungal Infection

Natamycin (Natacyn)	Susp: 5%	**Adults: Keratitis:** 1 gtt q1-2h x 3-4d, then 1 gtt 6-8x/d x 14-21d. **Blepharitis/Conjunctivitis:** 1 gtt 4-6x/d.	◐C ❄>

Glaucoma

ADRENERGIC AGONISTS

Dipivefrin (Propine)	Sol: 0.1%	**Adults: Usual:** 1 gtt q12h.	◐B ❄>

ALPHA ADRENERGIC AGONISTS

Apraclonidine Hydrochloride (Iopidine)	Sol: 0.5%, 1%	**Adults: 0.5%:** 1-2 gtts tid. **1%:** 1 gtt 1h pre-op & 1 gtt post-op.	◐C ❄v (1%) ❄> (0.5%)

BETA BLOCKERS

Betaxolol (Betoptic S)	Susp: 0.25%	**Adults:** 1-2 gtts bid.	◐C ❄>

Carteolol HCl (Ocupress)	Sol: 1%	Adults: 1 gtt bid.	◉C ✿>
Levobunolol HCl (Betagan, Betagan C Cap)	Sol: (Betagan C Cap) 0.25%, (Betagan) 0.5%	Usual: 0.5%: 1-2 gtts qd. 0.25%: 1-2 gtts bid. Severe/Uncontrolled: >0.5%: 1-2 gtts bid.	◉C ✿>
Metipranolol (Optipranolol)	Sol: 0.3%	Adults: 1 gtt bid.	◉C ✿v
Timolol Maleate (Timoptic, Timoptic-XE)	Sol: 0.25%, 0.5%; Sol, gel forming: (Timoptic XE) 0.25%, 0.5%	Timoptic: 1 gtt 0.25% bid, may increase to 1 gtt 0.5% bid. Maint: 1 gtt 0.25%/0.5% qd. Timoptic-XE: 1 gtt 0.25%/0.5% qd. Max: 1 gtt 0.5% qd.	◉C ✿v

CARBONIC ANHYDRASE INHIBITOR/BETA BLOCKER

Dorzolamide/Timolol Maleate (Cosopt)	Sol: 2%-0.5%	Adults: 1 gtt bid.	◉C ✿v

CARBONIC ANHYDRASE INHIBITORS

Acetazolamide (Diamox)	Cap,ER: 500 mg; Inj: 500 mg; Tab: 125 mg, 250 mg	Inj/Tab: Open Angle Glaucoma: 250 mg-1 gm/24h in divided doses. Secondary/Angle Closure Glaucoma: 250 mg q4h, or 500 mg followed by 125-250 mg q4h. Cap,ER: Glaucoma: 500 mg qam & qpm.	◉C ✿v
Brinzolamide (Azopt)	Susp: 1%	Adults: 1 gtt tid.	◉C ✿v
Dichlorphenamide (Daranide)	Tab: 50 mg	Initial: 100-200 mg, then 100 mg q12h until response. Maint: 25-50 mg qd-tid.	◉C ✿>

NAME	FORM/STRENGTH	DOSAGE	COMMENTS
Dorzolamide (Trusopt)	**Sol:** 2%	**Adults:** 1 gtt tid.	▣C ❄v
Methazolamide (Neptazane)	**Tab:** 25 mg, 50 mg	**Adults:** 50-100 mg bid-tid.	▣C ❄v

CHOLINERGIC AGONISTS

NAME	FORM/STRENGTH	DOSAGE	COMMENTS
Carbachol (Isopto Carbachol)	**Sol:** 0.75%, 1.5%, 2.25%, 3%	**Adults:** 2 gtts up to tid.	▣C ❄>
Echothiophate Iodide (Phospholine Iodide)	**Sol:** 0.03%, 0.06%, 0.125%, 0.25%	**Adults: Early Chronic Simple Glaucoma:** (0.3%) 1 gtt qam & qhs. **Advanced Chronic Simple Glaucoma/ Glaucoma 2° to Cataract Surgery: Initial:** (0.3%) 1 gtt qam & qhs. **Titrate:** Increase to higher strength as needed. **Peds: Accommodative Esotropia: Diagnosis:** (0.125%) 1 gtt qhs x 2-3 wks. **Treatment:** Decrease to 1 gtt (0.125%) qod or (0.6%) 1 gtt qd. **Titrate:** Decrease strength gradually. **Max:** (0.125%) 1 gtt qd.	▣C ❄v
Pilocarpine (Isopto Carpine, Pilocar, Pilopine HS)	**Gel:** 4%; **Sol:** 0.25%, 0.5%, 1%, 2%, 3%, 4%, 5%, 6%, 8%	**Usual:** 2 gtts tid-qid. Apply gel 1/2 inch ribbon qhs.	▣C ❄>

PROSTAGLANDIN ANALOGUES

NAME	FORM/STRENGTH	DOSAGE	COMMENTS
Bimatoprost (Lumigan)	**Sol:** 0.03%	**Usual/Max:** 1 gtt qpm.	▣C ❄>
Latanoprost (Xalatan)	**Sol:** 0.005%	**Usual/ Max:** 1 gtt qpm.	▣C ❄>

Travaprost (Travatan)	Sol: 0.004%	Adults: 1 gtt qpm.	⬤C ✿>
Unoprostone (Rescula)	Sol: 0.15%	Adults: 1 gtt bid.	⬤C ✿>

SYMPATHOMIMETICS

Brimonidine (Alphagan, Alphagan P)	Sol: (Alphagan P) 0.15%, (Alphagan) 0.2%	Adults & Peds: ≥2 yo: 1 gtt tid (q8h). Separate other topical products that lower IOP by at least 5 min.	⬤B ✿v
Epinephrine (Epifrin)	Sol: 0.5%, 1%, 2%	Adults: 1 gtt qd-bid.	⬤C ✿>

Mydriatics/Cycloplegics

ANTICHOLINERGICS

Atropine Sulfate	Oint: 1%; Sol: 1%	1-2 gtts tid or small amount of oint qd-bid.	⬤C ✿>
Cyclopentolate HCl (Cyclogyl, Cylate, Ocu-Pentolate)	Sol: 0.5%, 1%, 2%	Adults: 1-2 gtts, may repeat in 5-10 min. Peds: 1-2 gtts, may repeat in 5-10 min with 0.5%-1%.	⬤C ✿>
Cyclopentolate HCl/ Phenylephrine (Cyclomydril)	Sol: 0.2%-1%	Adults & Peds: 1 gtt q5-10min, up to 3x.	⬤N ✿>
Homatropine HBr (Isopto Homatropine)	Sol: 2%, 5%	Refraction: 1-2 gtts, may repeat in 5-10 min. Uveitis: 1-2 gtts up to q3-4h. Only use 2% in peds.	⬤C ✿>
Phenylephrine/ Scopolamine HBr (Murocoll 2)	Sol: 10%-0.3%	Mydriasis: 1-2 gtts, may repeat in 5 min. Post-op: 1-2 gtts tid-qid.	⬤N ✿>

NAME	FORM/STRENGTH	DOSAGE	COMMENTS
Scopolamine HBr (Isopto Hyoscine)	Sol: 0.25%	**Refraction:** 1-2 gtts 1h prior to refracting. **Uveitis:** 1-2 gtts up to 4x/d.	◉N ✿>
Tropicamide (Mydral, Mydriacyl, Ocu-Tropic, Tropicacyl)	Sol: 0.5%, 1%	**Refraction: 1%:** 1-2 gtts, may repeat in 5 min. **Fundal Exam: 0.5%:** 1-2 gtts 15-20 min before exam.	◉N ✿>

SYMPATHOMIMETICS

NAME	FORM/STRENGTH	DOSAGE	COMMENTS
Phenylephrine (Neo-Synephrine)	Sol: 2.5%, 10%; Sol, viscous: 10%	**Glaucoma/Vasocontriction/Pupil Dilation:** 1 gtt 10%. **Uveitis:** 1 gtt 10%. May continue the following day. **Surgery:** 2.5% or 10% 30-60 min pre-op. **Refraction: Adults & Peds:** 1 gtt 2.5% after cyclopegic. **Ophtho Exam:** 1 gtt 2.5%. **Diagnostic Procedure:** 1 gtt 2.5%.	◉C ✿> 10% is Cl in infants.

NSAIDs

NAME	FORM/STRENGTH	DOSAGE	COMMENTS
Diclofenac Sodium (Voltaren)	Sol: 1%	**Cataract Surgery:** 1 gtt qid, begin 24h post-op x 2wks. **Corneal Refractive Surgery:** 1-2 gtts within 1h pre-op, & 15 min post-op. Continue app up to 3d.	◉C ✿> Avoid during late pregnancy.
Flurbiprofen Sodium (Ocufen)	Sol: 0.03%	**Inhibit Intraoperative Miosis:** 1 gtts q30min x 4 doses, beginning 2h prior to surgery.	◉C ✿v
Ketorolac Tromethamine (Acular, Acular PF)	Sol: 0.5%	**Adults & Peds: ≥3 yo: Acular: Ocular Itching:** 1 gtt qid. **Post-Op Inflammation:** 1 gtt qid. Begin 24h post-op & continue x 2wks. **Acular PF: Pain/Photophobia:** 1 gtt post-op qid prn up to 3d.	◉C ✿>

Ocular Decongestant/Allergic Conjunctivitis

ANTIHISTAMINES

Emedastine Difumarate (Emadine)	**Sol:** 0.05%	**Adults & Peds:** ≥3 yo: 1 gtt up to qid.	B ❀>

H₁ ANTAGONIST/MAST CELL STABILIZERS

Ketotifen Fumarate (Zaditor)	**Sol:** 0.025%	**Adults & Peds:** ≥3 yo: 1 gtt bid, q8-12h.	C ❀>
Olopatadine HCl (Patanol)	**Sol:** 0.1%	**Adults & Peds:** ≥3 yo: 1-2 gtts bid, q6-8h.	C ❀>

H₁ RECEPTOR ANTAGONISTS

Azelastine (Optivar)	**Sol:** 0.05%	**Adults & Peds:** ≥3 yo: 1 gtt bid.	C ❀>
Epinastine HCl (Elestat)	**Sol:** 0.05%	**Adults & Peds:** ≥3 yo: 1 gtt in each eye bid.	C ❀>
Levocabastine (Livostin)	**Susp:** 0.05%	**Adults & Peds:** ≥12 yo: 1 gtt qid.	C ❀>

MAST CELL STABILIZERS

Cromolyn Sodium (Crolom, Opticrom)	**Sol:** 4%	**Adults & Peds:** ≥4 yo: 1-2 gtts 4-6x/d.	B ❀>

NAME	FORM/STRENGTH	DOSAGE	COMMENTS
Lodoxamide Tromethamine (Alomide)	Sol: 0.1%	**Adults & Peds: >2 yo:** 1-2 gtts qid up to 3 mths.	⬤B ❋>
Nedocromil Sodium (Alocril)	Sol: 2%	**Adults & Peds: ≥3 yo:** 1-2 gtts bid.	⬤B ❋>
SYMPATHOMIMETIC/H₁ ANTAGONISTS			
Naphazoline HCl/ Pheniramine Maleate (Naphcon-A)	Sol: 0.3%-0.025%	**Adults & Peds: ≥6 yo:** 1-2 gtts up to qid.	⬤N ❋>
SYMPATHOMIMETICS			
Naphazoline (AK-Con, Albalon, Allersol, Ocu-zoline)	Sol: 0.1%	**Adults:** 1-2 gtts q3-4h prn.	⬤C ❋>

Viral Infection

Trifluridine (Viroptic)	Sol: 1%	**Adults: ≥6 yo: Usual:** 1 gtt q2h w/a until re-epithelialization. **Max:** 9 gtts/d. **Following Re-epithelialization:** 1 gtt q4h w/a, min 5 gtts/d x 7d.	⬤C ❋v
Vidarabine (Vira-A)	Oint: 3%	**Adults: ≥2 yo: Usual:** Apply 1/2 in 5x/d q3h x 7d until re-epithelialization. **Following Re-epithelialization:** Apply 1/2 inch bid x 7d.	⬤C ❋v

Miscellaneous

Chondroitin Sulfate/Sodium Hyaluronate (Viscoat)	Sol: 40 mg-30 mg/ml	**Cataract Surgery/Intraocular Implantation:** Insert into anterior chamber.	⬤N ❋>

Cyclosporine (Restasis)	**Emulsion:** 0.05%	**Keratoconjunctivitis sicca: Adults:** 1 gtt bid, q12h.	◎C ❄>
Dapiprazole (Rev-Eyes)	**Sol:** 0.5%	**Reversal of Diagnostic Mydriasis:** 2 gtts, repeat after 5 min.	◎B ❄>
Sodium Hyaluronate (Biolon, Provisc, Vitrax)	**Liq:** 10 mg/ml, 30 mg/ml	**Cataract Surgery/Intraocular Lens Implant:** Insert during procedure into interior chamber. **Corneal Transplant:** Insert into anterior chamber. **Glaucoma Filtration:** Inject through corneal paracentesis to restore & maintain anterior chamber.	◎N ❄>

EENT/OTIC PREPARATIONS
Anesthetics

Antipyrine/Benzocaine (Aurodex, Auroto, Dolotic)	**Sol:** 54 mg-14 mg/ml	**Otitis Media:** Fill ear canal, then insert moistened pledget. Repeat q1-2h until relief. **Cerumen Removal:** Instill tid x 2-3d, then insert moistened pledget.	◎C ❄>
Antipyrine/Benzocaine/ Phenylephrine (Ear-Gesic, Tympagesic)	**Sol:** 5%-5%-0.25%	**Adults & Peds: ≥12 yo:** Fill ear canal & insert saturated cotton, re-wet q2-4h until pain relieved.	◎N ❄>
Benzocaine (Americaine Otic)	**Sol:** 20%	**Adults & Peds ≥1 yo:** Instill 4-5 gtts in external auditory canal, then insert cotton pledget into meatus. May repeat q1-2h.	◎C ❄>

NAME	FORM/STRENGTH	DOSAGE	COMMENTS
Antibacterial/Antifungal Combinations			
Acetic Acid/ Aluminum Acetate (Borofair, Domeboro)	**Sol:** 2%-0.79%	**Adults:** 4-6 gtts into ear, repeat q2-3h.	▶N ☼ ▼<
Acetic Acid (Vosol)	**Sol:** 2%	**Adults:** Insert saturated wick in ear & keep moist x 24h, remove wick & instill 5 gtts tid-qid. **Peds:** Insert wick & keep moist x 24h, remove wick & instill 3-4 gtts tid-qid.	▶N ☼ ▼<
Antibacterial/Corticosteroid Combinations			
Acetic Acid/Hydrocortisone (Acetasol HC, Oticot HC, Vosol HC)	**Sol:** 2%-1%	**Adults:** Insert cotton saturated w/med & keep moist w/ 3-5 gtts q4-6h x 24h, then remove. Continue to instill 5 gtts tid-qid. **Peds:** Insert cotton saturated w/med & keep moist w/3-4 gtts q4-6h x 24h, then remove. Continue to instill 3-4 gtts tid-qid.	▶N ☼ ▼>
Ciprofloxacin HCl/ Hydrocortisone (Cipro HC Otic)	**Susp:** 0.2%-1%	**Adults & Peds ≥1 yo:** 3 gtts bid x 7d.	▶C ☼ ▼v
Ciprofloxacin HCl/ Dexamethasone (Ciprodex)	**Susp:** 0.3%-0.1%	**Adults & Peds ≥6 mo:** 4 gtts bid x 7d.	▶C ☼ ▼v

| Colistin Sulfate/ Hydrocortisone Acetate/ Neomycin Sulfate/ Thonzonium Bromide (Coly-Mycin S, Cortisporin-TC) | **Susp:** 3 mg-10 mg-3.3 mg-0.5 mg/ml | **Adults:** 4-5 gtts tid-qid. **Peds:** 3-4 gtts tid-qid. | ◉N ❄> |
| Neomycin Sulfate/Polymyxin B Sulfate/Hydrocortisone (Cortisporin) | **Sol, Susp:** 1%-0.35%-10,000 U/ml | **Adults:** 4 gtts tid-qid up to 10d. **Peds:** 3 gtts tid-qid up to 10d. | ◉C ❄> |

Antibiotic Agents

| Chloramphenicol | **Sol:** 0.5% | **Adults:** 2-3 gtts tid. | ◉N ❄> |
| Ofloxacin (Floxin Otic, Floxin Otic Singles) | **Sol:** 0.3% | **Otitis Externa: 6 mo-13 yo:** 5 gtts or 1 single-dispensing container (SDC) qd x 7d. **≥13 yo:** 10 gtts or 2 SDCs qd x 7d. **Acute Otitis Media with Tympanostomy Tubes: 1-12 yo:** 5 gtts or 1 SDC bid x 10d. **Chronic Suppurative Otitis Media with Perforated Tympanic Membranes: ≥12 yo:** 10 gtts or 2 SDCs bid x 14d. | ◉C ❄v |

Surfactants

| Triethanolamine Polypeptide (Cerumenex) | **Sol:** 10% | **Adults:** Fill ear canal & insert cotton plug x 15-30 min. Flush w/warm water. May repeat. | ◉C ❄> |

NAME	FORM/STRENGTH	DOSAGE	COMMENTS

ENDOCRINE/METABOLIC

Androgens

NAME	FORM/STRENGTH	DOSAGE	COMMENTS
Danazol (Danocrine)	**Cap:** 50 mg, 100 mg, 200 mg	**Adults: Hereditary Angioedema: Initial:** 200 mg bid-tid. After favorable response, decrease up to 50% at intervals of ≥1-3 mths depending on frequency of attacks. Increase up to 200 mg if attack occurs.	◙X ❄v Cl in nursing. Begin during menses. [25]
Methyltestosterone CIII (Android, Testred)	**Cap:** 10 mg	**Adults: Androgen-Deficient Males:** 10-50 mg/d. **Breast Cancer in Females:** 50-200 mg/d. **Peds: Delayed Puberty:** Use lower range of 10-50 mg/d x 4-6mths.	◙X ❄v
Oxandrolone CIII (Oxandrin)	**Tab:** 2.5 mg, 10 mg	**Adults: Usual:** 2.5-20 mg/day given bid-qid x 2-4wks. **Pediatrics:** ≤0.1 mg/kg/d. Repeat intermittently as indicated.	◙X ❄v
Stanozolol CIII (Winstrol)	**Tab:** 2 mg	**Adults & Peds: Hereditary Angioedema: Initial:** 2 mg tid. After favorable response, decrease the dosage at intervals of 1-3 mths. **Maint:** 2 mg/d.	◙X ❄v
Testosterone CIII (Androderm, Testim, Testoderm, Testoderm TTS)	**Inj:** 50 mg/ml, 100 mg/ml; **Patch:** 2.5 mg/24h, 4 mg/24h, 5 mg/24h, 6 mg/24h; **Gel:** 1% [5 g (50 mg)/tube]	**≥15 yo: Inj:** 25-50 mg BIW-TIW. **Testoderm TTS:** 1 patch q24h on arm, back, or upper buttocks. **Testoderm: Initial:** 6 mg/d. Apply to scrotal skin x 22-24h. **Androderm: Initial:** 5 mg qhs x 24h on back, abdomen, upper arm, or thigh. **Maint:** 2.5-7.5 mg/d. **Testim: ≥18 yo: Initial:** Apply 5 g qd in am to shoulder or upper arm. **Titrate:** May increase to 10 g qd.	◙X ❄v

Testosterone CIII (Striant)	Tab, Buccal: 30 mg	**Adults:** 30 mg q12h to gum region above incisor tooth on either side of mouth. Rotate sites with each application. Hold in place for 30 sec.	◙X ❀v
Testosterone Cypionate CIII (Depo-Testosterone)	Inj: 100 mg/ml, 200 mg/ml	**Adults & Peds: ≥12 yo:** 50-400 mg IM q2-4wks.	◙X ❀v
Testosterone Enanthate CIII (Delatestryl, Everone)	Inj: 200 mg/ml	**Adults & Peds: Male Hypogonadism: Usual:** 50-400 mg IM q2-4wks. **Delayed Puberty:** 50-200 mg q2-4wks for a limited duration (eg, 4-6 mths). Caution in children.	◙X ❀v
Testosterone Propionate CIII	Inj: 100 mg/ml	**Adults & Peds: Usual:** 25-50 mg IM BIW-TIW.	◙X ❀v

Antidiabetic Agents

BIGUANIDES

| Metformin (Glucophage, Glucophage XR, Riomet) | **Sol:** (Riomet) 500 mg/5 ml; **Tab:** 500 mg, 850 mg, 1000 mg; **Tab,ER:** 500 mg, 750 mg | **Adults: Sol, Tab: Initial:** 500 mg bid or 850 mg qd w/meals. **Titrate:** Increase by 500 mg qwk, or 850 mg q2wks, or from 500 mg bid to 850 mg bid q2wks. **Max:** 2550 mg/d. **Tab,ER: (XR) Initial:** 500 mg qd w/pm meal. **Titrate:** Increase by 500 mg qwk. **Max:** 2 gm/d. **With Insulin:** Initial: 500 mg qd. **Titrate:** Increase by 500 mg/wk. **Max:** 2500 mg/d and 2000 mg/d (XR). Decrease insulin dose by 10-25% when FPG <120 mg/dL. **Peds: 10-16 yo: Tab: Initial:** 500 mg bid w/meals. **Titrate:** Increase by 500 mg qwk. **Max:** 2000 mg/d. | ◙B ❀v **H R** Lactic acidosis is rare, but can occur. |

25 Benign intracranial HTN. Thromboembolic events.

NAME	FORM/STRENGTH	DOSAGE	COMMENTS
GLUCOSIDASE INHIBITORS			
Acarbose (Precose)	**Tab:** 25 mg, 50 mg, 100 mg	**Adults: Initial:** 25 mg tid w/meals. **Titrate:** Adjust at 4-8 wk intervals. **Maint:** 50-100 mg tid. **Max: ≤60 kg:** 50 mg tid. **>60 kg:** 100 mg tid.	◑B ❋∨ R
Miglitol (Glyset)	**Tab:** 25 mg, 50 mg, 100 mg	**Adults: Initial:** 25 mg tid w/meals. **Titrate:** Increase after 4-8 wks to 50 mg tid x approx. 3 mths, then may further increase to 100 mg tid. **Max:** 100 mg tid.	◑B ❋∨ R
INSULIN			
Insulin Glargine Human (Lantus)	**Inj:** 100 U/ml (OptiPen) 100 U/ml	**Adults & Peds: ≥6 yo:** Dose per requirement. Give same time qd.	◑C ❋∨<
Insulin Lispro, Human (Humalog)	**Inj:** 100 U/ml	**Adults & Peds: ≥3 yo:** Dose per requirement.	◑B ❋∨<
Insulin, NPH (Humulin N)	**Inj:** 100 U/ml	**Adults & Peds:** Dose per requirement.	◑N ❋∨<
Insulin, Regular	**Inj:** 100 U/ml	**Adults & Peds:** Dose per requirement.	◑N ❋∨<
MEGLITINIDES			
Nateglinide (Starlix)	**Tab:** 60 mg, 120 mg	**Adults:** 120 mg tid w/meals (with or without metformin or thiazolidinedione). Take 1-30 min before meals. May use 60 mg tid (with or without metformin or thiazolidinedione) near goal HbA1c. Skip dose if meal is skipped.	◑C ❋∨

Repaglinide (Prandin)	Tab: 0.5 mg, 1 mg, 2 mg	Take within 15-30 min ac. Skip dose if skip meal & add dose if add meal. **Adults: Initial: Treatment-Naive or HbA1c <8%:** 0.5 mg with each meal. **Previous Oral Antidiabetic Therapy/Combination Therapy and HbA$_{1c}$ ≥8%:** 1-2 mg w/meals. **Titrate:** May adjust wkly by doubling preprandial dose up to 4 mg (bid-qid). **Maint:** 0.5-4 mg w/meals. **Max:** 16 mg/d.	●C ❄v H R

SULFONYLUREA/BIGUANIDE

Glipizide/Metformin HCl (Metaglip)	Tab: 2.5-250 mg, 2.5-500 mg, 5-500 mg	**Adults: Initial:** 2.5-250 mg qd. If FBG 280-320 mg/dL, give 2.5-500 mg bid. **Titrate:** Increase by 1 tab/d q2wks. **Max:** 10 mg-1 gm/d or 10 mg-2gm/d in divided doses. **2nd-Line Therapy: Initial:** 2.5-500 mg or 5-500 mg bid; do not exceed daily metformin or glipizide dose already being taken. **Titrate:** Increase by ≤5 mg-500 mg/d. **Max:** 20 mg-2 gm/d. Take with meals.	●C ❄v H R Lactic acidosis is rare, but can occur.
Glyburide/Metformin HCl (Glucovance)	Tab: 1.25-250 mg, 2.5-500 mg, 5-500 mg	**Adults: Initial:** 1.25-250 mg qd-bid w/meals. If HbA$_{1c}$ >9% or FPG >200 mg/dL, give 1.25-250 mg bid. **Titrate:** Increase by 1.25 mg-250 mg/d q2wks. **2nd Line Therapy: Initial:** 2.5-500 mg or 5-500 mg bid. **Titrate:** Increase by ≤5-500 mg/d. **Max:** 20 mg-2000 mg/d. **Concomitant Thiazolidinedione (TZD):** Initiate and titrate TZD as recommended.	●B ❄v H R Lactic acidosis is rare, but can occur.

SULFONYLUREAS-1ST GENERATION

Acetohexamide	Tab: 250 mg, 500 mg	**Adults:** 250 mg-1.5 gm/d ac.	●C ❄v H R

NAME	FORM/STRENGTH	DOSAGE	COMMENTS
Chlorpropamide (Diabinese)	**Tab:** 100 mg, 250 mg	**Adults: Initial:** 250 mg qd. **Titrate:** After 5-7d, adjust by 50-125 mg/d q3-5d. **Maint:** 100-500 mg qd. **Max:** 750 mg/d.	▣C ✿v H R
Tolazamide (Tolinase)	**Tab:** 100 mg, 250 mg, 500 mg	**Adults: Initial:** 100-250 mg qd w/food. **Titrate:** May increase by 100-250 mg/wk. **Maint:** 100-1000 mg/d. **Max:** 1000 mg/d. Divide dose if >500 mg.	▣C ✿v H R
Tolbutamide (Tol-Tab)	**Tab:** 500 mg	**Adults: Usual/Initial:** 1-2 gm/d. **Maint:** 0.25-3 gm/d. **Max:** 3 gm/d.	▣C ✿v H R

SULFONYLUREAS-2ND GENERATION

NAME	FORM/STRENGTH	DOSAGE	COMMENTS
Glimepiride (Amaryl)	**Tab:** 1 mg, 2 mg, 4 mg	**Adults: Initial:** 1-2 mg qd w/ a meal. **Titrate:** Increase ≤2 mg at 1-2 wk intervals. **Maint:** 1-4 mg qd.	▣C ✿v H R
Glipizide (Glucotrol, Glucotrol XL)	**Tab:** 5 mg, 10 mg; **Tab,ER:** 2.5 mg, 5 mg, 10 mg	**Adults: Glucotrol XL: Initial/Combination Therapy:** 5 mg qd w/ breakfast. Lower dose if sensitive to hypoglycemics. **Usual:** 5-10 mg qd. **Max:** 20 mg/d. **Glucotrol: Initial:** 5 mg qd 30 min ac. **Titrate:** Increase by 2.5-5 mg; divide if above 15 mg. **Max:** 40 mg/d.	▣C ✿v H R
Glyburide, Micronized (Glycron, Glynase Pres-Tab)	**Tab:** 1.5 mg, 3 mg, 4.5 mg, 6 mg	**Adults: Initial:** 1.5-3 mg qd with a meal. **Titrate:** Increase by no more than 1.5 mg at wkly intervals; >6 mg may give bid. **Maint:** 0.75-12 mg/d. **Max:** 12 mg/d.	▣B ✿v H R
Glyburide (Diabeta, Micronase)	**Tab:** 1.25 mg, 2.5 mg, 5 mg	**Adults: Initial:** 2.5-5 mg qd with a meal. **Titrate:** Increase by no more than 2.5 mg at wkly intervals, give bid if >10 mg/d. **Maint:** 1.25-20 mg/d. **Max:** 20 mg/d.	▣B (Micronase) ▣C (Diabeta) ✿v H R

THIAZOLIDINEDIONES

Pioglitazone (Actos)	Tab: 15 mg, 30 mg, 45 mg	Adults: Initial: 15-30 mg qd. Max: 45 mg/d.	●C ✿v H Monitor liver enzymes.
Rosiglitazone (Avandia)	Tab: 2 mg, 4 mg, 8 mg	≥18 yo: Initial: 2 mg bid or 4 mg qd. Titrate: May increase after 8-12 wks to 4 mg bid or 8 mg qd. Max: 8 mg/d as monotherapy or with metformin; 4 mg/d with sulfonylureas or insulin. Decrease insulin by 10-25% if hypoglycemic or FPG <100 mg/dL; individualize further adjustments based on glucose lowering response.	●C ✿v H Monitor liver enzymes.

THIAZOLIDINEDIONES/BIGUANIDE

| Rosiglitazone Maleate/ Metformin HCl (Avandamet) | Tab: 1 mg-500 mg, 2 mg-500 mg, 4 mg-500 mg, 2 mg-1000 mg, 4 mg-1000 mg | Adults: Prior Metformin 1 gm/d: Initial: 2 mg-500 mg tab bid. Prior Metformin 2 gm/d: Initial: 2 mg-1 gm tab bid. Prior Rosiglitazone 4 mg/d: Initial: 2 mg-500 mg tab bid. Prior Rosiglitazone 8 mg/d: 4 mg-500 mg tab bid. Titrate: May increase by 4 mg rosiglitazone and/or 500 mg metformin. Max: 8 mg-2 gm/d. Take with meals. | ●C ✿v H R Monitor liver enzymes. |

Antithyroid Agents

| Methimazole (Tapazole) | Tab: 5 mg, 10 mg | Adults: Initial: 5 mg q8h for mild hyperthyroidism; 30-40 mg/d given q8h for moderately severe hyperthyroidism, 20 mg q8h for severe hyperthyroidism. Maint: 5-15 mg/d. Peds: Initial: 0.4 mg/kg/d divided q8h. Maint: 1/2 of initial dose. | ●D ✿v CI in nursing. |

NAME	FORM/STRENGTH	DOSAGE	COMMENTS
Propylthiouracil (PTU)	Tab: 50 mg	**Adults:** 100 mg q8h, 400 mg/d as q8h for severe hyperthyroidism/large goiters, up to 600-900 mg/d if needed. **Maint:** 100-150 mg/d. **Peds: 6-10 yo: Initial:** 50-150 mg/d. **≥10 yo:** 150-300 mg/d. **Maint:** Determine dose by response.	⬛D ✿v CI in nursing.
Sodium Iodide I 131 (Iodotope)	Cap: 8, 15, 30, 50, or 100 MCI; Sol: 7.0 SMCI/ml	**Usual:** 4-10 MCI. Dose varies for clinical remission without entire thyroid destruction.	⬛X ✿v

SYSTEMIC CORTICOSTEROIDS

CORTICOSTEROID	EQUIVALENT POTENCY	MINERALOCORTICOID POTENCY	FORM/STRENGTH	DOSAGE RANGE
Betamethasone (Celestone)	0.6 mg	0	Syr: 0.6 mg/5 ml	Initial: 0.6-7.2 mg/d PO.
Betamethasone Sodium Phosphate & Betamethasone Acetate (Celestone Soluspan)	0.6 mg	0	Inj: 3 mg-3 mg/ml	Initial: 0.5-9 mg/d IM.
Cortisone Acetate	25 mg	2	Tab: 25 mg	Initial: 25-300 mg/d PO.
Dexamethasone (Decadron)	0.5 mg	0	Sol: 0.5 mg/5 ml Tab: 0.25 mg, 0.5 mg, 0.75 mg, 1 mg, 1.5 mg, 2 mg, 4 mg, 6 mg	Initial: 0.75-9 mg/d PO.

Drug	Dose equiv	Rating	Forms	Dosing
Dexamethasone Sodium Phosphate (Decadron Phosphate)	0.5 mg	0	**Inj:** 4 mg/ml	**Initial:** 0.5-9 mg/d IM/IV.
Hydrocortisone (Cortef)	20 mg	2	**Tab:** 5 mg, 10 mg, 20 mg	**Initial:** 20-240 mg/d PO.
Hydrocortisone Cypionate (Cortef)	20 mg	2	**Susp:** 10 mg/5 ml	**Initial:** 20-240 mg/d PO.
Hydrocortisone Sodium Phosphate	20 mg	2	**Inj:** 50 mg/ml	**Initial:** 15-240 mg/d IM/IV/SC.
Hydrocortisone Sodium Succinate (Solu-Cortef)	20 mg	2	**Inj:** 100 mg, 250 mg, 500 mg, 1000 mg	**Initial:** 100-500 mg IM/IV.
Methylprednisolone (Medrol)	4 mg	0	**Tab:** 2 mg, 4 mg, 8 mg, 16 mg, 24 mg, 32 mg	**Initial:** 4-48 mg/d PO.
Methylprednisolone Acetate (Depo-Medrol)	4 mg	0	**Inj:** 20 mg/ml, 40 mg/ml, 80 mg/ml	**Initial:** 40-120 mg/wk IM.
Methylprednisolone Sodium Succinate (Solu-Medrol)	4 mg	0	**Inj:** 40 mg, 125 mg, 500 mg, 1 gm, 2 gm	**Initial:** 10-40 mg IV.
Prednisolone (Prelone)	5 mg	1	**Syr:** 5 mg/5 ml, 15 mg/5 ml;	**Initial:** 5-60 mg/d PO.
Prednisolone Sodium Phosphate (Pediapred)	5 mg	1	**Sol:** 5 mg/5 ml	**Initial:** 5-60 mg/d PO.

CORTICOSTEROID	EQUIVALENT POTENCY	MINERALOCORTICOID POTENCY	FORM/STRENGTH	DOSAGE RANGE
Prednisone (Deltasone)	5 mg	1	**Sol:** 5 mg/ml, 5 mg/5 ml; **Tab:** 1 mg, 2.5 mg, 5 mg, 10 mg, 20 mg, 50 mg	**Initial:** 5-60 mg/d PO.
Triamcinolone (Aristocort)	4 mg	0	**Tab:** 4 mg	**Initial:** 4-60 mg/d PO.
Triamcinolone Acetonide (Kenalog-10)	4 mg	0	**Inj:** 10 mg/ml	**Intra-articular/ Intrabursal:** 2.5-20 mg/d.
Triamcinolone Acetonide (Kenalog-40)	4 mg	0	**Inj:** 40 mg/ml	**Initial:** 2.5-60 mg/d IM or intra-articular.
Triamcinolone Diacetate (Aristocort Forte)	4 mg	0	**Inj:** 40 mg/ml	**Initial:** 3-48 mg/d IM.
Triamcinolone Hexacetonide (Aristospan Intra-lesional, Aristospan Intra-articular)	4 mg	0	**Inj:** 5 mg/ml (intralesional), 20 mg/ml (intra-articular)	**Intra-articular:** 2-48 mg. **Intra-lesional:** Up to 0.5 mg/in^2 of area affected.

Gout

URICOSURICS

NAME	FORM/STRENGTH	DOSAGE	COMMENTS
Probenecid	Tab: 500 mg	**Adults:** 250 mg bid x 1 wk. **Titrate:** Increase by 500 mg q4wks. **Maint:** 500 mg bid. **Max:** 2 gm/d.	◉N ❄> R
Sulfinpyrazone	Tab: 100 mg	**Initial:** 100-200 mg bid w/meals or milk x 1 wk. **Maint:** 200 mg bid, increase to 300 mg/d if needed. **Max:** 800 mg/d.	◉N ❄>

XANTHINE OXIDASE INHIBITORS

NAME	FORM/STRENGTH	DOSAGE	COMMENTS
Allopurinol (Zyloprim)	Tab: 100 mg, 300 mg	**Adults: Usual:** 200-300 mg/d. **Prevention of Uric Acid Nephropathy with Chemotherapy: Usual:** 600-800 mg/d for 2-3d w/ high fluid intake.	◉C ❄> R

MISCELLANEOUS

NAME	FORM/STRENGTH	DOSAGE	COMMENTS
Colchicine	Inj: 0.5 mg/ml; Tab: 0.5 mg, 0.6 mg	**Acute Gouty Arthritis:** 1-1.2 mg, then 0.5-0.6 mg/h or 1-1.2 mg q2h until pain relieved or diarrhea ensues up to 4-8 mg; wait 3d between courses to avoid colchicine toxicity. **Prophylaxis:** (<1 attack/yr) 0.5-0.6 mg/d 3-4x/wk; (>1 attack/wk) 0.5-0.6 mg/d, severe cases may need 2-3 tabs/d.	◉C ❄> H R
Probenecid/Colchicine	Tab: 500-0.5 mg	**Adults: Initial:** 1 tab qd x 1 wk, then 1 tab bid. **Titrate:** May increase by 1 tab/d q4wks. **Max:** 4 tabs/d. Not for acute gouty attacks. May reduce dose by 1 tab q6mths if acute attacks have been absent ≥6 mths.	◉N ❄> R CI in pregnancy.

NAME	FORM/STRENGTH	DOSAGE	COMMENTS

Hypoglycemia

| Glucagon (GlucaGen) | Inj: 1 mg | **Adults & Peds: Severe Hypoglycemia: ≥25kg:** 1 mg IM/IV/SC. **<25 kg or <6-8 yo:** 0.5 mg IM/IV/SC. May repeat x1 dose after 15 min if no response while waiting for emergency assistance. | ▣B ❄> |

Obesity

CENTRALLY ACTING ADRENERGIC AGENTS

Benzphetamine HCl CIII (Didrex)	Tab: 50 mg	**Adults & Peds: ≥12 yo: Initial:** 25-50 mg qd. **Maint:** 25-50 mg qd-tid.	▣X ❄v
Diethylpropion HCl CIV (Tenuate)	Tab: 25 mg; Tab,ER: 75 mg	**Adults & Peds: ≥16 yo:** (Tab) 25 mg tab tid 1h ac & mid-evening prn. (Tab,ER) 75 mg qd mid-morning.	▣B ❄>
Methamphetamine HCl CII (Desoxyn)	Tab: 5 mg	**Adults & Peds ≥12 yo:** 5 mg 1/2 hr before each meal.	▣C ❄v High potential for abuse.
Phendimetrazine CIII (Prelu-2, Bontril)	Cap,ER: 105 mg; Tab: 35 mg	**Adults & Peds: ≥12 yo:** (Tab) 35 mg tab bid-tid 1h ac. May decrease to 17.5 mg/dose. (Cap,ER) 105 mg qam 30-60 min ac.	▣N ❄>
Phentermine HCl CIV (Adipex-P, Phentercot)	Cap: 15 mg, 18.75 mg, 30 mg, 37.5 mg; Tab: 8 mg, 37.5 mg	**Adults & Peds ≥16 yo:** 30 mg 2h before breakfast, 37.5 mg before breakfast or 1-2h after breakfast, or 18.75 mg qd-bid.	▣N ❄>
Phentermine Resin CIV (Ionamin)	Cap: 15 mg, 30 mg	**Adults & Peds: ≥16 yo:** 15-30 mg before breakfast or 10-14h before retiring.	▣N ❄>

| Sibutramine (Meridia) | Cap: 5 mg, 10 mg, 15 mg | Adults & Peds: ≥16 yo: Initial: 10 mg qd. Titrate: May increase after 4 wks to 15 mg qd. Max: 15 mg/d. May continue for up to 2 yrs. | ⊞C ❊v Do not give if severe renal/hepatic impairment. |

LIPASE INHIBITOR

| Orlistat (Xenical) | Cap: 120 mg | Adults & Peds: ≥12yo: 120 mg tid w/meals containing fat. Take during or up to 1h after meals. Omit dose if miss meal. Take a MVI w/fat-soluble vitamins at least 2h before or after dose. | ⊞B ❊v |

Osteoporosis
BISPHOSPHONATE

| Alendronate Sodium (Fosamax) | Sol: 70 mg/75 ml; Tab: 5 mg, 10 mg, 35 mg, 40 mg, 70 mg | Treatment in Females/Bone Mass Increase in Men: 10 mg qd or 70 mg qwk. Prevention in Females: 5 mg qd or 35 mg qwk. Take tab w/6-8 oz of water or sol w/2 oz of water at least 30 min before 1st food, beverage, or medication of the day. Do not lie down x 30 min after dose. | ⊞C ❊> R |

| Risedronate (Actonel) | Tab: 5 mg, 30 mg, 35 mg | Treatment/Prevention: Postmenopausal: 5 mg qd or 35 mg once wkly. Glucocorticoid-Induced: 5 mg qd. Take at least 30 min before 1st food or drink of day other than water. Swallow in upright position w/ 6-8 oz of water. Do not lie down x 30 min after dose. | ⊞C ❊v R |

NAME	FORM/STRENGTH	DOSAGE	COMMENTS
CALCITONIN			
Calcitonin-Salmon (Miacalcin)	**Inj:** 200 IU/ml; **Nasal Spray:** 200 IU/spray	**Treatment: Female:** 200 IU/day (1 spray) intranasally, alternate nostrils daily; 100 IU IM/SC qod.	▧C ✿v
ESTROGEN/PROGESTIN COMBINATION			
Estradiol/ Norethindrone (Activella)	**Tab:** 1-0.5 mg	**Prevention: Female:** 1 tab qd.	▧X ✿>
Estradiol/Norgestimate (Ortho-Prefest)	**Tab:** 1 mg-none, 1 mg-0.09 mg	**Prevention: Female:** 1 mg estradiol x 3d; alternate with 1 mg-0.09 mg tab x 3d on continuous schedule.	▧X ✿v 4
Estrogens, Conjugated/ Medroxyprogesterone Acetate (Premphase, Prempro)	**Tab:** (Premphase) 0.625 mg conjugated estrogens & 0.625-5 mg; (Prempro) 0.3-1.5 mg, 0.45-1.5 mg, 0.625-2.5 mg, 0.625-5 mg	**Prevention: Female:** Treat with lowest effective dose. Adjust dose based on response.	▧X ✿> 28
Ethinyl Estradiol/ Norethindrone (Femhrt)	**Tab:** 5 mcg-1 mg .	**Prevention: Female: Usual:** 1 tab qd.	▧X ✿> 4
ESTROGENS			
Estradiol (Estrace, Gynodiol)	**Tab:** (Estrace) 0.5 mg, 1 mg, 2 mg; (Gynodiol) 0.5 mg, 1 mg, 1.5 mg, 2 mg	**Prevention: Female:** 0.5mg qd (23 days on and 5 days off)	▧X ✿v 4,10

Estradiol (Alora, Climara, Vivelle, Vivelle-Dot)	**Patch:** (Alora) 0.025 mg/d, 0.05 mg/d, 0.075 mg/d, 0.1 mg/d; (Climara) 0.025 mg/d, 0.0375 mg/d, 0.05 mg/d, 0.06 mg/d, 0.075 mg/d, 0.1 mg/d; (Vivelle, Vivelle-Dot) 0.025 mg/d, 0.0375 mg/d, 0.05 mg/d, 0.075 mg/d, 0.1 mg/d	**Prevention: Female:** (Climara) Apply 0.025 mg/d patch qwk. (Vivelle, Vivelle-Dot) 0.025 mg/d patch BIW is minimum effective dose. (Alora) Apply 0.025 mg/d patch BIW. Titrate: May increase depending on bone mineral density and adverse events.	⊙X ❄> 4
Estrogens, Conjugated (Premarin)	**Tab:** 0.3 mg, 0.45 mg, 0.625 mg, 0.9 mg, 1.25 mg, 2.5 mg	**Prevention: Female:** 0.625 mg qd given continuously or cyclically (eg, 25d on, 5d off).	⊙X ❄> 4,28
Estropipate (Ogen, Ortho-Est)	**Tab:** (Ogen, Ortho-Est) 0.625 mg (0.75 mg estropipate), 1.25 mg (1.5 mg estropipate); (Ogen) 2.5 mg (3 mg estropipate)	**Prevention: Female:** 0.625 mg (0.75 mg estropipate) qd x 25d of a 31d cycle per mth.	⊙X ❄> 4

4 Contraindicated in pregnancy. Increased risk of endometrial carcinoma in postmenopausal women.

10 Attempt to taper or d/c at 3-6 mth intervals.

28 Not for CV disease prevention. The WHI reported increased risks of MI, stroke, invasive breast cancer, pulmonary emboli, & DVT in postmenopausal women. Prescribe at lowest effective doses for shortest duration.

NAME	FORM/STRENGTH	DOSAGE	COMMENTS

PARATHYROID HORMONE

NAME	FORM/STRENGTH	DOSAGE	COMMENTS
Teriparatide [rDNA origin] (Forteo)	**Inj:** 250 mcg/ml	**Treatment in Females/Bone Mass Increase in Men:** 20 mcg qd SQ into thigh or abdominal wall. Discard pen after 28d. Use for >2 yrs is not recommended. Administer initially under circumstances where patient can sit or lie down.	●C ❄v Avoid if risk of osteosarcoma.

SERM (SELECTIVE ESTROGEN RECEPTOR MODULATOR)

NAME	FORM/STRENGTH	DOSAGE	COMMENTS
Raloxifene HCl (Evista)	**Tab:** 60 mg	**Treatment/Prevention: Female:** 60 mg qd.	●X ❄v

Thyroid Agents
THYROID HORMONES

NAME	FORM/STRENGTH	DOSAGE	COMMENTS
Levothyroxine Sodium, T4 (Levoxyl, Synthroid)	**Inj:** 0.2 mg, 0.5 mg; **Tab:** 0.025 mg, 0.05 mg, 0.075 mg, 0.088 mg, 0.1 mg, 0.112 mg, 0.125 mg, 0.137 mg, 0.15 mg, 0.175 mg, 0.2 mg, 0.3 mg	**Adults & Peds: >12 yo:** Levoxyl: 1.7 mcg/kg/d. >200 mcg/d (seldom). **Synthroid:** 1.7 mcg/kg/d. May increase by 12.5-25 mcg q6-8wks until euthyroid. >200 mcg/d (seldom). **Peds:** Synthroid/Levoxyl: 0-3 mths: 10-15 mcg/kg/d. **3-6 mths:** 8-10 mcg/kg/d. **6-12 mths:** 6-8 mcg/kg/d. **1-5 yo:** 5-6 mcg/kg/d. **6-12 yo:** 4-5 mcg/kg/d. **>12 yo:** 2-3 mcg/kg/d.	●A ❄>
Liothyronine, T3 (Cytomel)	**Tab:** 0.005 mg, 0.025 mg, 0.05 mg	**Adults: Initial:** 25 mcg qd. **Titrate:** Increase up to 25 mcg q1-2wks. **Maint:** 25-75 mcg qd. **Peds: Initial:** 5 mcg qd. **Titrate:** Increase by 5 mcg qd q3-4d until desired response. **Maint: <1 yo:** 20 mcg qd. **1-3 yo:** 50 mcg qd. **>3 yo:** 25-75 mcg/d.	●A ❄>

Liotrix, T4/T3 in 4:1 ratio (Thyrolar)	**Tab:** (1/4) 3.1-12.5 mcg, (1/2) 6.25-25 mcg, (1) 12.5-50 mcg, (2) 25-100 mcg, (3) 37.5-150 mcg	**Adults: Initial:** 6.25-25 mcg qd. **Titrate:** Increase by 3.1-12.5 mcg q2-3wks. **Usual:** 12.5-50 mcg to 25-100 mcg/d. **Peds: >12 yo:** 18.75-75 mcg qd. **6-12 yo:** 12.5-50 mcg to 18.75-75 mcg qd. **1-5 yo:** 9.35-37.5 mcg to 12.5-50 mcg qd. **6-12 mths:** 6.25-25 mcg to 9.35-37.5 mcg qd. **0-6 mths:** 3.1-12.5 mcg to 6.25-25 mcg qd.	ⓒA ❄>
Thyroid, Desiccated (Armour Thyroid)	**Tab:** 15 mg, 30 mg, 60 mg, 90 mg, 120 mg, 180 mg, 240 mg, 300 mg	**Adults: Initial:** 30 mg qd. **Titrate:** Increase by 15 mg q2-3wks. **Maint:** 60-120 mg/d. **Peds: 0-6 mths:** 4.8-6 mg/kg/d. **6-12 mths:** 3.6-4.8 mg/kg/d. **1-5 yo:** 3-3.6 mg/kg/d. **6-12 yo:** 2.4-3 mg/kg/d. **>12 yo:** 1.2-1.8 mg/kg/d.	ⓒA ❄>
Thyrotropin alfa (Thyrogen)	**Inj:** 1.1 mg	**Adults & Peds: ≥16 yo: Thyroglobulin Testing:** 0.9 mg IM q24h x 2 doses or q72h x 3 doses into buttock.	ⓒC ❄>

Miscellaneous
BONE RESORPTION INHIBITOR

Pamidronate Disodium (Aredia)	**Inj:** 30 mg, 90 mg	**Adults: Moderate Hypercalcemia:** 60-90 mg IV single dose over 4-24h. **Severe Hypercalcemia:** 90 mg IV single dose over 24h. **Retreatment:** May repeat after 7d. **Paget's Disease:** 30 mg IV over 4h x 3d. **Osteolytic Bone Lesions of Multiple Myeloma:** 90 mg IV over 4h once monthly. **Osteolytic Bone Metastases of Breast Cancer:** 90 mg IV over 2h q3-4wks. **Max:** 90 mg/single dose for all indications.	ⓒD ❄> R

NAME	FORM/STRENGTH	DOSAGE	COMMENTS

XANTHINE OXIDASE INHIBITORS

NAME	FORM/STRENGTH	DOSAGE	COMMENTS
Allopurinol Sodium (Aloprim)	**Inj:** 500 mg	**Elevated Serum/Urinary Uric Acid Levels: Adults:** **Initial:** 200-400 mg/m²/d IV as qd or in divided doses every 6, 8, or 12h. **Max:** 600 mg/d. **Ped: Initial:** 200 mg/m²/d IV as qd or in divided doses every 6, 8, or 12h.	●C ❄> R

GASTROINTESTINAL AGENTS

Antidiarrheal Agents

NAME	FORM/STRENGTH	DOSAGE	COMMENTS
Atropine Sulfate/Difenoxin HCl CIV (Motofen)	**Tab:** 0.025-1 mg	**Adults & Peds:** ≥12 yo: **Usual:** 2 tabs, then 1 tab after each loose BM or q3-4h prn. **Max:** 8 tabs/24h.	●C ❄v
Atropine Sulfate/ Diphenoxylate HCl CV (Lomotil)	**Liq:** 0.025 mg-2.5 mg/5 ml; **Tab:** 0.025 mg-2.5 mg	**Adults: Initial:** 2 tabs or 10 ml qid. **Maint:** 2 tabs or 10 ml tid. **Max:** 20 mg diphenoxylate/d. **2-12 yo: Initial:** 0.3-0.4 mg/kg/d given qid. **13-16 yo: Initial:** 2 tabs or 10 ml qd. **Maint:** 1/4 of initial daily dose.	●C ❄>
Attapulgite (Kaopectate)	**Liq:** 750 mg/15 ml; **Tab:** 750 mg	≥12 yo: 1500 mg after loose BM. **Max:** 6 doses/d. 6-12 yo: 750 mg after loose BM. **Max:** 6 doses/d.	●N ❄>
Bismuth Subsalicylate (Pepto-Bismol)	**Chewtab:** 262 mg; **Susp:** 262 mg/15 ml, 525 mg/15 ml; **Tab:** 262 mg	**Adults:** 2 tabs or 30 ml q0.5-1h. **9-12 yo: Tab:** 1 tab q0.5-1h or 15 ml q1h. **6-9 yo:** 2/3 tab q0.5-1h or 10 ml q1h. **3-6 yo:** 1/3 tab q0.5-1h or 5 ml q1h. **Max:** 8 doses/d (reg str.), 4 doses/d (max str.).	●N ❄>

| Loperamide (Imodium A-D) | **Liq:** 1 mg/ 5 ml; **Tab:** 2 mg | **≥12 yo:** 4 mg after 1st loose BM, then 2 mg after loose BM. **Max:** 8 mg/d. **9-11 yo (60-95 lbs):** 2 mg after 1st loose BM, then 1 mg after loose BM. **Max:** 6 mg/d. **6-8 yo (48-59 lbs):** 2 mg after 1st loose BM, then 1 mg after loose BM. **Max:** 4 mg/d. **2-5 yo (24-47 lbs):** 1 mg after 1st loose BM, then 1 mg after loose BM. **Max:** 3 mg/d. | ◉N ✿> |

Antiemetics

5-HT₃ ANTAGONISTS

| Dolasetron Mesylate (Anzemet) | **Inj:** 20 mg/ml; **Tab:** 50 mg, 100 mg | **Prevent Chemo N/V: Adults:** 1.8 mg/kg IV or 100 mg IV/PO. **2-16 yo:** 1.8 mg/kg IV/PO, up to 100 mg IV/PO. Give IV 30 min before or PO within 1h before chemo. **Prevent Post-op N/V: Adults:** 12.5 mg IV or 100 mg PO. **2-16 yo:** 0.35 mg/kg IV, up to 12.5 mg IV; or 1.2 mg/kg PO, up to 100 mg PO. Give PO within 2h pre-op, IV 15 min before anesthesia cessation or at start of n/v. **Treat Post-op N/V: Adults:** 12.5 mg IV. **2-16 yo:** 0.35 mg/kg IV up to 12.5 mg IV. | ◉B ✿> |
| Granisetron HCl (Kytril) | **Inj:** 1 mg/ml; **Sol:** 2 mg/10 ml; **Tab:** 1 mg | **Prevent Chemo N/V: Adults & Peds 2-16 yo: IV:** 10 mcg/kg within 30 min before chemo. **Adults: PO:** 2 mg qd up to 1h before chemo or 1 mg bid (up to 1h before chemo & 12h later). **Prevent Radiation N/V: Adults: PO:** 2 mg qd within 1h of radiation. **Prevent Post-Op N/V: Adults: IV:** 1 mg over 30 sec before anesthesia induction or immediately before anesthesia reversal. **Treat Post-Op N/V: Adults: IV:** 1 mg over 30 sec. | ◉B ✿> |

NAME	FORM/STRENGTH	DOSAGE	COMMENTS
Ondansetron HCl (Zofran)	**Inj:** 2 mg/ml, 32 mg/50 ml; **Sol:** 4 mg/5 ml; **Tab:** 4 mg, 8 mg, 24 mg; **Tab, Dissolve:** 4 mg, 8 mg	**Prevent Chemo N/V: Adults (>18 yo):** single 32 mg dose IV over 15 min, 30 min before chemo or three 0.15 mg/kg doses IV over 15 min, 1st dose 30 min before chemo with subsequent doses given 4 & 8h after 1st dose. **4-18 yo:** Three 0.15 mg/kg doses IV over 15 min, 1st dose 30 min before chemo with subsequent doses given 4 & 8h after 1st dose. **Prevent Highly Emetogenic Chemo N/V: Adults:** 24 mg tab PO 30 min before chemo. **Prevent Moderate Emetogenic Chemo N/V: ≥12 yo:** 8 mg PO 30 min before chemo, then 8h after 1st dose, then 8 mg bid x 1-2d. **4-11 yo:** 4 mg PO 30 min before chemo, then 4 & 8h after 1st dose, then 4 mg tid x 1-2d. **Prevent Post-Op N/V: Adults:** 16 mg PO 1h before anesthesia. **>12 yo:** 4 mg IV/IM immediately before anesthesia or post-op. **2-12 yo:** 0.1 mg/kg IV single dose for ≤40 kg, and 4 mg IV single dose for >40 kg. **Prevent Radiation N/V: Adults: Usual:** 8 mg PO tid. **Total Body Irradiation:** 8 mg PO 1-2h before therapy daily. **Single High-Dose Therapy To Abdomen:** 8 mg PO 1-2h before therapy then q8h after 1st dose x 1-2d after complete therapy. **Daily Fractionated Therapy To Abdomen:** 8 mg PO 1-2h before therapy then q8h after 1st dose. **Severe Hepatic Dysfunction: Max:** 8 mg/d IV single dose 30 min before chemo or 8 mg/d PO.	▣B ❄> H

Palonosetron HCl (Aloxi)	Inj: 0.25 mg/5 ml	Adults: 0.25 mg IV single dose 30 mins before chemo. Repeated dosing within a 7d interval is not recommended.	▣B ❀v

ANTICHOLINERGICS

Scopolamine (Transderm Scop)	Patch: 0.33 mg/24h	Adults: Motion Sickness: 1 patch behind ear 4h prior to event. Replace after 3d. Prevent Post-op N/V: 1 patch x 24h post-op.	▣C ❀>
Trimethobenzamide (Tigan)	Cap: 300 mg; Inj: 100 mg/ml; Sup: 100 mg, 200 mg	Nausea in Gastroenteritis/Post-op N/V: Adults: Cap: 300 mg tid-qid. Inj: 200 mg IM tid-qid. Sup: 200 mg tid-qid. Pediatrics: Sup: 30-90 lbs: 100-200 mg tid-qid. <30 lbs: 100 mg tid-qid.	▣N ❀>

ANTIHISTAMINES

Dimenhydrinate (Dramamine)	Chewtab: 50 mg; Tab: 50 mg	Motion Sickness: Adults: 1-2 tabs q4-6h. Max: 400 mg/24h. 6-12 yo: 1/2-1 tab q6-8h. Max: 150 mg/24h. 2-6 yo: 1/4-1/2 tab q6-8h. Max: 75 mg/24h.	▣N ❀>
Hydroxyzine Pamoate (Vistaril)	Inj: 50 mg/ml	Prevent Post-op N/V: Adults: 25-100 mg IM. Peds: 0.5 mg/lb IM.	▣N ❀v Cl in early pregnancy.
Meclizine HCl (Antivert)	Tab: 12.5 mg, 25 mg, 50 mg	Adults & Peds: ≥12 yo: Vertigo: Usual: 25-100 mg/d in divided doses. Motion Sickness: 25-50 mg 1h before trip/departure; repeat q24h prn.	▣B ❀>

NAME	FORM/STRENGTH	DOSAGE	COMMENTS
Prochlorperazine (Compazine)	**Cap,ER:** 10 mg, 15 mg; **Inj:** 5 mg/ml; **Sup:** 2.5 mg, 5 mg, 25 mg; **Syr:** 5 mg/5 ml; **Tab:** 5 mg, 10 mg	**Severe N/V: Adults: PO:** 5-10 mg tab tid-qid; 10 mg cap q12h; 15 mg cap on arising. **PR:** 25 mg sup bid. **IM:** 5-10 mg 3-4h prn. **IV:** 2.5-10 mg (slow push). **Max:** 10 mg/IV single dose; 40 mg/d PO/IM/IV. **Peds: >2 yo & >20lbs: PO/PR: 20-29 lbs:** 2.5 mg qd-bid. **Max:** 7.5 mg/d. **30-39 lbs:** 2.5 mg bid-tid. **Max:** 10 mg/d. **40-85 lbs:** 2.5 mg tid or 5 mg bid. **Max:** 15 mg/d. **IM:** 0.06 mg/lb. **N/V with Surgery: Adults: IM/IV:** 5-10 mg IM 1-2h or 5-10 mg IV 15-30 min before anesthesia, or during or after surgery; repeat once if needed.	⊙N ✲>
Promethazine (Phenergan)	**Inj:** 25 mg/ml, 50 mg/ml; **Sup:** 12.5 mg, 25 mg, 50 mg; **Syr:** 6.25 mg/5 ml; **Tab:** 12.5 mg, 25 mg, 50 mg	**Prevent N/V & Post-op N/V: Adults:** 12.5-25 mg IM/IV q4h; 25 mg PO/PR initially, then 12.5-25 mg q4-6h prn. **Peds: ≥2 yo:** 0.5 mg/lb PO/PR/IM/IV q4-6h prn.	⊙C ✲>

DOPAMINE ANTAGONIST/PROKINETIC

NAME	FORM/STRENGTH	DOSAGE	COMMENTS
Metoclopramide (Reglan)	**Inj:** 5 mg/ml; **Syr:** 5 mg/5 ml; **Tab:** 5 mg, 10 mg	**Adults: Prevent Chemo N/V:** 1-2 mg/kg 30 min before chemo, then q2h x 2 doses, then q3h x 3 doses. **Prevent Post-op N/V:** 10-20 mg IM near end of surgery.	⊙B ✲> R

SUBSTANCE P/NEUROKININ 1 RECEPTOR ANTAGONIST

| Aprepitant (Emend) | Tab: 80 mg, 125 mg | Adults: Day 1: 125 mg 1h prior to chemotherapy. Days 2 & 3: 80 mg qam. Regimen should include a corticosteroid and a 5-HT$_3$ antagonist. Concomitant Corticosteroid: Reduce dexamethasone PO or methylprednisolone PO by 50% and methylprednisolone IV by 25%. | ◉B ❋> |

MISCELLANEOUS

| Dronabinol CIII (Marinol) | Cap: 2.5 mg, 5 mg, 10 mg | Adults & Peds: Prevent Chemo N/V: 5 mg/m² 1-3h before chemo, then 2-4h after chemo, up to 4-6 doses/d. Titrate: May increase by 2.5 mg/m² increments. Max: 15 mg/m²/dose. | ◉C ❋v |
| Droperidol (Inapsine) | Inj: 2.5 mg/ml | Premed for Surgery/Diagnostic Procedures: Adults: Initial (Max): 2.5 mg IM/IV. May give additional 1.25 mg cautiously for desired effect. Peds: 2-12 yo: Initial (Max): 0.1 mg/kg IM/IV. May give additional dose cautiously. | ◉C ❋> QT prolongation. Torsade de pointes. Arrhythmias. |

Antispasmodics

| Atropine Sulfate/ Hyoscyamine Sulfate/ Phenobarbital/Scopolamine (Donnatal) | Tab/Eli (per 5 ml): 0.0194 mg-0.1037 mg-16.2 mg-0.0065 mg | Adults: 1-2 tabs or 5-10 ml tid-qid. Peds: 10 lbs: 0.5 ml q4h or 0.75 ml q6h. 20 lbs: 1 ml q4h or 1.5 ml q6h. 30 lbs: 1.5 ml q4h or 2 ml q6h. 50 lbs: 2.5 ml q4h or 3.75 ml q6h. 75 lbs: 3.75 ml q4h or 5 ml q6h. 100 lbs: 5 ml q4h or 7.5 ml q6h. | ◉C ❋> H |

NAME	FORM/STRENGTH	DOSAGE	COMMENTS
Atropine Sulfate/ Hyoscyamine Sulfate/ Phenobarbital/Scopolamine (Donnatal Extentabs)	**Tab:** 0.0582 mg- 0.3111 mg-48.6 mg- 0.0195 mg	**Adults:** 1 tab q8-12h.	▣C ❄> H
Atropine/Hyoscyamine/ Phenobarbital (Arco-Lase Plus)	**Tab:** 0.02 mg-0.10 mg- 1/8 gr	**Adults:** 1 tab after meals.	▣N ❄>
Chlordiazepoxide HCl/ Clidinium (Librax)	**Tab:** 5 mg-2.5 mg	**Adults: Usual:** 1-2 caps tid-qid ac & qhs.	▣N ❄>
Dicyclomine HCl (Bentyl)	**Cap:** 10 mg; **Inj:** 10 mg/ml; **Syr:** 10 mg/ 5 ml; **Tab:** 20 mg	**Adults: Initial: PO:** 20 mg qid. **Maint:** 40 mg qid if tolerated. **IM:** 20 qid x 1-2d, followed by PO dose.	▣B ❄v
Hyoscyamine Sulfate (Cystospaz)	**Tab:** 0.15 mg	**Adults:** 0.15-0.3 mg qid prn.	▣C ❄>
Hyoscyamine Sulfate (IB-Stat)	**Spray:** 0.125 mg/spray	**Adults & Peds:** ≥ 12 yo: 1-2 sprays q4h or prn. **Max:** 12 sprays/24h.	▣C ❄>
Hyoscyamine Sulfate (Levbid, Levsin, Levsinex, NuLev)	**(Levbid) Tab,ER:** 0.375 mg; **(Levsin) Drops:** 0.125 mg/ml; **Eli:** 0.125 mg/5 ml; **Inj:** 0.5 mg/ml; **Tab:** 0.125 mg; **Tab,SL:** 0.125 mg; **(Levsinex) Cap,ER:**	**Adults & Peds** ≥12 yo: Drops/Eli/ODT/Tab/Tab, SL: 0.125-0.25 mg q4h or prn. **Max:** 1.5 mg/24h. **Cap, Tab,ER:** 0.375-0.75 mg q12h; or 1 cap q8h. **Max:** 1.5 mg/24h. **2 to <12 yo:** ODT/Tab/Tab,SL: 0.0625-0.125 mg q4h or prn. **Max:** 0.75 mg/24h. **Eli:** Give q4h or prn. **10 kg:** 1.25 ml. **20 kg:** 2.5 ml. **40 kg:** 3.75 ml. **50 kg:** 5 ml. **Max:** 30 ml/24h. **Drops:** 0.25-1 ml q4h or prn. **Max:** 6 ml/24h.	▣C ❄>

	0.375 mg; (NuLev) Tab,Dissolve (ODT): 0.125 mg	<2 yo: Drops: Give q4h or prn. 3.4 kg: 4 drops. Max: 24 drops/24h. 5 kg: 5 drops. Max: 30 drops/24h. 7 kg: 6 drops. Max: 36 drops/24h. 10 kg: 8 drops. Max: 48 drops/24h.	
Propantheline Bromide	Tab: 15 mg	Adults: 15 mg (tid 30 min ac), & 30 mg qhs (total 75 mg/d).	◙C ❄>

Antiulcer Agents

Helicobacter pylori TREATMENT REGIMENS*

MEDICATION/DOSE	FREQUENCY
PPI**+ 1 gm amoxicillin bid + 500 mg clarithromycin bid	10-14d (7d with rabeprazole)
PPI+ 500 mg metronidazole + 500 mg clarithromycin	bid x 2 wks
RBC (400 mg ranitidine bismuth citrate) + 500 mg clarithromycin +1 gm amoxicillin OR 500 mg metronidazole OR 500 mg tetracycline	bid x 2 wks
BSS*** qid + 500 mg metronidazole tid + 500 mg tetracycline qid + PPI qd	as indicated x 2 wks
BSS + 250 mg metronidazole qid + 500 mg tetracycline qid + H$_2$ receptor antagonist qd	as indicated x 2 wks, & continue H$_2$R antagonist x 2 wks

*Suggested regimens for the treatment of *H. pylori* infection. Not all of the above regimens are FDA-approved.
Am J Gastroenterol 1998; 93: 2330-2338.
**PPI= esomeprazole 40 mg qd, lansoprazole 30 mg bid, omeprazole 20 mg bid, rabeprazole 20 mg bid, or pantoprazole 40 mg bid
***BSS=bismuth subsalicylate 525 mg

NAME	FORM/STRENGTH	DOSAGE	COMMENTS
ANTICHOLINERGICS			
Methscopolamine Bromide (Pamine, Pamine Forte)	**Tab:** (Pamine) 2.5 mg; (Pamine Forte) 5 mg	**Adults:** 2.5 mg 1/2 hr before meals and 2.5-5 mg hs. **Severe Symptoms:** 5 mg 1/2 hr before meals and 5 mg hs. May increase to 30 mg daily. Reduce dose to eliminate/modify side effects.	■C ✿>
DUODENAL ULCER ADHERENT COMPLEX			
Sucralfate (Carafate)	**Susp:** 1 gm/10 ml; **Tab:** 1 gm	**Adults: Active Ulcer:** Sus/Tab: 1 gm qid x 4-8 wks. **Maint:** Tab: 1 gm bid.	■B ✿>
H₂ ANTAGONISTS			
Cimetidine (Tagamet)	**Cap:** 150 mg, 300 mg; **Inj:** 150 mg/ml, 300 mg/50 ml; **Sol:** 300 mg/5 ml; **Tab:** 200 mg, 300 mg, 400 mg, 800 mg	**≥16 yo: PO: Active DU:** 800 mg qhs or 300 mg qid or 400 mg bid x 4-8 wks. **Maint:** 400 mg qhs. **Active Benign GU:** 800 mg qhs or 300 mg qid x 6 wks. **IM/IV:** 300 mg q6-8h. **Max:** 2400 mg/d.	■B ✿v R
Famotidine (Pepcid, Pepcid RPD)	**Inj:** 0.4 mg/ml, 10 mg/ml; **Susp:** 40 mg/5 ml; **Tab:** 20 mg, 40 mg; **Tab, Dissolve:** 20 mg, 40 mg	**Adults: DU:** 20 mg IV q12h; 20 mg PO bid or 40 mg PO qhs x 4-8 wks. **Maint:** 20 mg PO bid up to 6 wks. **1-16 yo: DU/GU:** 0.25 mg/kg IV/PO q12h or 0.5 mg/kg/d PO qhs. **Max:** 40 mg/d.	■B ✿v R
Nizatidine (Axid)	**Cap:** 150 mg, 300 mg	**Adults:** 150 mg bid or 300 mg qhs up to 8 wks. **Maint:** 150 mg qhs up to 1 yr.	■B ✿v R

| **Ranitidine HCl** (Zantac) | **Cap:** 150 mg, 300 mg;
Inj: 1 mg/ml, 25 mg/ml;
Pkt: 150 mg;
Syr: 15 mg/ml;
Tab: 150 mg, 300 mg;
Tab,Eff: 25 mg, 150 mg | **Adults: GU/DU: PO:** 150 mg bid, or (DU) 300 mg after evening meal or qhs. **Maint:** 150 mg qhs. **IV/IM:** 50 mg q6-8h. **Continuous IV:** 6.25 mg/h. **Max:** 400 mg/d.
1 mth-16 yo: GU/DU: PO: 2-4 mg/kg bid.
Max: 300 mg/d. **Maint:** 2-4 mg/kg qd. **Max:** 150 mg/d.
DU: IV: 2-4 mg/kg/d given q6-8h. **Max:** 50 mg q6-8h. | ⊙B ❄> R |

NSAID/PROTON PUMP INHIBITOR

| **Lansoprazole-Naproxen**
(Prevacid NapraPAC) | **Cap, Delay:** 15 mg-375 mg; 15 mg-500 mg | **Adults:** 1 tab Naproxen + 1 cap Lansoprazole qam, before eating + 1 tab Naproxen qpm. **Max:** 1000 mg Naproxen/day. Take naproxen with full glass of water. Swallow lansoprazole whole. | ⊙B ❄v H R |

PROSTAGLANDIN E₁ ANALOG

| **Misoprostol** (Cytotec) | **Tab:** 100 mcg, 200 mcg | **Adults: NSAID Ulcer Prevention:** 200 mcg qid w/ food. May use 100 mcg dose if 200 mcg not tolerated. | ⊙X ❄v
Abortifacient. |

PROTON PUMP INHIBITORS

| **Lansoprazole**
(Prevacid) | **Cap, Delay:** 15 mg, 30 mg; **Susp:** 15 mg, 30 mg (granules/pkt);
Tab, Disintegrating (SoluTab): 15 mg, 30 mg. | **Adults: DU:** 15 mg qd x 4 wks. **Maint:** 15 mg qd.
GU: 30 mg qd up to 8 wks. | ⊙B ❄v H |
| **Omeprazole** (Prilosec) | **Cap,Delay:** 10 mg, 20 mg, 40 mg | **Adults: DU:** 20 mg qd x 4-8 wks.
GU: 40 mg qd x 4-8 wks. | ⊙C ❄v |

NAME	FORM/STRENGTH	DOSAGE	COMMENTS
Rabeprazole Sodium (Aciphex)	Tab, Delay: 20 mg	Adults: DU Treatment: 20 mg qd up to 4 wks.	⊙B ✿v

GERD

DOPAMINE ANTAGONIST/PROKINETIC

Metoclopramide (Reglan)	Syr: 5 mg/5 ml; Tab: 5 mg, 10 mg	Adults: 10-15 mg qid 30 min ac & qhs. Max: 12 wks of therapy. Intermittent Symptoms: Up to 20 mg single dose prior to provoking situation.	⊙B ✿> R

H₂ ANTAGONISTS

Cimetidine (Tagamet)	Sol: 300 mg/5 ml; Tab: 200 mg, 300 mg, 400 mg, 800 mg	≥16 yo: 400 mg PO qid, or 800 mg PO bid x 12 wks.	⊙B ✿v R
Famotidine (Pepcid)	Inj: 0.4 mg/ml, 10 mg/ml; Susp: 40 mg/5 ml; Tab: 20 mg, 40 mg; Tab, Dissolve: 20 mg, 40 mg	Adults: 20 mg IV q12h; 20 mg PO bid up to 6 wks. Esophagitis: 20-40 mg PO bid up to 12 wks. Peds: 1-16 yo: 0.25 mg/kg IV q12h (up to 40 mg/d) or 0.5 mg/kg PO bid (up to 40 mg bid). GERD: 3 mths-1 yo: 0.5 mg/kg PO bid for up to 8 wks. <3 mths: 0.5 mg/kg PO qd for up to 8 wks.	⊙B ✿v R
Nizatidine (Axid, Axid Oral Solution)	Cap: 150 mg, 300 mg; Sol: 15 mg/ml	Adults: 150 mg bid up to 12 wks. Peds: ≥12 yo: Erosive Esophagitis/GERD: Sol: 150 mg bid up to 8 wks. Max: 300 mg/d.	⊙B ✿v R

| Ranitidine HCl (Zantac) | Cap: 150 mg, 300 mg; Inj: 1 mg/ml, 25 mg/ml; Pkt: 150 mg; Syr: 15 mg/ml; Tab: 150 mg, 300 mg; Tab,Eff: 25 mg, 150 mg | Adults: PO: Symptomatic: 150 mg bid. Erosive Esophagitis: 150 mg qid. Maint: 150 mg bid. IV/IM: 50 mg q6-8h. Continuous IV: 6.25 mg/h. Max: 400 mg/d. 1 mth-16 yo: Symptomatic/Erosive Esophagitis: 2.5-5 mg/kg PO bid. | ▣B ❄> R |

PROTON PUMP INHIBITORS

Esomeprazole Magnesium (Nexium)	Cap,Delay: 20 mg, 40 mg	Adults: Symptomatic: 20 mg qd x 4 wks; additional 4 wks with continued symptoms. Erosive Esophagitis: 20-40 mg qd x 4-8 wks; additional 4-8 wks if not healed. Maint: 20 mg qd up to 6 mths.	▣B ❄v H
Lansoprazole (Prevacid, Prevacid I.V.)	Cap, Delay: 15 mg, 30 mg; Inj: 30 mg; Susp: 15 mg, 30 mg (granules/pkt); Tab, Disintegrating (SoluTab): 15 mg, 30 mg.	Adults: PO: Symptomatic: 15 mg qd up to 8 wks. Erosive Esophagitis: 30 mg qd up to 8 wks. May repeat x 8 wks if needed. Maint: 15 mg qd. Peds: 1-11 yo: Symptomatic/Erosive Esophagitis: ≤30 kg: 15 mg qd for up to 12 wks. >30 kg: 30 mg qd for up to 12 wks. Titrate: May increase up to 30 mg bid after 2 wks prn. IV: Erosive Esophagitis: 30 mg/d for up to 7d. Switch to PO when possible.	▣B ❄v H
Omeprazole (Prilosec)	Cap,Delay: 10 mg, 20 mg, 40 mg	Adults: Symptomatic: 20 mg qd up to 4 wks. Erosive Esophagitis: 20 mg qd x 4-8 wks. Maint: 20 mg qd. Peds: ≥2 yo: GERD/Erosive Esophagitis: >20 kg: 20 mg qd. <20 kg: 10 mg qd.	▣C ❄v

NAME	FORM/STRENGTH	DOSAGE	COMMENTS
Pantoprazole Sodium (Protonix)	**Inj:** 40 mg; **Tab,Delay:** 20 mg, 40 mg	**Adults: PO: Erosive Esophagitis:** 40 mg qd up to 8 wks. May repeat course. **Maint:** 40 mg qd. **IV: GERD:** 40 mg qd x 7-10d.	⬤B ❄v
Rabeprazole Sodium (Aciphex)	**Tab, Delay:** 20 mg	**Adults: Erosive/Ulcerative GERD: Healing:** 20 mg qd x 4-8 wks. May repeat x 8 wks if needed. **Maint:** 20 mg qd. **Symptomatic GERD:** 20 mg qd x 4 wks. May repeat x 4 wks if needed.	⬤B ❄v

Laxatives

BOWEL EVACUANTS

NAME	FORM/STRENGTH	DOSAGE	COMMENTS
Polyethylene Glycol with Electrolytes (Colyte)	**Pow for Sol:** 3754 ml, 4000 ml	**Adults: GI Exam Prep: PO** 240 ml q10min until fecal discharge is clear. **NG Tube:** 20-30 ml/min (1.2-1.8 L/h).	⬤C ❄>
Sodium Phosphate/ Disodium Phosphate (Visicol)	**Tab:** 1.102-0.398 gm	**Adults: Colonoscopy:** Evening before exam, 3 tabs with 8 oz clear liquids q15min for total of 20 tabs (last dose is 2 tabs). Repeat day of exam 3-5h before procedure. May retreat after 7d.	⬤C ❄>

BULK-FORMING AGENTS

NAME	FORM/STRENGTH	DOSAGE	COMMENTS
Calcium Polycarbophil (FiberCon)	**Tab:** 625 mg	**Adults & Peds: ≥12 yo:** 2 tabs qd. **Max:** 2 tabs qid. **6-12 yo:** 1 tab qd. **Max:** 1 tab qid.	⬤N ❄>
Methylcellulose (Citrucel)	**Pow:** 2 gm/heaping tbs; **Tab:** 500 mg	**Adults & Peds ≥12 yo:** 1 heaping tbs up to tid, or 2 tabs up to 6x/d. **6-12 yo:** 1/2 tbs qd or 1 tab up to 6x/d. Dissolve pow in 8 oz of cold water & follow pow/tabs with additional glass of water.	⬤N ❄>

Psyllium (Metamucil)	**Pow:** 3.4 gm psyllium husk/dose	**Adults & Peds ≥12 yo:** 1 tsp, 1 tbs, or 1 pkt (depending on product). **6-12 yo:** 1/2 adult dose. May take qd-tid. Mix with 8 oz of liquid.	◉N ❄>

COLONIC ACIDIFIER

Lactulose (Constulose, Enulose)	**Sol:** 10 gm/15 ml	**Adults:** 15-30 ml qd. **Max:** 60 ml/d.	◉B ❄>

EMOLLIENT LAXATIVE

Mineral Oil (Fleet Mineral Oil Enema)	**Enema:** 118 ml/bottle	**Adults & Peds: ≥12 yo:** 1 dose/bottle PR. **2-12 yo:** 1/2 dose/bottle PR.	◉N ❄>

OSMOTIC AGENT

Polyethylene Glycol (MiraLax)	**Powder:** 17 gm/tbs	**Adults:** Dissolve 17 gm in 8 oz of water, juice, soda, coffee, or tea x drink qd up to 2 wks.	◉C ❄>

SALINE LAXATIVES

Magnesium Citrate (Citrate of Magnesia)	**Liq:** 10 oz bottle	**Adults:** Drink 240 ml prn. **Peds:** Drink 120 ml; repeat if necessary.	◉N ❄>
Magnesium Hydroxide (Milk of Magnesia)	**Liq:** 400 mg/5 ml	**Adults & Peds: ≥12 yo:** 30-60 ml qhs or qam. **6-11 yo:** 15-30 ml. **2-5 yo:** 5-15 ml.	◉N ❄>

NAME	FORM/STRENGTH	DOSAGE	COMMENTS
Sodium Biphosphate (Fleet Phospho-Soda, Fleet Enema)	**Sol:** (Phospho-Soda) 1.5 oz, 3 oz; **Enema:** (Adult) 4.5 oz, (Ped) 2.25 oz	**Phospho-Soda: Adults & Peds: ≥12 yo:** 20-45 ml. **10-11 yo:** 10-20 ml. **5-9 yo:** 5-10 ml. Dilute dose w/ 4 oz clear liquid, then follow w/ 8 oz clear liquid. Take on empty stomach in the morning at least 30 min before a meal or hs. **Enema: ≥12 yo:** (Adult Enema) 1 bottle PR. **5-11 yo:** (Ped Enema) 1 bottle PR. **2 to <5 yo:** (Ped Enema) Use 1/2 bottle PR.	●N ✿>

STIMULANT/STOOL SOFTENERS

NAME	FORM/STRENGTH	DOSAGE	COMMENTS
Casanthranol/Docusate Sodium (Peri-Colace)	**Cap:** 30 mg-100 mg; **Syr:** 10 mg-20 mg/5 ml	**Adults:** 1-2 caps or 15-30 ml qhs. **Severe:** 2 caps or 30 ml bid, or 3 caps qhs. **Peds:** 5-15 ml qhs.	●N ✿>

STIMULANTS

NAME	FORM/STRENGTH	DOSAGE	COMMENTS
Bisacodyl (Dulcolax)	**Sup:** 10 mg; **Tab:** 5 mg	**Adults & Peds ≥12 yo:** 2-3 tabs or 1 sup qd as single dose. **6-12 yo:** 1 tab or 1/2 sup qd.	●N ✿>
Cascara Sagrada	**Liq:** 120 ml; **Tab:** 325 mg	**Adults:** 1 tab or 5 ml qhs.	●N ✿>
Castor Oil (Purge)	**Liq:** (Purge) 95%	**Adults: Usual:** 15-60 ml. **Peds: 2-12 yo:** 5-15 ml.	●N ✿>
Senna (Senokot, SenokotXTRA)	**Granules:** 15 mg/tsp; **Tab:** 8.6 mg, 17 mg	**Adults & Peds ≥12 yo:** 2 tabs or 1 tsp qd. **Max:** 4 tabs or 2 tsp bid. **6-12 yo:** 1 tab or 1/2 tsp qd. **Max:** 2 tabs or 1 tsp bid. **2-6 yo:** 1/2 tab or 1/4 tsp qd. **Max:** 1 tab or 1/2 tsp bid. SenokotXTRA dose is 1/2 of reg str tab.	●N ✿>

Docusate Calcium (Surfak)	Cap: 240 mg	Adults & Peds ≥12 yo: 240 mg qd until bowel movement.	ⓒN ❄>
Docusate Sodium (Colace)	Cap: 50 mg, 100 mg; Liq: 10 mg/ml; Syr: 20 mg/5 ml	Adults & Peds ≥12 yo: 50-200 mg qd. 6-12 yo: 40-120 mg/d Liq. 3-6 yo: 2 ml Liq tid. Mix Liq/Syr with 6-8 oz of milk, juice or formula. Retention/Flushing Enemas: Add 5-10 ml Liq to enema fluid.	ⓒN ❄>
Glycerin (Fleet Glycerin Suppositories, Fleet Babylax, Fleet Liquid Glycerin Suppository)	Enema: (Babylax) 2.3 gm; Sup: (Child) 1 gm, (Adult) 2 gm, (Adult Max Strength) 3 gm; Liquid Glycerin Sup: 5.6 gm	Adults & Peds: ≥6 yo: 1 Liq Sup (5.6 gm) or 1 sup (2 or 3 gm) PR. 2-6 yo: 1 Babylax (2.3 gm) or 1 sup (1 gm) PR.	ⓒN ❄>

Ulcerative Colitis

ANTI-INFLAMMATORY/IMMUNOMODULATORY AGENTS

| Sulfasalazine (Azulfidine, Azulfidine EN-tabs) | Tab: 500 mg; Tab,Enteric: 500 mg | Adults: Initial: 1-4 gm/d in divided doses. Maint: 2 gm/d. ≥2 yo: 40-60 mg/kg/24h divided in 3-6 doses. Maint: 7.5 mg/kg qid. | ⓒB ❄> |

SALICYLATES

| Balsalazide Disodium (Colazal) | Cap: 750 mg | Adults: 2250 mg tid x 8 wks (up to 12 wks if needed). | ⓒB ❄> |

NAME	FORM/STRENGTH	DOSAGE	COMMENTS
Mesalamine (Asacol, Canasa, Pentasa, Rowasa)	Cap,ER: (Pentasa) 250 mg; Enema: (Rowasa) 4 gm/60 ml; Sup: (Canasa) 500 mg; Tab: (Asacol) 400 mg	**Adults: Asacol: Active Ulcerative Colitis:** 800 mg PO tid x 6 wks. **Remission Maint:** 1.6 gm/d in divided doses. **Canasa:** 500 mg PR bid; retain x 1-3h. Increase to tid after 2 wks if inadequate response. **Rowasa:** 4 gm enema qhs x 3-6 wks; retain x 8h. **Pentasa:** 1 gm PO qid up to 8 wks.	▣B ❀>
Olsalazine Sodium (Dipentum)	Cap: 250 mg	**Adults:** 500 mg bid.	▣C ❀>

Zollinger-Ellison Agents

H_2 ANTAGONISTS

NAME	FORM/STRENGTH	DOSAGE	COMMENTS
Cimetidine (Tagamet)	Inj: 150 mg/ml, 300 mg/50ml; Sol: 300 mg/5 ml; Tab: 200 mg, 300 mg, 400 mg, 800 mg	**Adults: PO:** 300 mg qid. **Max:** 2400 mg/d. **IM/IV:** 300 mg q6-8h. **Max:** 2400 mg/d.	▣B ❀v R
Famotidine (Pepcid)	Inj: 0.4 mg/ml, 10 mg/ml; Susp: 40 mg/5 ml; Tab: 20 mg, 40 mg; Tab, Dissolve: 20 mg, 40 mg	**Adults: PO: Initial:** 20 mg q6h. **Max:** 160 mg q6h. **IV:** 20 mg IV q12h or greater if required.	▣B ❀v R

| Ranitidine HCl (Zantac) | Cap: 150 mg, 300 mg; Inj: 1 mg/ml, 25 mg/ml; Pkt: 150 mg; Syr: 15 mg/ml; Tab: 150 mg, 300 mg; Tab,Eff: 150 mg | Adults: PO: 150 mg bid. May give up to 6 gm/d with severe disease. IM/IV (Intermittent): 50 mg q6-8h. IV (Continuous): 1 mg/kg/h IV. Titrate: May increase after 4 hrs by 0.5 mg/kg/h increments. Max: 2.5 mg/kg/h or 220 mg/h. | ⊞B ✿> R |

PROTON PUMP INHIBITORS

Lansoprazole (Prevacid)	Cap, Delay: 15 mg, 30 mg; Susp: 15 mg, 30 mg (granules/pkt); Tab, Disintegrating (SoluTab): 15 mg, 30 mg.	Adults: 60 mg qd. Max: 90 mg bid. Divide dose if >120 mg/d.	⊞B ✿v H
Omeprazole (Prilosec)	Cap,Delay: 10 mg, 20 mg, 40 mg	Adults: 60 mg qd, then adjust as needed. Divide dose if >80 mg/d. Doses up to 120 mg tid have been given.	⊞C ✿v
Pantoprazole Sodium (Protonix)	Inj: 40 mg; Tab,Delay: 20 mg, 40 mg	Adults: PO: 40 mg bid. Max: 240 mg/d. IV: 80 mg q12h, adjust based on acid output. Max: 240 mg/d.	⊞B ✿v
Rabeprazole Sodium (Aciphex)	Tab, Delay: 20 mg	Adults: Initial: 60 mg qd, then adjust as needed. Maint: Up to 100 mg qd or 60 mg bid.	⊞B ✿v

NAME	FORM/STRENGTH	DOSAGE	COMMENTS
Miscellaneous			
Alosetron HCl (Lotronex)	Tab: 0.5 mg, 1 mg	Diarrhea-Predominant Irritable Bowel Syndrome (Women): Adults: Initial: 1 mg qd x 4 wks. Titrate: May increase to 1 mg bid. D/C after 4 wks if symptoms unconrolled on 1 mg bid.	OB ✤ v>: Serious GI adverse events reported. D/C if constipation or ischemic colitis symptoms develop.
Cromolyn Sodium (Gastrocrom)	Sol: 100 mg/5 ml	Mastocytosis: Adults & Peds ≥13 yo: 200 mg qid. 2-12 yo: 100 mg qid. Max: 40 mg/kg/d. Maint: Reduce to minimum dose required to maintain low degree of symptomatology. Take 30 min ac & qhs.	OB ✤ <:
Infliximab (Remicade)	Inj: 100 mg	Crohn's Disease (Reducing Signs/Symptoms & Inducing/Maintaining Remission): Induction: 5 mg/kg IV at 0, 2, & 6 wks. Maint: 5 mg/kg q8wks.	OB ✤ v> TB, & other fungal, & other opportunistic infections reported.
Tegaserod Maleate (Zelnorm)	Tab: 2 mg, 6 mg	Constipation-Predominant Irritable Bowel Syndrome (Women): ≥18 yo: 6 mg bid x 4-6 wks. If respond, may repeat course.	OB ✤ v>
Ursodiol (Actigall)	Cap: 300 mg	Gallstone Dissolution: 8-10 mg/kg/d in 2-3 divided doses. Prevention: 300 mg bid.	OB ✤ <:

Anti-Infective Agents

ANTIBACTERIALS

Clindamycin Phosphate (Cleocin Vaginal, Cleocin Vaginal Ovules)	**Cre:** 2%; **Sup:** (Ovules) 100 mg	**Bacterial Vaginosis: Ovules: Post-menarchal Females:** 1 sup intravaginally qhs x 3d. **Cre: Adults:** 1 applicatorful intravaginally qhs x 3-7d (non-pregnant) or x 7d (pregnant).	◧B ❖>
Metronidazole (Flagyl, Flagyl ER)	**Cap:** 375 mg; **Tab:** 250 mg, 500 mg; **Tab,ER:** 750 mg	**Adults: Flagyl: Trichomoniasis:** 375 mg (cap) bid or 250 mg (tab) tid x 7d. **Alternate Regimen:** If non-pregnant, 2 gm (tab) single or divided dose. **Flagy ER: Bacterial Vaginosis:** 750 mg qd x 7d on empty stomach.	◧B ❖v **H** Cl in 1st trimester.
Metronidazole (MetroGel-Vaginal)	**Gel:** 0.75%	**Adults: Bacterial Vaginosis:** 1 applicatorful intravaginally qd-bid x 5d.	◧B ❖v
Sulfanilamide (AVC)	**Cre:** 15%; **Sup:** 1.05 gm	**Adults: Vulvovaginal Candidiasis:** 1 applicatorful or 1 sup intravaginally qd-bid. Continue x 30d.	◧B ❖v
Tinidazole (Tindamax)	**Tab:** 250 mg, 500 mg	**Adults: Trichomoniasis:** 2 gm single dose with food. Treat sexual partner with same dose.	◧X (1st trimester) ◧C (2nd/3rd trimester) ❖v **R** Avoid unnecessary use.

ANTIFUNGALS

Butoconazole Nitrate (Gynazole-1, Mycelex-3)	**Cre:** 2%	**Adults: Vulvovaginal Candidiasis:** **Gynazole-1:** 1 applicatorful intravaginally once. **Mycelex-3:** 1 applicatorful intravaginally qhs x 3d.	◧C ❖>

NAME	FORM/STRENGTH	DOSAGE	COMMENTS
Clotrimazole (Gyne-Lotrimin Combination, Gyne-Lotrimin 3)	**Gyne-Lotrimin 3 Cre:** 2%; **Sup:** 200 mg; **Gyne-Lotrimin Combination Cre:** 1%; **Sup:** 100 mg	**Adults & Children: ≥12 yo: Vulvovaginal Candidiasis: Gyne-Lotrimin 3:** 1 applicatorful or 1 insert intravaginally qhs x 3d. **Combination:** 1 sup intravaginally qhs for 7d. Apply cre prn.	◉N ❄>
Clotrimazole (Mycelex 7)	**Cre:** 1%	**Adults & Children: ≥12 yo: Vulvovaginal Candidiasis:** 1 applicatorful intravaginally qhs x 7d.	◉N ❄>
Fluconazole (Diflucan)	**Tab:** 150 mg	**Adults: Vaginal Candidiasis:** 150 mg single dose.	◉C ❄v
Miconazole Nitrate (Monistat 3, Monistat 7, Monistat Dual-Pak)	**Monistat-7 Cre:** 2%, **Sup:** 100 mg; **Monistat-3 Cre:** 4%, **Sup:** 200 mg; **Dual-Pak Cre:** 2%; **Insert:** 1200 mg	**Adults & Children: ≥12 yo: Vulvovaginal Candidiasis: Monistat 3:** 100 mg sup or 2% intravaginally qhs x 3d. **Monistat 7:** 200 mg sup or 4% intravaginally qhs x 7d. **Monistat Dual-Pak:** 1200 mg intravaginally qhs. Apply 2% cream bid up to 7d for external itching.	◉C ❄>
Miconazole Nitrate (Femizol-M)	**Cre:** 2%	**Adults & Children: ≥12 yo: Vulvovaginal Candidiasis:** 1 applicatorful intravaginally qhs x 7d. May apply small amount to vulva bid up to 7d for external itching.	◉N ❄>
Terconazole (Terazol 3, Terazol 7)	**Terazol-7 Cre:** 0.4%; **Terazol-3 Cre:** 0.8%; **Sup:** 80 mg	**Adults: Vulvovaginal Candidiasis:** 1 applicatorful of 0.8% or 80 mg sup intravaginally qhs x 3d. 1 applicatorful of 0.4% intravaginally qhs x 7d.	◉C ❄>
Tioconazole (Monistat 1, Vagistat 1)	**Oint:** 6.5%	**Adults & Children: ≥12 yo: Vulvovaginal Candidiasis:** Insert contents of applicator intravaginally once hs.	◉N ❄>

Contraceptives

Estradiol Cypionate/ Medroxyprogesterone Acetate (Lunelle)	**Susp:** 5-25 mg/0.5 ml	**Adults:** 0.5 ml IM monthly.	⊕X ✿v
Ethinyl Estradiol/ Levonorgestrel (Seasonale)	**Tab:** 0.03 mg/0.15 mg	**Adults:** 1 tab qd x 91d, then repeat. Start 1st Sunday after menses begin.	⊕X ✿v
Levonorgestrel (Mirena)	**IUD:** 52 mg	**Adults:** Insert intravaginally initially within 7d of menses onset. May replace any time in the cycle. May insert 6 wks postpartum or until involution of uterus is complete, & immediately after 1st trimester abortion. Replace q5yrs.	⊕X ✿v
Levonorgestrel (Norplant)	**Implant:** 36 mg	**Adults:** Implant 216 mg (6 implants) during 1st 7d of menses onset. Replace by end of 5th year.	⊕X ✿>
Medroxyprogesterone Acetate (Depo-Provera)	**Inj:** 150 mg/ml	**Adults:** 150 mg IM q3mths. Give 1st inj during 1st 5d of menses; within 1st 5d postpartum if not nursing; or 6 wks postpartum if nursing.	⊕X ✿>
Mifepristone (Mifeprex)	**Tab:** 200 mg	**Day 1:** 600 mg single dose. **Day 3:** If treatment fails, 400 mcg misoprostol. **Day 14:** Confirm complete termination.	⊕X ✿v

ORAL CONTRACEPTIVES

DRUG	ESTROGEN	PROGESTIN	STRENGTH (ESTROGEN-PROGESTIN)
MONOPHASIC			
Alesse, Levlite, Aviane, Lessina	Ethinyl Estradiol	Levonorgestrel	20 mcg-0.1 mg
Apri, Desogen, Ortho-Cept	Ethinyl Estradiol	Desogestrel	30 mcg-0.15 mg
Brevicon, Modicon, Necon 0.5/35	Ethinyl Estradiol	Norethindrone	35 mcg-0.5 mg
Demulen 1/35, Zovia 1/35E	Ethinyl Estradiol	Ethynodiol Diacetate	35 mcg-1 mg
Demulen 1/50, Zovia 1/50E	Ethinyl Estradiol	Ethynodiol Diacetate	50 mcg-1 mg
Levlen, Levora, Nordette, Portia	Ethinyl Estradiol	Levonorgestrel	30 mcg-0.15 mg
Loestrin 1/20, Loestrin Fe 1/20, Microgestin Fe 1/20, Junel 1/20	Ethinyl Estradiol	Norethindrone Acetate	20 mcg-1 mg
Loestrin 21 1.5/30, Loestrin Fe 1.5/30, Microgestin 1.5/30, Junel 1.5/30	Ethinyl Estradiol	Norethindrone Acetate	30 mcg-1.5 mg
Lo/Ovral, Low-Ogestrol, Cryselle	Ethinyl Estradiol	Norgestrel	30 mcg-0.3 mg
Necon 1/35, Norinyl 1/35, Ortho-Novum 1/35	Ethinyl Estradiol	Norethindrone	35 mcg-1 mg
Necon 1/50, Norinyl 1/50, Ortho-Novum 1/50	Mestranol	Norethindrone	50 mcg-1 mg

Ortho-Cyclen, Sprintec, Mononessa	Ethinyl Estradiol	Norgestimate	35 mcg-0.25 mg
Ovcon 35	Ethinyl Estradiol	Norethindrone	35 mcg-0.4 mg
Ovcon 50	Ethinyl Estradiol	Norethindrone	50 mcg-1 mg
Ovral-21, Ovral-28, Ogestrel-28	Ethinyl Estradiol	Norgestrel	50 mcg-0.5 mg
Seasonale	Ethinyl Estradiol	Levonorgestrel	30 mcg-0.15 mg
Yasmin	Ethinyl Estradiol	Drospirenone	30 mcg-3 mg
BIPHASIC			
Necon 10/11 Ortho-Novum 10/11	Ethinyl Estradiol	Norethindrone	**Phase 1:** 35 mcg-0.5 mg **Phase 2:** 35 mcg-1 mg
Mircette, Kariva	Ethinyl Estradiol	Desogestrel	**Phase 1:** 20 mcg-0.15 mg **Phase 2:** 10 mcg-NONE
TRIPHASIC			
Cyclessa	Ethinyl Estradiol	Desogestrel	**Phase 1:** 25 mcg-0.1 mg **Phase 2:** 25 mcg-0.125 mg **Phase 3:** 25 mcg-0.15 mg
Ortho-Novum 7/7/7, Necon 7/7/7, Nortrel 7/7/7	Ethinyl Estradiol	Norethindrone	**Phase 1:** 35 mcg-0.5 mg **Phase 2:** 35 mcg-0.75 mg **Phase 3:** 35 mcg-1 mg
Ortho Tri-Cyclen	Ethinyl Estradiol	Norgestimate	**Phase 1:** 35 mcg-0.18 mg **Phase 2:** 35 mcg-0.215 mg **Phase 3:** 35 mcg-0.25 mg

DRUG	ESTROGEN	PROGESTIN	STRENGTH (ESTROGEN-PROGESTIN)
Ortho Tri-Cyclen Lo	Ethinyl Estradiol	Norgestimate	**Phase 1:** 25 mcg-0.18 mg **Phase 2:** 25 mcg-0.215 mg **Phase 3:** 25 mcg-0.25 mg
Tri-Levlen, Triphasil, Trivora	Ethinyl Estradiol	Levonorgestrel	**Phase 1:** 30 mcg-0.05 mg **Phase 2:** 40 mcg-0.075 mg **Phase 3:** 30 mcg-0.125 mg
Tri-Norinyl	Ethinyl Estradiol	Norethindrone	**Phase 1:** 35 mcg-0.5 mg **Phase 2:** 35 mcg-1 mg **Phase 3:** 35 mcg-0.5 mg
PROGESTIN ONLY			
Ortho-Micronor, Nor-Q.D, Camila, Errin		Norethindrone	0.35 mg
Ovrette		Norgestrel	0.075 mg
EMERGENCY			
Plan B		Levonorgestrel	0.75 mg
Preven	Ethinyl Estradiol	Levonorgestrel	50 mcg-0.25 mg

Dysmenorrhea

NSAIDS

NAME	FORM/STRENGTH	DOSAGE	COMMENTS
Celecoxib (Celebrex)	**Cap:** 100 mg, 200 mg	**Adults: Day 1:** 400 mg, then 200 mg if needed. **Maint:** 200 mg bid prn.	⊙C ❄v H
Diclofenac Potassium (Cataflam)	**Tab:** 50 mg	**Adults:** 50 mg tid or 100 mg x 1 dose, then 50 mg tid. **Max:** 150 mg/d (200 mg/d on d1).	⊙B ❄v
Ibuprofen (Motrin)	**Susp:** 100 mg/5 ml; **Tab:** 400 mg, 600 mg, 800 mg	**Adults:** 400 mg q4h prn.	⊙B ❄v R Avoid use during late pregnancy.
Ketoprofen	**Cap:** 50 mg, 75 mg	**Adults:** 25-50 mg q6-8h prn. **Max:** 300 mg/d.	⊙B ❄v H R
Meclofenamate Sodium	**Cap:** 50 mg, 100 mg	**≥14 yo:** 100 mg tid for up to 6d starting at onset of menstrual flow.	⊙N ❄v
Mefenamic Acid (Ponstel)	**Cap:** 250 mg	**≥14 yo:** 500 mg, then 250 mg q6h, up to 3d.	⊙C ❄v
Naproxen (Naprosyn)	**Susp:** 25 mg/ml; **Tab:** 250 mg, 375 mg, 500 mg	**Adults: Initial:** 500 mg, then 250 mg q6-8h prn.	⊙B ❄v
Naproxen Sodium (Anaprox, Anaprox DS, Naprelan)	**Tab:** (Anaprox) 275 mg, (Anaprox DS) 550 mg; **Tab,ER:** (Naprelan) 375 mg, 500 mg	**Adults: Tab: Initial:** 550 mg, then 550 mg q12h or 275 mg q6-8h prn. **Max:** 1100 mg/d for maint. **Tab,ER: Intial:** 1000-1500 mg qd. **Max:** 1000 mg/d for maint.	⊙B ❄v

NAME	FORM/STRENGTH	DOSAGE	COMMENTS
Rofecoxib (Vioxx)	**Susp:** 12.5 mg/5 ml, 25 mg/5 ml; **Tab:** 12.5 mg, 25 mg, 50 mg	**≥18 yo:** 50 mg qd prn up to 5d.	◐C ❁v H
Valdecoxib (Bextra)	**Tab:** 10 mg, 20 mg	**≥18 yo:** 20 mg bid.	◐C ❁v

Endometriosis
ANDROGEN

NAME	FORM/STRENGTH	DOSAGE	COMMENTS
Danazol (Danocrine)	**Cap:** 50 mg, 100 mg, 200 mg	**Adults: Mild:** 100-200 mg bid. **Moderate-Severe:** 400 mg bid. Start during menstruation & continue x 3-6 mths; may extend to 9 mths.	◐X ❁v

GONADOTROPINS

NAME	FORM/STRENGTH	DOSAGE	COMMENTS
Goserelin Acetate (Zoladex)	**Implant:** 3.6 mg	**Adults:** 3.6 mg SC in upper abdominal wall q28d for up to 6 mths.	◐X ❁v
Leuprolide Acetate (Lupron Depot)	**Inj:** (Depot) 3.75 mg, (Depot-3 Month) 11.25 mg	**Adults:** 11.25 mg IM q3mths or 3.75 mg IM monthly, alone or w/norethindrone acetate 5 mg/d. Max: 6 mths of therapy. May retreat with the combo up to 6 mths if symptoms recur.	◐X ❁v
Nafarelin Acetate (Synarel)	**Spray:** 200 mcg/inh	**Adults: ≥18 yo:** 1 spray into one nostril qam and 1 spray into other nostril qpm. Initiate b/w d2-4 of menstrual cycle. Increase to 1 spray/nostril qam & qpm after 2 mths if amenorrhea has not occurred. Treat x 6 mths.	◐X ❁v

| Norethindrone Acetate (Aygestin) | **Tab:** 5 mg | **Adults:** Assume interval between menses is 28d. **Initial:** 5 mg qd x 2 wks. **Titrate:** Increase by 2.5 mg/d q2wks until 15 mg/d. Continue x 6-9 mths or until breakthrough bleeding demands temporary termination. | ⊡X ❀> H |

Hormone Replacement Therapy

| Estradiol Acetate (Femring) | **Vaginal Ring:** 0.05 mg/day, 0.10 mg/day | **Adults: Initial:** Use lowest effective dose. Insert ring vaginally. Replace q3mths. Reevaluate periodically. | ⊡X ❀> [4,28] |
| Estradiol (Alora, Climara, Vivelle, Vivelle-Dot) | **Patch:** (Alora) 0.025 mg/d, 0.05 mg/d, 0.075 mg/d, 0.1 mg/d; (Climara) 0.025 mg/d, 0.0375 mg/d, 0.05 mg/d, 0.06 mg/d, 0.075 mg/d, 0.1 mg/d; (Vivelle, Vivelle-Dot) 0.025 mg/d, 0.0375 mg/d, 0.05 mg/d, 0.075 mg/d, 0.1 mg/d | **Vasomotor Symptoms, Vulval/Vaginal Atrophy, Hypoestrogenism: Alora: Initial:** Apply 0.05 mg/d 2x/wk. **Vivelle, Vivelle-Dot: Initial:** 0.0375 mg/d 2x/wk. **Alora, Vivelle, Vivelle-Dot:** Use continuously without intact uterus. **Climara: Initial:** 0.025 mg/d qwk. **Titrate:** Adjust dose. Use cyclic schedule (3 wks on, 1 wk off) with intact uterus. | ⊡X ❀> [4,10] |

[4] Contraindicated in pregnancy. Increased risk of endometrial carcinoma in postmenopausal women.

[10] Attempt to taper or d/c at 3-6 mth intervals.

[28] Not for CV disease prevention. The WHI reported increased risks of MI, stroke, invasive breast cancer, pulmonary emboli, & DVT in postmenopausal women. Prescribe at lowest effective doses for shortest duration.

NAME	FORM/STRENGTH	DOSAGE	COMMENTS
Estradiol (Estrace, Gynodiol)	**Tab:** (Estrace) 0.5 mg, 1 mg, 2 mg; (Gynodiol) 0.5 mg, 1 mg, 1.5 mg, 2 mg; **Vag Cre:** (Estrace) 0.01 mg/gm	**Adults: Cre: Estrace: Vulval/Vaginal Atrophy:** 2-4 g/d x 1-2 wks, then 1-2 g/d x 1-2 wks. **Maint:** 1 g 1-3 times/wk. **Tab: Estrace, Gynodiol: Menopause/Vulval/Vaginal Atrophy:** 1-2 mg/d (3 wks on, 1 wk off). **Maint:** Minimum effective dose. **Hypoestrogenism:** 1-2 mg/d. **Maint:** Minimum effective dose.	◑X ❄v 4,10
Estradiol (Estrasorb)	**Emulsion:** 0.025 mg/d/pouch	**Adults: Vasomotor Symptoms:** 2 pouches (0.05 mg/d) qam. Apply 1 pouch to each leg from the upper thigh to the calf. Rub in for 3 mins.	◑X ❄> 4,10
Estradiol (EstroGel)	**Gel:** 0.06%	**Adults: Vasomotor Symptoms, Vulvar/Vaginal Atrophy:** Apply 1 compression (1.25 g) to one arm from wrist to shoulder qd.	◑X ❄> 4, 28
Estradiol/Levonorgestrel (Climara Pro)	**Patch:** 0.045 mg-0.015 mg/d	**Adults: Vasomotor Symptoms:** Apply 1 patch qwk to lower abdomen (avoid breasts/waistline). Rotate application site; allow 1 wk between same site.	◑ X ❄> 4, 10, 28
Estradiol/Norethindrone Acetate (CombiPatch)	**Patch:** 0.05-0.14 mg/d, 0.05-0.25 mg/d	**Adults: Menopause, Vulval/Vaginal Atrophy, Hypoestrogenism: Intact Uterus: Continuous Combined Regimen:** 0.05-0.14 mg 2x/wk. **Continuous Sequential Regimen:** Wear estradiol-only patch for 1st 14d of 28d cycle, replace 2x/wk. 0.05-0.14 mg 2x/wk. for remaining 14d.	◑X ❄v 10
Estradiol/Norethindrone (Activella)	**Tab:** 1-0.5 mg	**Adults: Vulval/Vaginal atrophy, Vasomotor Symptoms: Intact Uterus:** 1-0.5 mg qd.	◑ X ❄>

Estradiol/Norgestimate (Ortho-Prefest)	Tab: 1 mg-none, 1 mg-0.09 mg	**Adults: Vasomotor symptoms, Vulvar/Vaginal Atrophy: Intact Uterus:** 1 mg estradiol x3d alternating with 1-0.09 mg x3d on continuous schedule.	⊙X ❀v
Estrogens, Conjugated (Cenestin)	Tab: 0.3 mg, 0.45 mg, 0.625 mg, 0.9 mg, 1.25 mg	**Adults: Vasomotor Symptoms: Initial:** 0.45 mg qd. Adjust dose based on response. **Vulvar/Vaginal Atrophy:** 0.3 mg qd.	⊙N ❀> CI in pregnancy. [4,10]
Estrogens, Conjugated (Premarin)	Tab: 0.3 mg, 0.45 mg, 0.625 mg, 0.9 mg, 1.25 mg, 2.5 mg; Vag Cre: 0.625 mg/gm	**Adults: Tab: Vasomotor Symptoms/Vulvar/Vaginal Atrophy:** 0.3 mg continuous or cyclically (eg, 25d on, 5d off). **Female Hypogonadism:** 0.3-0.625 mg qd cyclically. **Female Castration/Primary Ovarian Failure:** 1.25 mg qd cyclically. **Cre: Atrophic Vaginitis/Kraurosis Vulvae:** 1/2-2 g intravaginally qd cyclically (3 wks on, 1 wk off).	⊙X ❀> [4,10,28]
Estrogens, Conjugated/ Medroxyprogesterone Acetate (Premphase, Prempro)	Tab: (Premphase) 0.625 mg conjugated estrogens & 0.625-5 mg; (Prempro) 0.3-1.5 mg, 0.45-1.5 mg, 0.625-2.5 mg, 0.625-5 mg	**Adults: Menopause/Atrophy:** Treat with lowest effective dose. Adjust dose based on response.	⊙X ❀> [10,28]

[4] Contraindicated in pregnancy. Increased risk of endometrial carcinoma in postmenopausal women.

[10] Attempt to taper or d/c at 3-6 mth intervals.

[28] Not for CV disease prevention. The WHI reported increased risks of MI, stroke, invasive breast cancer, pulmonary emboli, & DVT in postmenopausal women. Prescribe at lowest effective doses for shortest duration.

NAME	FORM/STRENGTH	DOSAGE	COMMENTS
Estrogens, Esterified (Menest)	**Tab:** 0.3 mg, 0.625 mg, 1.25 mg, 2.5 mg	**Vasomotor Symptoms:** 1.25 mg qd cyclically (3 wks on, 1 wk off). **Atrophic Vaginitis/Kraurosis Vulvae:** 0.3-1.25 mg qd cyclically. **Female Hypogonadism:** 2.5-7.5 mg/d in divided doses for 20d, then 10d off therapy; repeat until menses occurs. **Female Castration/Primary Ovarian Failure:** 1.25 mg qd cyclically. **Maint:** Lowest effective dose.	⊙X ❄v 4,10
Estrogens, Esterified/ Methyltestosterone (Estratest, Estratest H.S.)	**Tab:** 1.25-2.5 mg, (HS) 0.625-1.25 mg	**Adults: Vasomotor Symptoms:** 0.625-1.25 mg or 1.25-2.5 mg qd cyclically (3 wks on, 1 wk off).	⊙X ❄v 4,10
Estropipate (Ogen, Ortho-Est)	**Tab:** (Ogen, Ortho-Est) 0.625 mg (0.75 mg estropipate), 1.25 mg (1.5 mg estropipate); (Ogen) 2.5 mg (3 mg estropipate)	**Adults: Vasomotor Symptoms:** 0.75-6 mg/d (as estropipate). **Vulval/Vaginal Atrophy:** 0.75-6 mg/d (as estropipate), cyclically. **Female Hypogonadism/Female Castration/Primary Ovarian Failure:** 1.5-9 mg/d (as estropipate) for 1st 3 wks of cycle, then 8-10d off.	⊙X ❄> 4,10
Ethinyl Estradiol/ Norethindrone Acetate (femhrt)	**Tab:** 5 mcg-1 mg	**Menopausal Symptoms: Intact Uterus:** 5 mcg-1 mg qd.	⊙X ❄> 10

Premenstrual Dysphoric Disorder

SSRIS

NAME	FORM/STRENGTH	DOSAGE	COMMENTS
Fluoxetine (Sarafem)	**Cap:** 10 mg, 20 mg	**Continuous: Initial:** 20 mg qd. **Maint:** 20 mg/d up to 6 mths. **Max:** 60 mg/d. **Intermittent: Initial:** 20 mg qd; start 14d before menses onset through 1st full day of menses. **Maint:** 20 mg/d up to 3 mths. **Max:** 60 mg/d.	⊙C ❄v H

Haemophilus b Conjugate Vaccine (ActHIB)	Inj: 10 mcg	**Peds: Reconstituted With DTP or Saline:** 0.5 ml IM at 2, 4, and 6 mths old; 4th dose at 15-18 mths; 5th dose at 4-6 yo. **Reconstituted With Tripedia (as 4th dose in series):** 0.5 ml IM at 15-18 mths; 5th dose at 4-6 yo. **Unvaccinated: 7-11 mths:** 2 doses at 8 wk intervals with a booster at 15-18 mths. **12-14 mths:** 1 dose followed by a booster 2 mths later.	◐C ✽>
Hepatitis A Inactivated, Hepatitis B Recombinant (Twinrix)	Inj: 720 U-20 mcg	**Adults:** 1 ml IM at 0-, 1- and 6-mth schedule.	◐C ✽>
Hepatitis A Vaccine, Inactivated (Havrix, Vaqta)	**Inj: Children:** (Havrix) 360 EL.U./0.5 ml, 720 EL.U./0.5 ml; (Vaqta) 25 U/0.5 ml. **Adults:** (Havrix) 1440 EL.U./ml (Vaqta) 50 U/ml	**Havrix: 2-18 yo:** 360 EL.U. IM qmth x 2 doses or 720 EL.U. IM once. **Adults:** 1440 EL.U. IM. All ages require booster dose at 6-12 mths following primary dose. **Vaqta: 2-18 yo:** 25 U IM, repeat 6-18 mths later. **≥19 yo:** 50 U IM, repeat 6-12 mths later.	◐C ✽>
Hepatitis B Immune Globulin (BayHep, Nabi-HB)	Inj: 0.5 ml, 1 ml, 5 ml.	**Percutaneous or Permucosal Exposure, BsAg-Positive or High Risk Source:** 0.06 ml/kg IM x 1 dose repeat in 1 mth if HB vaccine is not given. Initiate HB vaccine series if unvaccinated person.	◐C ✽>
Hepatitis B Vaccine, Recombinant (Engerix-B, Recombivax HB)	**Inj: Engerix-ped:** 10 mcg/0.5 ml, **Recombivax HB-ped:** 5 mcg/0.5 ml, **Engerix-adult:** 20 mcg/ml, **Recombivax HB adult:** 10 mcg/ml	**Engerix: >19 yo:** 20 mcg/ml IM at 0, 1, 6 mths. **≤19 yo:** 10 mcg/0.5 ml IM at 0, 1, 6 mths. **Booster: ≥11 yo:** 20 mcg IM. **≤10 yo:** 10 mcg IM. **Recombivax: ≥20 yo:** 10 mcg IM at 0, 1, 6 mths. **0-19 yo:** 5 mcg IM at 0, 1, 6 mths.	◐C ✽>

NAME	FORM/STRENGTH	DOSAGE	COMMENTS
Influenza Virus Vaccine Live, Intranasal (FluMist)	Nasal Spray: 0.5 ml/spray	**Adults & Peds ≥9 yo:** 0.25 ml per nostril. **5-8 yo: Not Previously Vaccinated With FluMist:** 0.25 ml per nostril x 2 doses 60d (+/- 14d) apart. **Previously Vaccinated With FluMist:** 0.25 ml per nostril.	◐C ❄>
Influenza Virus Vaccine, Subvirion (Fluvirin)	Inj: 45 mcg/0.5 ml	**≥4 yo:** 0.5 ml IM. **<9 yo (Not Previously Vaccinated):** Repeat dose min 1 mth apart. Administer in deltoid muscle to older children & thigh muscle in young children.	◐C ❄>
Influenza Virus Vaccine, Subvirion (FluShield, Fluzone)	Inj: 45 mcg/0.5 ml	**6-35 mths:** 0.25 ml IM. **≥3 yrs:** 0.5 ml IM. **<9 yo (Not Previously Vaccinated):** Repeat dose min 1 mth apart. Administer in deltoid muscle to older children & thigh muscle in infants & young children.	◐C ❄>
Measles Virus Vaccine Live (Attenuvax)	Inj: 1000 TCID$_{50}$	**12-15 mths:** 0.5 ml SQ in upper arm. If vaccinated <12 mths old, revaccinate at 12-15 mths old. Revaccinate prior to school entry.	◐C ❄>
Measles/Mumps/Rubella Virus Vaccine Live (M-M-R II)	Inj: 0.5 ml/dose	**Adults & Peds >12 mths:** 0.5 ml SQ in upper arm. Recommended primary vaccination is at 12-15 mths; repeat before elementary school entry. If vaccinated at 6-12 mths due to outbreak, give another dose at 12-15 mths & before elementary school entry.	◐C ❄>
Meningitis Vaccine (Menomune-A/c/y/w-135)	Inj: 0.05 mg	**Adults & Peds ≥2 yo:** 0.05 ml SC.	◐C ❄>

Mumps Virus Vaccine (Mumpsvax)	**Inj:** 20,000 TCID$_{50}$	**≥12 mths:** 0.5 ml SQ in outer aspect of upper arm. Give primary vaccine at 12-15 mths. Revaccinate prior to elementary school.	⬤C ❄>
Pneumococcal Vaccine, Diphtheria Protein (Prevnar)	**Inj:** 16 mcg/0.5 ml	**Peds:** *S. pneumoniae*/Otitis Media: 0.5 ml IM. 1st dose at 6 wks-2 mths old, then q2mths x 2 more doses. 4th dose given at 12-15 mths. **Unvaccinated: 7-11 mths:** 0.5 ml IM. 1st 2 doses at least 4 wks apart, then 3rd dose after 1 yo birthday at least 2 mths after 2nd dose. **12-23 mths:** 0.5 ml IM x 2 doses given at least 2 mths apart. **≥24 mths-9 yo:** 0.5 ml IM single dose.	⬤C ❄v
Pneumococcal Vaccine (Pneumovax 23, Pnu-Imune 23)	**Inj:** 0.5 ml/dose	**≥2 yo:** Usual: 0.5 ml SQ/IM in deltoid muscle or lateral mid-thigh.	⬤C ❄>
Polio Vaccine, inactivated (Ipol)	**Inj:** 80 D Antigen U/ 0.5 ml	**Children: Primary Immunization:** 0.5 ml SC/IM at 2 mths, 4 mths, and 6-18 mths. Give booster at 4-6 yo if 1st dose received at ≤6 wks.	⬤C ❄>
Rabies Immune Globulin, Human (BayRab, Imogam)	**Inj:** 150 IU/ml	**Adults:** 20 IU/kg infiltrated in the area around the wound & the rest IM in gluteal area.	⬤C ❄>
Rabies Vaccine (Imovax, RabAvert)	**Inj:** 2.5 IU	**Adults: Pre-exposure:** 1 ml IM on Days 0, 7 & either 21 or 28 (3 total doses), booster shots as needed based on titers. **Post-exposure:** (Imovax) 1 ml IM on Days 0, 3, 7, 14 & 30 (ACIP recommendations). (Rabavert) 1 ml IM on Days 0, 3, 7, 14 & 28.	⬤C ❄>

NAME	FORM/STRENGTH	DOSAGE	COMMENTS
Rubella Virus Vaccine Live (Meruvax)	Inj: 1000 TCID$_{50}$	**12-15 mths:** 0.5 ml SQ in outer aspect of upper arm. Revaccinate with MMR II prior to elementary school entry.	◐C ❄> CI in pregnancy.
Tetanus & Diphtheria Toxoids Adsorbed (Td)	Inj: 5 LFU-2 LFU/0.5 ml	**>7 yo:** 0.5 ml IM in the vastus lateralis or deltoid. Repeat 4-8 wks later. Give 3rd dose 6-12 mths after 2nd dose. **Booster:** 0.5 ml IM q10yrs.	◐C ❄>
Tetanus Immunoglobulin (BayTet)	Inj: 250 U	**Prophylactic:** **≥7 yo:** 750 U IM. **<7 yo:** 4 U/kg or 250 U. **Active Case:** Adjust dose to severity of infection.	◐C ❄>
Tetanus Toxoid (Tetanus Toxoid Adsorbed Purogenated)	Inj: 0.5 ml/dose	**≥1 yo:** 0.5 ml IM. Repeat at 4-8 wks then 6-12 mths after 2nd dose. **Booster:** 0.5 ml IM q10yrs. **<1 yo:** 3 doses of 0.5 ml IM 4-8 wks apart, then 4th dose (0.5 ml) 6-12 mths after 3rd dose. Last dose before 4 yo. **Booster:** 0.5 ml at 4-6 yo.	◐C ❄>
Typhoid Vi Polysaccharide Vaccine (Typhim Vi)	Inj: 25 mcg of purified Vi polysaccharide/ 0.5 ml	**≥2 yo:** 0.5 ml IM.	◐C ❄>
Varicella Virus Vaccine Live (Varivax)	Inj: 1350 PFU/vial	**1-12 yo:** 0.5 ml SC x 1 dose. **≥13 yo:** 0.5 ml SC, repeat in 4-8 wks.	◐C ❄> CI in pregnancy.
Varicella-Zoster Immune Globulin	Inj: 125 U/vial, 625 U/vial	**IM (gluteal): 0-10 kg:** 125 U. **10.1-20 kg:** 250 U. **20.1-30 kg:** 375 U. **30.1-40 kg:** 500 U. **>40 kg:** 625 U.	◐C ❄>

IMMUNIZATIONS

RECOMMENDED CHILDHOOD IMMUNIZATION SCHEDULE UNITED STATES, 2004*

Vaccine	Birth	1 mo	2 mos	4 mos	6 mos	12 mos	15 mos	18 mos	24 mos	4-6 yrs	11-12 yrs	13-18 yrs
Hepatitis B[1]	Hep B #1	only if mother HBsAg (−)			Hep B #2	Hep B #3					Hep B series	
Diphtheria, Tetanus, Pertussis[2]			DTaP	DTaP	DTaP		DTaP			DTaP	Td	Td
Haemophilus influenzae Type b[3]			Hib	Hib	Hib[3]	Hib						
Inactivated Polio[4]			IPV	IPV		IPV				IPV		
Measles, Mumps, Rubella[5]						MMR #1				MMR #2	MMR #2	
Varicella[6]						Varicella					Varicella	
Pneumococcal[7]			PCV	PCV	PCV	PCV				PCV	PPV	
Influenza[8]					Influenza (yearly)						Influenza (yearly)	
Hepatitis A[9]											Hepatitis A series	

Vaccines below this line are for selected populations

☐ Range of recommended ages   ⬭ Catch-up vaccination   ▓ Preadolescent assessment

233 KEY: ◉ PREGNANCY RATING; ✿ BREASTFEEDING SAFETY; H HEPATIC ADJUSTMENT; R RENAL ADJUSTMENT

This schedule indicates the recommended ages for routine administration of currently licensed childhood vaccines, as of April 1, 2004, for children through age 18 years. Any dose not given at the recommended age should be given at any subsequent visit when indicated and feasible. ⬭ Indicates age groups that warrant special effort to administer those vaccines not previously given. Additional vaccines may be licensed and recommended during the year. Licensed combination vaccines may be used whenever any components of the combination are indicated and the vaccine's other components are not contraindicated. Providers should consult the manufacturers' package inserts for detailed recommendations.

1. **Hepatitis B vaccine (Hep B).** All infants should receive the first dose of hepatitis B vaccine soon after birth and before hospital discharge; the first dose may also be given by age 2 months if the infant's mother is HBsAg-negative. Only monovalent hepatitis B vaccine can be used for the birth dose. Monovalent or combination vaccine containing hepatitis B may be used to complete the series; 4 doses of vaccine may be administered when birth dose is given. The second dose should be given at least 4 weeks after the first dose, except for combination vaccines which cannot be administered before age 6 weeks. The third dose should be given at least 16 weeks after the first dose and at least 8 weeks after the second dose. The last dose in the immunization series (third or fourth dose) should not be administered before age 24 weeks.

Infants born to HBsAg-positive mothers should receive hepatitis B vaccine and 0.5mL hepatitis B immune globulin (HBIG) within 12 hours of birth at separate sites. The second dose is recommended at age 1-2 months. The last dose in the series should not be given before age 24 weeks. These infants should be tested for HBsAg and anti-HBs at age 9-15 months of age.

Infants born to mothers whose HBsAg status is unknown should receive the first dose of the hepatitis B vaccine series within 12 hours of birth. Maternal blood should be drawn as soon as possible to determine the mother's HBsAg status; if the HBsAg test is positive, the infant should receive HBIG as soon as possible (no later than age 1 week). The second dose is recommended at age 1-2 months. The last dose in the series should not be given before age 24 weeks.

2. **Diphtheria and tetanus toxoids and acellular pertussis vaccine (DTaP).** The fourth dose of DTaP may be administered at age 12 months, provided 6 months have elapsed since the third dose and the child is unlikely to return at age 15-18 months. The final dose in the series should be given at age ≥4 years. **Tetanus and diphtheria toxoids (Td)** is recommended at age 11-12 years if at least 5 years have elapsed since the last dose of tetanus and diphtheria toxoid-containing vaccine. Subsequent routine Td boosters are recommended every 10 years.

3. **Haemophilus influenzae type b (Hib) conjugate vaccine.** Three Hib conjugate vaccines are licensed for infant use. If PRP-OMP (PedvaxHIB® or ComVax® [Merck]) is administered at ages 2 and 4 months, a dose at age 6 months is not required. DTaP/Hib combination products should not be used for primary immunization in infants at age 2, 4 or 6 months, but can be used as boosters following any Hib vaccine. The final dose in the series should be given at age ≥12 months.

4. **Inactivated poliovirus vaccine (IPV).** An all-IPV schedule is recommended for routine childhood poliovirus vaccination in the United States. All children should receive 4 doses of IPV at age 2 months, 4 months, 6-18 months, and 4-6 years.

5. **Measles, mumps, and rubella vaccine (MMR).** The second dose of MMR is recommended routinely at age 4-6 years but may be administered during any visit, provided at least 4 weeks have elapsed since the first dose and that both doses are administered beginning at or after age 12 months. Those who have not previously received the second dose should complete the schedule by the visit at age 11-12 years.

6. **Varicella vaccine.** Varicella vaccine is recommended at any visit at or after age 12 months for susceptible children (ie, those who lack a reliable history of chickenpox). Susceptible persons aged ≥13 years should receive 2 doses, given at least 4 weeks apart.

7. **Pneumococcal vaccine.** The heptavalent **pneumococcal conjugate vaccine (PCV)** is recommended for all children aged 2-23 months and for certain children aged 24-59 months. The final dose in the series should be given at age ≥12 months. **Pneumococcal polysaccharide vaccine (PPV)** is recommended in addition to PCV for certain high-risk groups.

8. **Influenza vaccine.** Influenza vaccine is recommended annually for children aged ≥6 months with certain risk factors (including but not limited to asthma, cardiac disease, sickle cell disease, HIV, and diabetes), healthcare workers, and other persons (including household members) in close contact with persons in groups at high risk and can be administered to all others wishing to obtain immunity.
   In addition, healthy children aged 6-23 months and close contacts of healthy children aged 0-23 months are encouraged to receive influenza vaccine because children in this age group are at substantially increased risk for influenza-related hospitalizations. For healthy persons aged 5-49 years, the intranasally administered live attenuated influenza vaccine (LAIV) is an acceptable alternative to the intramuscular trivalent inactivated influenza vaccine (TIV). Children receiving TIV should receive a dosage appropriate for their age (0.25mL if age 6-35 months or 0.5mL if age ≥3 years). Children aged ≤8 years who are receiving influenza vaccine for the first time should receive two doses (separated by at least 4 weeks for TIV and at least 6 weeks for LAIV).

9. **Hepatitis A vaccine.** Hepatitis A vaccine is recommended for children and adolescents in selected states and regions, and for certain high-risk groups; consult your local public health authority.

*Source: *MMWR*, Advisory Committee on Immunization Practices (ACIP), American Academy of Pediatrics (AAP), and the American Academy of Family Physicians (AAFP).

NEUROLOGY/PSYCHOTHERAPEUTICS

NAME	FORM/STRENGTH	DOSAGE	COMMENTS

ADHD/Narcolepsy Agents

NOREPINEPHRINE REUPTAKE INHIBITOR

Atomoxetine HCl (Strattera)	**Cap:** 10 mg, 18 mg, 25 mg, 40 mg, 60 mg	**Adults & Peds: ≥6 yo & >70 kg: Initial:** 40 mg/d given qam or evenly divided doses in am and late afternoon/early pm. **Titrate:** Increase after minimum of 3d to target dose of about 80 mg/d. After 2-4 wks, may increase to max of 100 mg/d. **Max:** 100 mg/d. **Peds: ≥6 yo & ≤70 kg: Initial:** 0.5 mg/kg/d given qam or evenly divided doses in am and late afternoon/early pm. **Titrate:** Increase after minimum of 3d to target dose of about 1.2 mg/kg/d. **Max:** 1.4 mg/kg/d or 100 mg, whichever is less. Adjust with CYP450 2D6 inhibitors.	◎C ✱✤ H

OXAZOLIDINONE

Pemoline CIV (Cylert)	**Chewtab:** 37.5 mg; **Tab:** 18.75 mg, 37.5 mg, 75 mg	**ADHD: ≥6 yo: Initial:** 37.5 mg qam. **Titrate:** Increase by 18.75 mg qwk. **Usual:** 56.25-75 mg/d. **Max:** 112.5 mg.	◎B ✱✤ H Hepatic failure reported.

| **Paroxetine** (Paxil CR) | **Tab,CR:** 12.5 mg, 25 mg, 37.5 mg | **Initial:** 12.5 mg qd continuous or limited to luteal phase. Titrate: Wait at least 1 wk between dose changes. | ⬤C ❀> H R |
| **Sertraline** (Zoloft) | **Tab:** 25 mg, 50 mg, 100 mg;
Sol: 20 mg/ml | **Initial:** 50 mg qd continuous or limit to luteal cycle phase. Titrate: Increase by 50 mg/cycle up to 150 mg/d for continuous or 100 mg/d for luteal phase dosing. If 100 mg/d is established for luteal phase dosing, then titrate by 50 mg/d x 3d at beginning of each luteal phase dosing period. | ⬤C ❀> H |

Miscellaneous

| **Danazol** (Danocrine) | **Cap:** 50 mg, 100 mg, 200 mg | **Fibrocystic Breast Disease: Adults:** 50-200 mg bid. Start during menstruation. | ⬤X ❀v |
| **Estradiol** (Estring) | **Vag Ring:** 2 mg/ring | **Postmenopausal Urogenital Symptoms:** Insert ring into upper 1/3 of the vaginal vault, remove & replace after 90d. | ⬤X ❀v [4,10] |

[4] Contraindicated in pregnancy. Increased risk of endometrial carcinoma in postmenopausal women.

[10] Attempt to taper or d/c at 3-6 mth intervals.

NAME	FORM/STRENGTH	DOSAGE	COMMENTS

HEMATOLOGY/IMMUNOLOGY
Hematopoietic Agents

NAME	FORM/STRENGTH	DOSAGE	COMMENTS
Darbepoetin Alfa (Aranesp)	**Inj:** 0.025 mg/ml, 0.04 mg/ml, 0.06 mg/ml, 0.1 mg/ml, 0.2 mg/ml, 0.3 mg/ml, 0.5 mg/ml	**Adults: CRF: Initial:** 0.45 mcg/kg IV/SC wkly. **Titrate:** Adjust to target Hgb <12 gm/dL. If Hgb increases >1 gm/dL in a 2-wk period or is approaching 12 gm/dL, decrease dose by 25%. If Hgb continues to increase, hold dose until Hgb begins to decrease, and reinitiate at 25% below previous dose. Do not increase more than once monthly. **Malignancy: Initial:** 2.25 mcg/kg SC wkly. **Titrate:** Increase to 4.5 mcg/kg if Hgb increase is <1 gm/dL after 6 wks of therapy. If Hgb increases >1 gm/dL in a 2-wk period or if Hgb >12 gm/dL, decrease dose by 25%. If Hgb >13 gm/dL, hold dose until Hgb falls to 12 gm/dL and reinitiate at 25% below previous dose.	▣C ✿>
Epoetin Alfa (Epogen, Procrit)	**Inj:** 2000 U/ml, 3000 U/ml, 4000 U/ml, 10,000 U/ml, 20,000 U/ml, 40,000 U/ml	**Adults: CRF: Initial:** 50-100 U/kg IV/SC TIW. **Maint:** Adjust to maintain target Hct range. **AZT Therapy:** 100 U/kg IV/SC TIW x 8 wks. **Titrate:** Increase by 50-100 U/kg TIW up to 300 U/kg TIW. **Maint:** Adjust based on AZT & Hct. **Chemotherapy: Initial:** 150 U/kg SC TIW x 8 wks. **Titrate:** May increase to 300 U/kg TIW after 8 wks of therapy. **Surgery:** 300 U/kg/d SC x 10d prior to surgery, on day of, and 4d after surgery; or 600 U/kg SC wkly on d21, d14, & d7 prior to surgery, & a 4th dose on day of surgery. **Peds: CRF: Initial:** 50 U/kg TIW IV/SC. **Maint:** Adjust to maintain target Hct range.	▣C ✿>

Filgrastim (Neupogen)	Inj: 300 mcg/0.5 ml, 300 mcg/ml, 480 mcg/0.8 ml, 480 mcg/1.6 ml	**Adults: Myelosuppressive Chemotherapy: Initial:** 5 mcg/kg/d IV/SC. **BMT Cancer: Initial:** 10 mcg/kg/d IV/SC. **Congenital Neutropenia: Initial:** 6 mcg/kg SC bid. **Idiopathic/Cyclic Neutropenia: Initial:** 5 mcg/kg SC qd. **Maint:** Adjust dose for above based on neutrophil count. **Peripheral Blood Progenitor Cell Collection: Initial:** 10 mcg/kg/d SC 4d before & x 6-7d with leukapheresis on d5, d6 & d7.	▣C ❆>
Oprelvekin (Neumega)	Inj: 5 mg	**Severe Thrombocytopenia Prevention: Adults:** 50 mcg/kg SC qd. Initiate 6-24h after chemo completion. Continue therapy until post-nadir platelets ≥50,000 cells/mcL. D/C at least 2d before next chemo cycle. **Max:** 21d of therapy.	▣C ❆v
Pegfilgrastim (Neulasta)	Inj: 6 mg/0.6 ml	**Infection/Febrile Neutropenia with Non-Myeloid Malignancies: Adults:** 6 mg SC, once per chemotherapy cycle. Do not administer in the period 14d before and 24h after chemotherapy.	▣C ❆>
Sargramostim (Leukine)	Inj: 250 mcg, 500 mcg/ml	**BMT Myeloid Reconstitution:** 250 mcg/m²/d IV post bone marrow infusion, continue until ANC >1500 cells/mm³ x 3d. **BMT Failure/Engraftment Delay:** 250 mcg/m²/d IV x 14d, repeat after 7d if needed; 500 mcg m²/d IV x 14d after another 7d off therapy, if needed. **Post Peripheral Blood Progenitor Cell (PBPC) Transplant:** 250 mcg m²/d SC until ANC >1500 cells/mm³ x 3d. **PBPC Mobilization:** 250 mcg/m²/d IV/SC, continue through PBPC collection period. **Post-Chemo in AML:** 250 mcg/m²/d IV until ANC >1500 cells/mm³ x 3d or max of 42d.	▣C ❆>

NAME	FORM/STRENGTH	DOSAGE	COMMENTS

Vaccines/Toxoids/Immunoglobulins

NAME	FORM/STRENGTH	DOSAGE	COMMENTS
Anthrax Vaccine Adsorbed (Biothrax)	**Inj:** 5 ml	**Pre-exposure Prophylaxis: 18-65 yo:** 0.5 ml SC at 0, 2, 4 wks, then 0.5 ml at 6, 12, 18 mths. **Booster:** 0.5 ml yearly.	◉D ❄>
Diphtheria Toxoid/ Tetanus Toxoid/Acellular Pertussis Vaccine Adsorbed (Daptacel, Infanrix, Tripedia)	**Inj: Daptacel:** 15 LFU-5 LFU-23 mcg/0.5 ml; **Infanrix:** 25 LFU-10 LFU-58 mcg/0.5 ml; **Tripedia:** 6.7 LFU-5 LFU-46.8 mcg/0.5 ml	**≥6 wks-up to 7 yo: Infanrix, Tripedia:** 3 doses of 0.5 ml IM at 4-8 wk intervals. **Booster:** Give at 15-20 mths, at least 6 mths after 3rd dose. **Daptacel:** 4 doses of 0.5 ml IM with 1st 3 doses at 6-8 wk intervals. The interval between 3rd & 4th dose should be at least 6 mths.	◉C ❄>
Diphtheria/Tetanus Toxoids Adsorbed	**Inj:** 2-5 LFU/0.5 ml, 6.6-5 LFU/0.5 ml, 10-5 LFU/0.5 ml	**>7 yo:** 0.5 ml IM in the vastus lateralis or deltoid. Repeat 4-8 wks later. Give 3rd dose 6-12 mths after 2nd dose. **Booster:** 0.5 ml IM every 10 yrs. **6 wks-12 mths:** 0.5 ml IM x 3 doses 4-8 wks apart. 4th dose 6-12 mths after 3rd dose. **1-6 yo:** 0.5 ml IM x 2 doses 4-8 wks apart. 3rd dose 6-12 mths after 2nd dose. **Booster: If received 4 doses:** 0.5 ml IM before entering school.	◉C ❄>
Haemophilus b Conjugate & Hepatitis B Vaccine Recombinant (Comvax)	**Inj:** 7.5 mcg-5 mcg-125 mcg/0.5 ml	**Peds: ≥6 wks:** 0.5 ml IM at 2, 4, & 12-15 mths of age. If cannot follow schedule, wait at least 6 wks between 1st 2 doses. 2nd & 3rd dose should be close to 8-11 mths apart.	◉C ❄>

Drug	Forms	Dosing	
Amphetamine & Dextroamphetamine Mixture CII (Adderall, Adderall XR)	**Cap,ER:** 5 mg, 10 mg, 15 mg, 20 mg, 25 mg, 30 mg; **Tab:** 5 mg, 7.5 mg, 10 mg, 12.5 mg, 15 mg, 20 mg, 30 mg	**ADHD: Adderall: ≥6 yo:** 5 mg qd-bid, increase qwk by 5 mg. **Max:** 40 mg/d. **3-5 yo:** 2.5 mg, increase qwk by 2.5 mg until optimal response. **Adderall XR: ≥6 yo: Initial:** 10 mg qam. **Titrate:** May increase qwk by 5-10 mg/d. **Max:** 30 mg/d. May switch from Adderall to Adderall XR at same total daily dose taken qd. **Narcolepsy: Adderall: ≥12 yo: Initial:** 10 mg/d. 5-60 mg/d. **6-12 yo: Initial:** 5 mg/d. May increase by 5 mg wkly.	●C ✾v High potential for abuse.
Dexmethylphenidate HCl CII (Focalin)	**Tab:** 2.5 mg, 5 mg, 10 mg	**≥6 yo:** Take bid at least 4h apart. **Methylphenidate Naive: Initial:** 2.5 mg bid. **Titrate:** Increase wkly by 2.5-5 mg/day. **Max:** 20 mg/day. **Currently on Methylphenidate: Initial:** Take 1/2 methylphenidate dose. **Max:** 20 mg/day. D/C if no improvement after 1-mth.	●C ✾>
Dextroamphetamine CII (Dexedrine, Dexedrine Spansules, DextroStat)	**Cap,ER:** (Spansules) 5 mg, 10 mg, 15 mg; **Tab:** (Dexedrine) 5 mg; (DextroStat) 5 mg, 10 mg	**ADHD: 3-5 yo: Initial:** 2.5 mg qd. **Titrate:** Increase qwk by 2.5 mg. **≥6 yo: Initial:** 5 mg qd-bid. **Titrate:** Increase qwk by 5 mg. **Max:** 40 mg/d. **Narcolepsy: 6-12 yo: Initial:** 5 mg/d. **Titrate:** Increase qwk by 5 mg. **≥12 yo: Initial:** 10 mg/d. **Titrate:** Increase qwk by 10 mg/d. **Usual:** 5-60 mg/d. Give Cap,ER qd & tab q4-6h.	●C ✾v High potential for abuse.
Methamphetamine HCl CII (Desoxyn)	**Tab:** 5 mg	**ADHD: ≥6 yo: Initial:** 5 mg qd-bid. **Titrate:** Increase by 5 mg qwk until optimum response. **Usual:** 20-25 mg/d given bid.	●C ✾v High potential for abuse.

NAME	FORM/STRENGTH	DOSAGE	COMMENTS
Methylphenidate CII (Concerta, Metadate CD, Metadate ER, Methylin, Methylin ER, Ritalin, Ritalin LA Ritalin-SR)	Cap,ER: (Metadate CD) 10 mg, 20 mg, 30 mg (Ritalin LA) 10 mg, 20 mg, 30 mg, 40 mg; Tab: (Methylin, Ritalin) 5 mg, 10 mg, 20 mg; Tab,ER: (Concerta) 18 mg, 27 mg, 36 mg, 54 mg; (Metadate ER, Methylin ER) 10 mg, 20 mg; (Ritalin-SR) 20 mg	ADHD: Concerta: ≥6 yo: Initial: 18 mg qam (12h duration of effect). Titrate: Adjust by 18 mg increments. Max: 54 mg/d. Metadate CD: ≥6 yo: 20 mg qd. Titrate: Adjust by 10-20 mg increments. Max: 60 mg/d. Ritalin, Methylin: Initial: Adults: 10-60 mg/d divided bid-tid 30-45 min ac. ≥6 yo: 5 mg bid. Titrate: Increase by 5-10 mg qwk. Max: 60 mg/d. Ritalin LA: ≥6 yo: Initial: 10-20 mg qam. Titrate: Adjust by 10 mg increments. Max: 60 mg/d. May use Ritalin-SR, Methylin ER, or Metadate ER when 8h extended release dose corresponds to titrated 8h immediate release dose.	◉C ✿> Caution with emotionally unstable patients & during drug withdrawal.

MISCELLANEOUS

| Modafinil CIV (Provigil) | Tab: 100 mg, 200 mg | Adults & Peds: ≥ 16 yo: 200 mg qd. Narcolepsy/OSAHS: Take in AM. SWSD: Take 1 hr prior to start of work shift. | ◉C ✿> H |

Alzheimer's Therapy
CHOLINESTERASE INHIBITORS

| Donepezil (Aricept) | Tab: 5 mg, 10 mg | Initial: 5 mg qhs x 4-6 wks. Maint: 10 mg qd. | ◉C ✿v |
| Galantamine (Reminyl) | Sol: 4 mg/ml; Tab: 4 mg, 8 mg, 12 mg | Initial: 4 mg bid. Titrate: Increase to 8 mg bid after 4 wks, then to 12 mg bid after 4 wks. Usual: 8-12 mg bid. Max: 24 mg/d. | ◉B ✿> H R |

| Rivastigmine (Exelon) | Cap: 1.5 mg, 3 mg, 4.5 mg, 6 mg; Sol: 2 mg/ml | Adults: Initial: 1.5 mg bid. Titrate: May increase by 1.5 mg bid q2wks. Max: 12 mg/d. Suspend therapy if not tolerated. If interrupt longer than several days, reinitiate w/ lowest daily dose. | ●B ✿v |
| Tacrine (Cognex) | Cap: 10 mg, 20 mg, 30 mg, 40 mg | Initial: 10 mg qid. Titrate: Increase to 20 mg qid after 4 wks, then increase at 4-wk intervals to 30 mg qid then to 40 mg qid if no significant transaminase elevations. | ●C ✿> H |

NMDA-RECEPTOR ANTAGONIST

| Memantine HCl (Namenda) | Tab: 5 mg, 10 mg | Adults: Initial: 5 mg qd. Maint: 10 mg bid. Titrate: Increase by 5 mg increments to 10 mg/d (5 mg bid), 15 mg/d (5 mg and 10 mg as separate doses), then 20 mg/d (10 mg bid). Minimum recommended interval between dose increases is 1 wk. | ●B ✿> R |

Antianxiety/Hypnotic Agents
BARBITURATES

Amobarbital CII (Amytal)	Inj: 500 mg	Adults: Sedative: 30-50 mg IM/IV bid-tid. Hypnotic: 65-200 IM/IV mg qhs. IV use restricted & should not exceed 50 mg/min. Peds >6 yo: 65 mg-500 mg IV.	●D ✿> H R
Amobarbital/Secobarbital CII (Tuinal)	Cap: 50 mg-50 mg	Adults: Insomnia: 1-2 caps qhs.	●D ✿> H R
Butabarbital CIII (Butisol)	Eli: 30 mg/5 ml; Tab: 30 mg, 50 mg	Adults: Daytime Sedative: 15-30 mg tid-qid. Bedtime Hypnotic/Pre-op Sedation: 50-100 mg. Peds: Pre-op Sedation: 2-6 mg/kg. Max: 100 mg.	●D ✿>

NAME	FORM/STRENGTH	DOSAGE	COMMENTS
Pentobarbital CII (Nembutal Sodium)	**Inj:** 50 mg/ml	**Adults:** 150-200 mg IM. **Peds: Usual:** 2-6 mg/kg/24h IM. **Max:** 100 mg IM. Avoid IV use if possible.	▣D ✲> H R
Phenobarbital CIV	**Eli:** 20 mg/5 ml; **Inj:** 30 mg/ml, 60 mg/ml, 65 mg/ml, 130 mg/ml; **Tab:** 15 mg, 30 mg, 32.4 mg, 60 mg, 64.8 mg, 97.2 mg, 100 mg	**Adults: Daytime Sedation:** 30-120 mg/d PO given in 2-3 doses, or IM/IV given in 2-9 doses. **Peds: Pre-op Sedation:** 1-3 mg/kg IM/IV.	▣D ✲>
Secobarbital CII (Seconal)	**Cap:** 100 mg	**Adults: Hypnotic:** 100 mg qhs. **Peds: Pre-op:** 2-6 mg/kg. **Max:** 100 mg.	▣D ✲> H R
BENZODIAZEPINES			
Alprazolam CIV (Xanax, Xanax XR)	**Tab:** 0.25 mg, 0.5 mg, 1 mg, 2 mg; **Tab,ER:** 0.5 mg, 1 mg, 2 mg, 3 mg	**Adults: Xanax: Anxiety: Initial:** 0.25-0.5 mg tid. Titrate: May increase q3-4d. **Max:** 4 mg/d. **Panic Disorder: Initial:** 0.5 mg tid. Titrate: Increase by 1 mg/d q3-4d. **Usual:** 1-10 mg/d. **Xanax XR: Panic Attack: Initial:** 0.5-1 mg qd, preferably in am. **Titrate:** Increase by 1 mg/d q3-4d. **Maint:** 1-10 mg/d. **Usual:** 3-6 mg/d.	▣D ✲v H
Chlordiazepoxide CIV (Librium)	**Cap:** 5 mg, 10 mg, 25 mg; **Inj:** 100 mg	**Adults: Mild-Moderate Anxiety:** 5-10 mg PO tid-qid. **Severe Anxiety: Initial:** 20-25 mg PO tid-qid or 50-100 mg IM/IV. **Maint:** 5-25 mg PO tid-qid or 25-50 mg IM/IV tid-qid. **Peds: ≥6 yo: Initial:** 5 mg PO bid-qid. **Max:** 10 mg PO bid-tid. **≥12 yo: Acute/Severe Anxiety:** 25-50 mg PO, then 12.5-50 mg tid-qid prn.	▣N ✲>

Clorazepate CIV (Tranxene T-Tab, Tranxene-SD)	**Tab:** (T-Tab) 3.75 mg, 7.5 mg, 15 mg; **Tab,ER:** (SD) 11.25 mg, 22.5 mg	**Adults & Peds >9 yo: Anxiety: Tab: Initial:** 15 mg qhs. **Usual:** 30 mg/d in divided doses. **Max:** 60 mg/d. **Tab,ER:** 22.5 mg qd if controlled on 7.5 mg tid or 11.25 mg qd if controlled on 3.75 mg tid.	◉N ❄v
Diazepam CIV (Valium)	**Inj:** 5 mg/ml; **Tab:** 2 mg, 5 mg, 10 mg	**Anxiety: Adults: PO:** 2-10 mg bid-qid. **IM/IV:** (moderate) 2-5 mg or (severe) 5-10 mg, repeat in 3-4h if needed. **Peds: ≥6 mths: Initial:** 1-2.5 mg PO tid-qid.	◉N ❄>
Estazolam CIV (ProSom)	**Tab:** 1 mg, 2 mg	**>18 yo: Insomnia: Initial:** 1 mg qhs. **Maint:** 1-2 mg qhs.	◉X ❄v
Flurazepam CIV (Dalmane)	**Cap:** 15 mg, 30 mg	**Adults & Peds ≥15 yo: Insomnia:** 15-30 mg qhs.	◉X ❄v
Lorazepam CIV (Ativan)	**Tab:** 0.5 mg, 1 mg, 2 mg	**Adults & Peds >12 yo: Anxiety: Initial:** 2-3 mg/d given bid-tid. **Usual:** 2-6 mg/d. **Insomnia:** 2-4 mg qhs.	◉N ❄v
Midazolam CIV (Versed)	**Inj:** 1 mg/ml, 5 mg/ml; **Syr:** 2 mg/ml	**Sedation & Anxiolysis: Pre-op: Adults: <60 yo: IM:** 0.07-0.08 mg/kg (approx. 5 mg) IM. **IV:** Individualize dose. Up to 2.5 mg over 2 min, titrate as needed. **Max:** 5 mg. **Peds: PO:** 0.25-1.0 mg/kg single dose. **Max:** 20 mg/dose. **IM:** 0.1-0.15 mg/kg, up to 0.5 mg/kg. **Max:** 10 mg/dose. **IV: 6 mths-5 yo:** 0.05-0.1 mg/kg, up to 0.6 mg/kg. **Max:** 6 mg/dose. **6-12 yo:** 0.025-0.05 mg/kg, up to 0.4 mg/kg. **Max:** 10 mg/dose. **12-16 yo:** Adult dose.	◉D ❄> Associated with respiratory depression & respiratory arrest.
Quazepam CIV (Doral)	**Tab:** 7.5 mg, 15 mg	**≥18 yo: Insomnia:** 7.5-15 mg qhs.	◉X ❄v

NAME	FORM/STRENGTH	DOSAGE	COMMENTS
Temazepam CIV (Restoril)	**Cap:** 7.5 mg, 15 mg, 30 mg	**≥18 yo: Insomnia:** 7.5-30 mg qhs. **Transient Insomnia:** 7.5 mg qhs.	◉X ❄>
Triazolam CIV (Halcion)	**Tab:** 0.125 mg, 0.25 mg	**≥18 yo: Insomnia: Usual:** 0.25 mg qhs. **Max:** 0.25 mg qhs. **Low-weight Patients:** 0.125 mg qhs. **Max:** 0.25 mg qhs.	◉X ❄v

SEROTONIN/NE REUPTAKE INHIBITORS

NAME	FORM/STRENGTH	DOSAGE	COMMENTS
Venlafaxine (Effexor XR)	**Cap,ER:** 37.5 mg, 75 mg, 150 mg	**Adults: Generalized Anxiety Disorder/Social Anxiety Disorder: Initial:** 75 mg/d, or 37.5 mg/d increase to 75 mg/d after 4-7d. **Titrate:** Increase by 75 mg/d at intervals of no less than 4 d. **Max:** 225 mg/d.	◉C ❄v H R

SSRIS

NAME	FORM/STRENGTH	DOSAGE	COMMENTS
Escitalopram Oxalate (Lexapro)	**Sol:** 5 mg/5 mL; **Tab:** 5 mg, 10 mg, 20 mg	**Adults: Generalized Anxiety Disorder: Initial:** 10 mg qd, in am or pm. **Titrate:** May increase to 20 mg after at least 1 wk. **Elderly:** 10 mg qd.	◉C ❄v H
Fluoxetine (Prozac)	**Cap:** 10 mg, 20 mg, 40 mg; **Sol:** 20 mg/5ml; **Tab:** 10 mg	**Adults: Panic Disorder: Initial:** 10 mg/d. May increase to 20 mg/d after 1 wk. May increase further after several wks if needed. **Max:** 60 mg/d.	◉C ❄v H
Paroxetine (Paxil, Paxil CR)	**Susp:** 10 mg/5 ml; **Tab:** 10 mg, 20 mg, 30 mg, 40 mg; **Tab,CR:** 12.5 mg, 25 mg, 37.5 mg	**Adults: Panic Disorder: Susp/Tab: Initial:** 10 mg qam. **Usual:** 40 mg/d. **Max:** 60 mg/d. **Social Anxiety Disorder: Susp/Tab: Initial/Usual:** 20 mg qam. **Tab,CR: Initial:** 12.5 mg/d. May increase wkly by 12.5 mg/d. **Max:** 37.5 mg/d. **GAD/PTSD: Initial:** 20 mg qam. **Usual:** 20-50 mg qam. May increase wkly by 10 mg/d. **Tab,CR: Panic Disorder: Initial:** 12.5 mg qam. May increase wkly by 12.5 mg/d. **Max:** 75 mg qam.	◉C ❄> H R

| Sertraline (Zoloft) | **Tab:** 25 mg, 50 mg, 100 mg; **Sol:** 20 mg/ml | **Adults: Panic Disorder/Social Anxiety Disorder/PTSD: Initial:** 25 mg qd. **Titrate:** Increase to 50 mg qd after 1 wk. Adjust wkly. **Max:** 200 mg/d. | ◉C ❋> H |

MISCELLANEOUS

Buspirone (BuSpar, Vanspar)	**Tab:** (Buspar) 5 mg, 10 mg, 15 mg; (Vanspar) 7.5 mg	**≥18 yo: Anxiety: Initial:** 7.5 mg bid. **Titrate:** Increase by 5 mg/d q2-3d. **Usual:** 20-30 mg/d. **Max:** 60 mg/d.	◉B ❋v
Chloral Hydrate CIV	**Cap:** 500 mg; **Sup:** 325 mg, 650 mg; **Syr:** 500 mg/5 ml	**Adults: Insomnia:** 500 mg-1 gm 15-30 min before retiring. **Sedative:** 250 mg tid. **Children: Insomnia:** 50 mg/kg or 1.5 gm/m². **Max:** 1 gm. **Sedative:** 8 mg/kg or 250 mg/m² tid. **Max:** 500 mg/d.	◉C ❋>
Ethchlorvynol CIV (Placidyl)	**Cap:** 500 mg, 750 mg	**Adults: Insomnia: Initial:** 500-750 mg qhs. **Max:** 1000 mg qhs.	◉C ❋v
Hydroxyzine (Atarax, Vistaril)	**(Vistaril) Cap:** 25 mg, 50 mg, 100 mg; **Inj:** 25 mg/ml, 50 mg/ml, 100 mg/ml; **Susp:** 25 mg/5 ml; **(Atarax) Syr:** 10 mg/5 ml; **Tab:** 10 mg, 25 mg, 50 mg, 100 mg	**Anxiety: Adults: PO:** 50-100 mg qid. **Peds: PO: <6 yo:** 50 mg/d in divided doses. **>6 yo:** 50-100 mg/d in divided doses. **Psych/Emotional Emergency: Adults: IM:** 50-100 mg stat, then q4-6h prn.	◉N ❋v CI in early pregnancy.
Meprobamate CIV (Miltown)	**Tab:** 200 mg, 400 mg	**Anxiety: Adults: Usual:** 1200-1600 mg/d given tid-qid. **Max:** 2400 mg/d. **6-12 yo:** 200-600 mg/d given bid-tid.	◉N ❋>

NAME	FORM/STRENGTH	DOSAGE	COMMENTS
Zaleplon CIV (Sonata)	Cap: 5 mg, 10 mg	**Adults: Insomnia:** 10 mg qhs. **Low-weight Patients: Initial:** 5 mg qhs. **Max:** 20 mg qhs. **Debilitated Patients:** 5 mg qhs. **Max:** 10 mg qhs.	▣C ❄v H
Zolpidem Tartrate CIV (Ambien)	Tab: 5 mg, 10 mg	**≥18 yo: Insomnia:** 10 mg qhs. **Debilitated Patients:** 5 mg qhs. Decrease dose w/ other CNS depressants.	▣B ❄v H

Anticonvulsants

BENZODIAZEPINES

NAME	FORM/STRENGTH	DOSAGE	COMMENTS
Clonazepam CIV (Klonopin)	Tab: 0.5 mg, 1 mg, 2 mg	**Seizure Disorder: Adults: Initial:** Up to 0.5 mg tid. **Titrate:** Increase by 0.5-1 mg q3d. **Max:** 20 mg/d. **Peds: Up to 10 yo or 30 kg: Initial:** 0.01-0.03 mg/kg/d (up to 0.05 mg/kg/d) given bid-tid. **Titrate:** Increase by 0.25-0.5 mg q3d. **Maint:** 0.1-0.2 mg/kg/d given tid.	▣D ❄v
Diazepam CIV (Diastat, Valium)	(Diastat) Rectal gel: 2.5 mg, 5 mg, 10 mg, 15 mg, 20 mg; (Valium) Inj: 5 mg/ml; Tab: 2 mg, 5 mg, 10 mg	**Diastat:** 0.2-0.5 mg/kg rounded upward. **2-5 yo:** 0.5 mg/kg. **6-11 yo:** 0.3 mg/kg. **≥12 yo:** 0.2 mg/kg. May give 2nd dose 4-12h later. **Max:** 5 episodes/mth or 1 episode q5d. **Valium: PO: Adults:** 2-10 mg bid-qid. **Peds: ≥6 mths: Initial:** 1-2.5 mg tid-qid. **Status Epilepticus: IV: Adults: Initial:** 5-10 mg, may repeat q10-15min. **Max:** 30 mg. **Peds: 30 days-5 yo:** 0.2-0.5 mg, q2-5min. **Max:** 5 mg. **≥5 yo:** 1 mg q2-5min. **Max:** 10 mg.	▣D (Diastat) ▣N (Valium) ❄v (Diastat) ❄> (Valium)
Lorazepam CIV (Ativan)	Inj: 2 mg/ml, 4 mg/ml	**Status Epilepticus: ≥18 yo:** 2 mg/min IV x 2 min, may repeat x 1 dose after 10-15 min. **Max:** 8 mg.	▣D ❄v

HYDANTOIN DERIVATIVES

Ethotoin (Peganone)	**Tab:** 250 mg	**Tonic-Clonic & Complex Partial Seizures: Adults:** Give q4-6h. **Initial:** 1 gm or less. **Titrate:** Increase over several days. **Maint:** 2-3 gm/d. **Peds:** Give q4-6h. **Initial:** Up to 750 mg/d. **Maint:** 500 mg-1 gm.	◉C ❋v
Fosphenytoin Sodium (Cerebyx)	**Inj:** 50 mg/ml	**Adults: LD:** 10-20 mg PE/kg IV/IM (≤150 mg PE/min). **Maint:** 4-6 mg PE/kg/d. **Status Epilepticus: LD:** 15-20 mg PE/kg; administer as 100-150 mg PE/min.	◉D ❋v H R
Phenytoin (Dilantin)	**Cap,ER:** 30 mg, 100 mg; **Chewtab:** 50 mg; **Susp:** 125 mg/5 ml	**Tonic-Clonic & Complex Partial Seizures/Seizure Treatment or Prevention w/Neurosurgery: Adults:** **Cap,ER: Initial:** 100 mg tid-qid. **Titrate:** Increase q7-10d. **Max:** 200 mg tid. May give ER qd if controlled on 300 mg/d. **LD:** 400 mg PO, then 300 mg q2h x 2 doses (total 1 gm). Start maint 24h later. **Chewtab: Initial:** 100 mg tid. **Titrate:** Increase q7-10d. **Usual:** 300-400 mg/d. **Max:** 600 mg/d. **Susp: Initial:** 125 mg tid. **Titrate:** Increase q7-10d. **Max:** 625 mg/d. **Peds: Initial:** 5 mg/kg/d given bid-tid. **Titrate:** Increase q7-10d. **Maint:** 4-8 mg/kg/d. **Max:** 300 mg/d. **>6 yo:** May require min adult dose (300 mg/d).	◉N ❋v

SUCCINIMIDES

Ethosuximide (Zarontin)	**Cap:** 250 mg; **Syr:** 250 mg/5 ml	**Absence Seizures: Adults & Peds ≥6 yo:** 500 mg qd. **3-6 yo: Initial:** 250 mg qd. **Titrate:** Increase daily dose by 250 mg q4-7d. Usual optimal dose for peds is 20 mg/kg/d. **Max:** 1.5 gm/d.	◉N ❋>

NAME	FORM/STRENGTH	DOSAGE	COMMENTS
Methsuximide (Celontin)	Cap: 150 mg, 300 mg	**Absence Seizures: Adults & Peds: Initial:** 300 mg qd x 7d. **Titrate:** Increase wkly by 300 mg/d wkly x 3 wks. **Max:** 1.2 gm/d.	⊙N ❀>

SULFONAMIDE

Zonisamide (Zonegran)	Cap: 25 mg, 50 mg, 100 mg	**Partial Seizures: ≥16 yo: Initial:** 100 mg qd. **Titrate:** Increase by 100 mg q2wks, given qd-bid. **Max:** 400 mg/d.	⊙C ❀v H R

MISCELLANEOUS

Carbamazepine (Carbatrol, Tegretol, Tegretol XR)	**Cap,ER:** (Carbatrol) 200 mg, 300 mg; **Chewtab:** 100 mg; **Susp:** 100 mg/5 ml; **Tab:** 200 mg; **Tab,ER:** (XR) 100 mg, 200 mg, 400 mg	**Partial/Tonic-Clonic/Mixed Seizures: ≥12 yo: Initial: Cap,ER/Chewtab/Tab/Tab,ER:** 200 mg bid. **Susp:** 100 mg qid. **Maint:** 800-1200 mg/d. **Max: >15 yo:** 1200 mg/d. **12-15 yo:** 1000 mg/d. **6 mths-12 yo: Cap,ER: Usual/Max:** ≤35mg/kg/d. **6-12 yo: Chewtab/Tab/Tab,ER: Initial:** 100 mg bid. **Susp:** 50 mg qid. **Maint:** 400-800 mg/d. **Max:** 1000 mg/d. **6 mths-6 yo: Chewtab/Tab: Initial:** 10-20 mg/kg/d given bid-tid. **Susp:** 10-20 mg/kg/d given qid. **Max:** 35 mg/kg/d.	⊙D ❀v H Aplastic anemia. Agranulocytosis.

Divalproex Sodium (Depakote)	**Cap:** 125 mg; **Tab:** 125 mg, 250 mg, 500 mg	**Complex Partial Seizures: Adults & Peds >10 yo:** **Initial:** 10-15 mg/kg/d. **Titrate:** Increase by 5-10 mg/kg/wk. **Max:** 60 mg/kg/d. **Absence Seizures: Adults: Initial:** 15 mg/kg/d. **Titrate:** Increase by 5-10 mg/kg/wk. **Max:** 60 mg/kg/d.	⊕D ✿v Hepatotoxic. Teratogenic. Pancreatitis.
Divalproex Sodium (Depakote ER)	**Tab,ER:** 250 mg, 500 mg	**Complex Partial Seizures: Adults & Peds >10 yo:** **Initial:** 10-15 mg/kg qd. **Titrate:** Increase by 5-10 mg/kg/wk. **Usual:** <60 mg/kg/d. **Absence** **Seizures: Adults & Peds >10 yo: Initial:** 15 mg/kg qd. **Titrate:** Increase by 5-10 mg/kg/wk. **Max:** 60 mg/kg/d.	⊕D ✿v Hepatotoxic. Teratogenic. Pancreatitis.
Felbamate (Felbatol)	**Susp:** 600 mg/5 ml; **Tab:** 400 mg, 600 mg	**Partial & Generalized Seizures: ≥14 yo: Initial:** 300 mg qid or 400 mg tid. **Max:** 3.6 gm/d. **Lennox-Gastaut Adjunct Therapy: 2-14 yo: Initial:** 15 mg/kg/d. **Titrate:** Increase wkly by 15 mg/kg/d to 45 mg/kg/d.	⊕C ✿> H R Hepatic failure. Aplastic anemia.
Gabapentin (Neurontin)	**Cap:** 100 mg, 300 mg, 400 mg; **Sol:** 250 mg/5 ml; **Tab:** 600 mg, 800 mg	**Partial Seizures: Adults & Peds ≥12 yo: Initial:** 300 mg tid. **Titrate:** Increase up to 1.8 gm/d. **Max:** 3.6 gm/d. **3-12 yo: Initial:** 10-15 mg/kg/d given tid. **Titrate:** Increase over 3d. **Usual: 3-4 yo:** 40 mg/kg/d given tid. **≥5 yo:** 25-35 mg/kg/d given tid. **Max:** 50 mg/kg/d.	⊕C ✿> R

NAME	FORM/STRENGTH	DOSAGE	COMMENTS
Lamotrigine (Lamictal, Lamictal CD)	**Chewtab:** (CD) 2 mg, 5 mg, 25 mg; **Tab:** 25 mg, 100 mg, 150 mg, 200 mg	**Lennox-Gastaut/Partial Seizures:** Special dosing requirements with VPA. **Adults & Peds >12 yo: Concomitant EIAEDs with VPA:** 25 mg qod x 2 wks, then 25 mg qd x 2 wks. **Titrate:** Increase q1-2 wks by 25-50 mg/d. **Maint:** 100-400 mg/d, given qd or bid. **Concomitant EIAEDs without VPA:** 50 mg qd x 2 wks, then 50 mg bid x 2 wks. **Titrate:** Increase q1-2wks by 100 mg/d. **Maint:** 150-250 mg bid. **Conversion to Monotherapy From Single EIAED:** ≥16 yrs: 50 mg qd x 2 wks, then 50 mg bid x 2 wks. **Titrate:** Increase q1-2 wks by 100 mg/day. **Maint:** 250 mg bid. Withdraw EIAED over 4 weeks. **Conversion to Monotherapy From VPA:** ≥16 yrs: **Step 1:** Follow Concomitant AEDs with VPA dosing regimen to achieve Lamictal dose of 200 mg/day. Maintain previous VPA dose. **Step 2:** Maintain Lamictal 200 mg/day. Decrease VPA to 500 mg/day by decrements of ≤500 mg/day per wk. Maintain VPA 500 mg/day x 1 wk. **Step 3:** Increase to Lamictal 300 mg/day x 1 wk. Decrease VPA simultaneously to 250 mg/day x 1 wk. **Step 4:** Discontinue VPA. Increase Lamictal 100 mg/day every wk to maint dose of 500 mg/day. **Peds: 2-12 yo:** ≥6.7 kg: **Concomitant EIAEDs without VPA:** 0.3 mg/kg bid x 2 wks, then 0.6 mg/kg bid x 2 wks. **Titrate:** Increase q1-2wks by 1.2 mg/kg/d. **Maint:** 2.5-7.5 mg/kg bid. **Max:** 400 mg/d. Round dose down to nearest whole tab.	ⓒC ❀v H R Serious rashes, Stevens-Johnson syndrome reported.

Levetiracetam (Keppra)	Sol: 100 mg/ml; Tab: 250 mg, 500 mg, 750 mg	Partial Onset Seizures: ≥16 yo: Initial: 500 mg bid. Titrate: Increase q2wks by 1000 mg/d. Max: 3 gm/d.	⬤C ✿> R
Magnesium Sulfate	Inj: 40 mg/ml, 80 mg/ml	Nephritic Seizures: Peds: 20-40 mg/kg IM to control seizures.	⬤A ✿>
Oxcarbazepine (Trileptal)	Susp: 300 mg/5 ml; Tab: 150 mg, 300 mg, 600 mg	Partial Seizures: Monotherapy: Adults: Initial: 300 mg bid. Titrate: Increase by 300 mg/d q3d. Maint: 1200 mg/d. 4-16 yo: Initial: 4-5 mg/kg bid. Titrate: Increase by 5 mg/kg/d q3d. Maint (mg/d): 20 kg: Initial: 600 mg. Max: 900 mg. 25-30 kg: Initial: 900 mg. Max: 1200 mg. 35-40 kg: Initial: 900 mg. Max: 1500 mg. 45 kg: Initial: 1200 mg. Max: 1500 mg. 50-55 kg: Initial: 1200 mg. Max: 1800 mg. 60-65 kg: Initial: 1200 mg. Max: 2100 mg. 70 kg: Initial: 1500 mg. Max: 2100 mg. Adjunct Therapy: Adults: Initial: 300 mg bid. Titrate: Increase wkly by max of 600 mg/d. Maint: 600 mg bid. 4-16 yo: Initial: 4-5 mg/kg bid. Max: 600 mg/d. Titrate: Increase over 2 wks. Maint (mg/d): 20-29 kg: 900 mg. 29.1-39 kg: 1200 mg. >39 kg: 1800 mg. Conversion to Monotherapy: Adults: Initial: 300 mg bid while reducing other AEDs. Titrate: Increase wkly by 600 mg/d. Maint: 2400 mg/d. 4-16 yo: Initial: 4-5 mg/kg bid while reducing other AEDs. Titrate: Increase wkly by max of 10 mg/kg/d to target dose. Withdraw other AEDs over 3-6 wks.	⬤C ✿v R

NAME	FORM/STRENGTH	DOSAGE	COMMENTS
Primidone (Mysoline)	**Tab:** 50 mg, 250 mg	**Grand Mal/Psychomotor/Focal Seizures: Adults and Peds ≥8 yo: Initial/Titrate: Days 1-3:** 100-125 mg qhs. **Days 4-6:** 100-125 mg bid. **Days 7-9:** 100-125 mg tid. **Day 10-Maint:** 250 mg tid. **Max:** 500 mg qid. **<8 yo: Initial/Titrate: Days 1-3:** 50 mg qhs. **Days 4-6:** 50 mg bid. **Days 7-9:** 100 mg bid. **Day 10-Maint:** 125-250 mg tid or 10-25 mg/kg/d in divided doses.	●N ❖✿
Tiagabine (Gabitril)	**Tab:** 2 mg, 4 mg, 12 mg, 16 mg, 20 mg	**Partial Seizures: Adults: Initial:** 4 mg qd. **Titrate:** Increase qwk up to 56 mg/d given bid-qid. **12-18 yo: Initial:** 4 mg qd. **Titrate:** Increase qwk up to 32 mg/d given bid-qid.	●C ❖✿
Topiramate (Topamax)	**Cap:** 15 mg, 25 mg; **Tab:** 25 mg, 100 mg, 200 mg	**Partial Onset/Tonic-Clonic Seizures: ≥17 yo: Initial:** 25-50 mg qpm. **Titrate:** Increase qwk by 25-50 mg. **Usual:** 200 mg bid. **Max:** 1600 mg/d. **2-16 yo: Initial:** 1-3 mg/kg/d qpm x 1 wk. **Titrate:** Increase by 1-3 mg/kg/d qwk. **Usual:** 5-9 mg/kg/d given as bid.	●C ❖> R
Valproate Sodium (Depacon)	**Inj:** 100 mg/ml	**Complex Partial Seizure: Adults & Peds ≥10 yo: IV: Initial:** 10-15 mg/kg/d. **Titrate:** Increase wkly by 5-10 mg/kg/d. **Max:** 60 mg/kg/d. **Simplex/Complex Absence Seizure: Adults: IV: Initial:** 15 mg/kg/d. **Titrate:** Increase wkly by 5-10 mg/kg/d. **Max:** 60 mg/kg/d.	●D ❖v H Hepatic failure. Teratogenic. Pancreatitis.

Valproic Acid (Depakene)	Cap: 250 mg; Syr: 250 mg/5 ml	Complex Partial Seizure: Adults & Peds ≥10 yo: Initial: 10-15 mg/kg/d. Titrate: Increase wkly by 5-10 mg/kg/d. Max: 60 mg/kg/d. Simplex/Complex Absence Seizure: Adults: Initial: 15 mg/kg/d. Titrate: Increase wkly by 5-10 mg/kg/d. Max: 60 mg/kg/d.	●D ❄v H Hepatic failure. Teratogenic. Pancreatitis.

Antidepressant Agents

5-HT$_2$/ALPHA$_1$ ANTAGONISTS

Nefazodone	Tab: 50 mg, 100 mg, 150 mg, 200 mg, 250 mg	≥18 yo: Initial: 100 mg bid. Titrate: Increase qwk by 100-200 mg/d. Usual: 300-600 mg/d.	●C ❄> Hepatic failure reported.

DOPAMINE/NOREPINEPHRINE REUPTAKE INHIBITOR

Bupropion HCl (Wellbutrin XL)	Tab,ER: 150 mg, 300 mg	≥18 yo: Initial: 150 mg qam, may increase to 300 mg qam after 3d. Usual: 300 mg qam. Max: 450 mg qam. Swallow whole.	●B ❄v H R
Bupropion (Wellbutrin, Wellbutrin SR)	Tab: 75 mg, 100 mg; Tab,ER: 100 mg, 150 mg, 200 mg	≥18 yo: Tab: Initial: 100 mg bid. Maint: 100 mg tid. Max: 450 mg/d. Tab,ER: Initial: 150 mg qam. Maint: 150 mg bid. Max: 200 mg bid.	●B ❄v H R

MAOIS

Isocarboxazid (Marplan)	Tab: 10 mg	≥16 yo: Initial: 10 mg bid. Titrate: Increase by 10 mg q2-4d to 40 mg/d by end of wk. Max: 60 mg/d.	●N ❄v
Phenelzine (Nardil)	Tab: 15 mg	≥16 yo: Initial: 15 mg tid. Titrate/Maint: Increase to 60-90 mg/d until max benefit, then reduce dose to 15 mg qd or 15 mg qod.	●N ❄>

NAME	FORM/STRENGTH	DOSAGE	COMMENTS
Tranylcypromine (Parnate)	**Tab:** 10 mg	**Adults: Initial:** 30 mg/d in divided doses. **Titrate:** Increase by 10 mg/d q1-3wks. **Max:** 60 mg/d.	◑N ❄>

SEROTONIN/NE REUPTAKE INHIBITORS

NAME	FORM/STRENGTH	DOSAGE	COMMENTS
Venlafaxine (Effexor, Effexor XR)	**Cap,ER:** 37.5 mg, 75 mg, 150 mg; **Tab:** 25 mg, 37.5 mg, 50 mg, 75 mg, 100 mg	**≥18 yo: Tab: Initial:** 37.5 mg bid or 25 mg tid. **Titrate:** Increase by 75 mg/d q4d to 150-225 mg/d. **Max:** 375 mg/d. **Cap,ER: Initial:** 75 mg/d. **Titrate:** Increase by 75 mg/d at intervals not less than 4d. **Max:** 225 mg/d.	◑C ❄v H R

SSRIS

NAME	FORM/STRENGTH	DOSAGE	COMMENTS
Citalopram (Celexa)	**Sol:** 10 mg/5 ml; **Tab:** 10 mg, 20 mg, 40 mg	**Adults: Initial:** 20 mg qd, in am or pm. **Titrate:** May increase by 20 mg at intervals ≥1 wk, to 40 mg/d. **Max:** 60 mg/d.	◑C ❄v H
Escitalopram Oxalate (Lexapro)	**Sol:** 5 mg/5 ml; **Tab:** 5 mg, 10 mg, 20 mg	**Adults: Initial:** 10 mg qd, in am or pm. **Titrate:** May increase to 20 mg after at least 1 wk. **Elderly:** 10 mg qd.	◑C ❄v H
Fluoxetine (Prozac Weekly)	**Cap,ER:** 90 mg	**Prozac Weekly: Initial:** One 90 mg capsule 7d after the last daily dose of Prozac 20 mg. Must be stabilized on 20 mg/d prior to initiation.	◑C ❄v H

Fluoxetine (Prozac)	Cap: 10 mg, 20 mg, 40 mg; Sol: 20 mg/5 ml; Tab: 10 mg	**Adults: Daily Dosing: Initial:** 20 mg qam. **Titrate:** Increase dose if no improvement after several wks. Doses >20 mg/d, give qam or bid (am and noon). **Max:** 80 mg/d. **Peds ≥8 yo: Higher Weight Peds: Initial:** 10 or 20 mg/d. After 1 wk at 10 mg/d, may increase to 20 mg/d. **Lower Weight Peds: Initial:** 10 mg/d. **Titrate:** May increase to 20 mg/d after several wks if clinical improvement not observed.	●C ❄v H
Paroxetine (Paxil, Paxil CR)	Susp: 10 mg/5 ml; Tab: 10 mg, 20 mg, 30 mg, 40 mg; Tab,CR: 12.5 mg, 25 mg, 37.5 mg	**Adults: Susp/Tab: Initial:** 20 mg qam. **Max:** 50 mg/d. **Tab,CR: Initial:** 25 mg/d. **Titrate:** May increase wkly by 12.5 mg/d. **Max:** 62.5 mg/d.	●C ❄> H R
Sertraline (Zoloft)	Sol: 20 mg/ml; Tab: 25 mg, 50 mg, 100 mg	**Adults: Initial:** 50 mg qd. **Titrate:** Adjust wkly. **Max:** 200 mg/d.	●C ❄> H

TETRACYCLICS

| Maprotiline | Tab: 25 mg, 50 mg, 75 mg | **Adults: Outpatients: Initial:** 25-75 mg qd x 2 wks. **Maint:** Increase by 25 mg. **Max:** 225 mg/d. **Adults: Hospitalized: Initial:** 100-150 mg qd. **Maint:** 150-225 mg/d. **Max:** 225 mg/d. | ●B ❄> |
| Mirtazapine (Remeron, Remeron SolTab) | Tab,Dissolve: 15 mg, 30 mg, 45 mg; Tab: 15 mg, 30 mg, 45 mg | **Adults: Initial:** 15 mg qhs. **Titrate:** Increase q1-2wks. **Maint:** 15-45 mg qd. **Max:** 45 mg qd. | ●C ❄> |

NAME	FORM/STRENGTH	DOSAGE	COMMENTS
TRICYCLIC ANTIDEPRESSANTS			
Amitriptyline	**Inj:** 10 mg/ml; **Tab:** 10 mg, 25 mg, 50 mg, 75 mg, 100 mg, 150 mg	**PO: Adults: Initial:** (Outpatient) 75 mg/d in divided doses or 50-100 mg qhs. (Inpatient) 100 mg/d. **Titrate:** (Outpatient) Increase by 25-50 mg qhs. (Inpatient) Increase to 200 mg/d. **Maint:** 50-100 mg qhs. **Max:** (Outpatient) 150 mg/d. (Inpatient) 300 mg/d. **≥12 yo:** 10 mg tid or 20 mg qhs. **Adults & Peds ≥12 yo: IM: Initial:** 20-30 mg qid. **Elderly:** 10mg tid or 20 mg qhs.	●C ❄v
Amoxapine	**Tab:** 25 mg, 50 mg, 100 mg, 150 mg	**≥16 yo: Initial:** 50 mg bid-tid. **Titrate:** Increase to 100 mg bid-tid. **Maint:** Effective dose given qhs. **Max:** 300 mg/d.	●C ❄>
Desipramine HCl (Norpramin)	**Tab:** 10 mg, 25 mg, 50 mg, 75 mg, 100 mg, 150 mg	**Adults: Usual:** 100-200 mg qd. **Max:** 300 mg/d. **Adolescents: Usual:** 25-100 mg qd. **Max:** 150 mg/d.	●N ❄>
Doxepin (Sinequan)	**Cap:** 10 mg, 25 mg, 50 mg, 75 mg, 100 mg, 150 mg; **Sol:** 10 mg/ml	**Adults & Peds ≥12 yo: Mild Illness: Usual:** 25-50 mg/d. **Mild-Moderate: Initial:** 75 mg/d. **Usual:** 75-150 mg/d. **Severely Ill:** Up to 300 mg/d.	●N ❄>
Imipramine HCl (Tofranil)	**Tab:** 10 mg, 25 mg, 50 mg	**Adults: Initial:** (Inpatients) 100 mg/d; may increase to 200 mg/d x 2 wks, then 250-300 mg/d if needed. (Outpatients) 75 mg/d; may increase to 150 mg/d, then to 200 mg/d if needed. **Maint:** 50-150 mg/d. **Adolescents: Initial:** 30-40 mg qhs. **Max:** 100 mg/d.	●N ❄v

Imipramine Pamoate (Tofranil-PM)	**Cap:** 75 mg, 100 mg, 125 mg, 150 mg	**Adults: Initial:** (Inpatients) 100-150 mg/d; may increase to 200 mg/d x 2 wks, then 250-300 mg/d if needed. (Outpatients) 75 mg/d; may increase to 150 mg/d, then to 200 mg/d if needed. **Maint:** 75-150 mg/d. **Adolescents:** May use if daily dose ≥75 mg.	⊙N ❄v
Nortriptyline HCl (Pamelor)	**Cap:** 10 mg, 25 mg, 50 mg, 75 mg; **Sol:** 10 mg/5 ml	**Adults: Usual:** 25 mg tid-qid. **Max:** 150 mg/d. **Adolescents:** 30-50 mg/d.	⊙N ❄>
Protriptyline HCl (Vivactil)	**Tab:** 5 mg, 10 mg	**Adults: Initial:** 15-40 mg/d given tid-qid. **Max:** 60 mg/d. **Adolescents: Initial:** 5 mg tid. **Maint:** Increase gradually if necessary.	⊙N ❄>
Trimipramine Maleate (Surmontil)	**Cap:** 25 mg, 50 mg, 100 mg	**Adults: Outpatients: Initial:** 75 mg/d in divided doses. **Maint:** 50-150 mg/d. **Max:** 200 mg/d. **Adults: Inpatients: Initial:** 100 mg/d in divided doses. **Titrate:** Increase gradually to 200 mg/d. **Max:** 250-300 mg/d. **Adolescents: Initial:** 50 mg/d. **Max:** 100 mg/d.	⊙C ❄>

MISCELLANEOUS

Trazodone (Desyrel)	**Tab:** 50 mg, 100 mg, 150 mg, 300 mg	**≥18 yo: Initial:** 150 mg/d in divided doses. **Titrate:** Increase by 50 mg/d q3-4d. **Max:** (Outpatients) 400 mg/d, (Inpatients) 600 mg/d.	⊙C ❄>

NAME	FORM/STRENGTH	DOSAGE	COMMENTS

Antidepressant/Anxiolytic Combinations

NAME	FORM/STRENGTH	DOSAGE	COMMENTS
Amitriptyline/ Chlordiazepoxide CIV (Limbitrol, Limbitrol DS)	**Tab:** 12.5 mg-5 mg, 25 mg-10 mg	**Adults & Peds ≥12 yo: Initial:** 3-4 tabs/d in divided doses. **Maint:** 2-6 tabs/d.	●N ✿v
Amitriptyline/Perphenazine (Etrafon, Triavil)	**Tab:** 10 mg-2 mg, 25 mg-2 mg, 25 mg-4 mg	**Adults: Initial:** 25-2 or 25-4 mg tab tid-qid or 50-4 mg bid. **Maint:** 25-2 or 25-4 mg bid-qid or 50-4 mg bid. **Max:** 4 tabs/d of 50-4 or 8 tabs/d any other strength.	●N ✿v

Antiparkinson's Agents

ANTICHOLINERGIC AGENTS

NAME	FORM/STRENGTH	DOSAGE	COMMENTS
Benztropine Mesylate (Cogentin)	**Inj:** 1 mg/ml; **Tab:** 0.5 mg, 1 mg, 2 mg	**Initial:** 0.5-1 mg PO/IV/IM qhs. **Usual:** 1-2 mg/d. **Max:** 6 mg/d.	●N ✿>
Trihexyphenidyl	**Eli:** 2 mg/5 ml; **Tab:** 2 mg, 5 mg	**Idiopathic:** 1 mg on d1. **Titrate:** Increase by 2 mg q3-5d. **Usual:** 6-10 mg/d. **Max:** 15 mg/d. **Drug-Induced: Initial:** 1 mg, increase until achieve control. **Usual:** 5-15 mg/d.	●N ✿>

COMT INHIBITOR

NAME	FORM/STRENGTH	DOSAGE	COMMENTS
Entacapone (Comtan)	**Tab:** 200 mg	**Adults:** 200 mg with each levodopa/carbidopa dose. **Max:** 1600 mg/d.	●C ✿>
Tolcapone (Tasmar)	**Tab:** 100 mg, 200 mg	**Adults: Initial:** 100 mg tid. Use 200 mg tid if clinical benefit justified. May need to decrease levodopa dose.	●C ✿> Risk of acute fulminant liver failure.

DOPAMINE AGONISTS

Drug	Forms	Dosage	
Bromocriptine Mesylate (Parlodel)	**Cap:** 5 mg; **Tab:** 2.5 mg	**Adults: Initial:** 1.25 mg bid. **Titrate:** Increase by 2.5 mg/d q2-4wks. **Max:** 100 mg/d.	●B ❄v
Pergolide Mesylate (Permax)	**Tab:** 0.05 mg, 0.25 mg, 1 mg	**Adults: Initial:** 0.05 mg/d for 1st 2d. **Titrate:** Increase by 0.1-0.15 mg/d q3d over next 12d, then increase by 0.25 mg/d q3d. **Max:** 5 mg/d. Give in 3 divided doses.	●B ❄v
Pramipexole (Mirapex)	**Tab:** 0.125 mg, 0.25 mg, 0.5 mg, 1 mg, 1.5 mg	**Initial:** 0.125 mg tid. **Titrate:** Increase q5-7d according to titration table. **Maint:** to 0.5-1.5 mg tid.	●C ❄v R
Ropinirole (Requip)	**Tab:** 0.25 mg, 0.5 mg, 1 mg, 2 mg, 3 mg, 4 mg, 5 mg	**Initial:** 0.25 mg tid. **Titrate/Maint:** Increase wkly by 0.25 mg tid x 4 wks. After wk 4, increase wkly by 1.5 mg/d up to 9 mg/d, then by 3 mg/d wkly to 24 mg/d.	●C ❄v

DOPAMINE PRECURSOR/DOPA-DECARBOXYLASE INHIBITOR/COMT INHIBITOR

Drug	Forms	Dosage	
Carbidopa/Levodopa/ Entacapone (Stalevo 50, Stalevo 100, Stalevo 150)	**Tab:** 12.5 mg/50 mg/ 200 mg; 25 mg/100 mg/ 200 mg; 37.5 mg/ 150 mg/200 mg	**Adults: Currently Taking Carbidopa/Levodopa and Entacapone:** May switch directly to corresponding strength of levodopa/carbidopa. **Currently Taking Carbidopa/Levodopa but not Entacapone:** First titrate individually with carbidopa/levodopa product and entacapone product then transfer to corresponding dose. **Max:** 8 tabs/d.	●C ❄>

MAOIS

Drug	Forms	Dosage	
Selegeline HCl (Eldepryl)	**Cap:** 5 mg	**Adults:** 5 mg bid, at breakfast & lunch. **Max:** 10 mg/d.	●C ❄v

NAME	FORM/STRENGTH	DOSAGE	COMMENTS

Antipsychotic Agents

BENZISOXAZOLE DERIVATIVE

NAME	FORM/STRENGTH	DOSAGE	COMMENTS
Risperidone (Risperdal, Risperdal Consta, Risperdal M-Tab)	**Inj:** 25 mg, 37.5 mg, 50 mg; **Sol:** 1 mg/ml; **Tab:** 0.25 mg, 0.5 mg, 1 mg, 2 mg, 3 mg, 4 mg; **Tab, Dissolve:** 0.5 mg, 1 mg, 2 mg	**Adults: Schizophrenia: Inj:** 25 mg IM q2wks. **Max:** 50 mg/dose. Give 1st inj with oral dosage form or other oral antipsychotic. Continue for 3 wks, then d/c oral. **Titrate:** Increase at intervals of no more than q4wks. **PO: Initial:** 1 mg bid. **Maint:** 2-8 mg/d given qd-bid. **Max:** 16 mg/d.	▣C ❄v H R
Ziprasidone (Geodon)	**Cap:** 20 mg, 40 mg, 60 mg, 80 mg; **Inj:** 20 mg/ml	**Adults: Initial: PO:** 20 mg bid w/food. **Max:** 80 mg bid. **Acute Agitation: IM:** 10 mg q2h or 20 mg q4h up to 40 mg/d x 3d.	▣C ❄v

BUTYROPHENONES

NAME	FORM/STRENGTH	DOSAGE	COMMENTS
Haloperidol (Haldol, Haldol Decanoate)	**Cnt:** 2 mg/ml; **Inj:** (lactate) 5 mg/ml; **Inj:** (decanoate) 50 mg/ml, 100 mg/ml; **Tab:** 0.5 mg, 1 mg, 2 mg, 5 mg, 10 mg, 20 mg	**Adults: Usual: PO:** 0.5-5 mg bid-tid. **IM:** (Lactate) 2-5 mg q4-8h or q1h prn. **Max:** 100 mg/d. (Decanoate) Give q4wks. 10-20x daily PO dose up to 100 mg. Give remainder of dose 3-7d later if initial dose >100 mg. **3-12 yo (15-40 kg): PO:** 0.05-0.15 mg/kg/d given bid-tid. **Max:** 6 mg/d.	▣C ❄v

DIBENZAPINE DERIVATIVE

Clozapine (Clozaril)	**Tab:** 12.5 mg, 25 mg, 100 mg	**Schizophrenia/Suicidal Behavior Risk Reduction:** **Adults: Initial:** 12.5 mg qd-bid. **Titrate:** Increase by 25-50 mg/d, up to 300-450 mg/d by end of 2nd wk, then increase wkly or bi-wkly by up to 100 mg. **Usual:** 100-900 mg/d given tid. **Max:** 900 mg/d. If at risk of suicial behavior then treat for at least 2 yrs then assess; reassess thereafter at regular intervals. To d/c, gradually reduce dose over 1-2 wks.	◕B ✿v [26]
Loxapine (Loxitane)	**Cap:** 5 mg, 10 mg, 25 mg, 50 mg; **Cnt:** 25 mg/ml; **Inj:** 50 mg/ml	**Adults: PO: Initial:** 10 mg bid, up to 50 mg/d for severely disturbed. **Titrate:** Increase rapidly over 7-10d. **Maint:** 60-100 mg/d. **Max:** 250 mg/d. **IM:** 12.5-50 mg q4-6h. Individualize dose.	◕N ✿v
Olanzapine (Zyprexa, Zyprexa Zydis, Zyprexa IntraMuscular)	**Inj:** 10 mg; **Tab:** 2.5 mg, 5 mg, 7.5 mg, 10 mg, 15 mg, 20 mg; **Tab,Dissolve:** 5 mg, 10 mg, 15 mg, 20 mg	**Adults: Schizophrenia: PO: Initial/Usual:** 5-10 mg qd. **Titrate:** Adjust wkly by 5 mg/d. **Agitation Associated with Schizophrenia: Inj: Initial:** 10 mg IM. **Range:** 2.5-10 mg IM. **Max:** 3 doses of 10 mg IM q2-4h. May initiate PO therapy when clinically appropriate.	◕C ✿v
Quetiapine Fumarate (Seroquel)	**Tab:** 25 mg, 100 mg, 200 mg, 300 mg	**Adults: Initial:** 25 mg bid. **Titrate:** Increase by 25-50 mg bid-tid daily up to 300-400 mg/d. May adjust by 25-50 mg bid q2d. **Max:** 800 mg/d.	◕C ✿v H

[26] Agranulocytosis, Seizures. Myocarditis. Other cardiovascular/respiratory effects.

NAME	FORM/STRENGTH	DOSAGE	COMMENTS
DIHYDROINDOLONE DERIVATIVES			
Molindone (Moban)	Syr: 20 mg/ml; Tab: 5 mg, 10 mg, 25 mg, 50 mg, 100 mg	≥12 yo: Initial: 50-75 mg/d; Titrate: Increase to 100 mg/d in 3-4d, & adjust to patient response. Maint: (mild) 5-15 mg bid-qid, (moderate) 10-25 mg tid-qid, (severe) 225 mg/d.	N⊛ ≋ ⟨H⟩
PARTIAL D2/5HT1A AGONIST/5HT2A ANTAGONIST			
Aripiprazole (Abilify)	Tab: 5 mg, 10 mg, 15 mg, 20 mg, 30 mg	Adults: Initial/Target: 10-15 mg qd. Titrate: Should not increase before 2 wks. Maint: Periodically reassess need for therapy. Adjust dose with CYP450 3A4 inducers and inhibitors, or with CYP450 2D6 inhibitors.	∨⊛ ≋ C⟨H⟩
PHENOTHIAZINES			
Chlorpromazine	Cap,ER: 30 mg, 75 mg; Inj: 25 mg/ml; Sup: 25 mg, 100 mg; Syr: 10 mg/5 ml; Tab: 10 mg, 25 mg, 50 mg, 100 mg, 200 mg	Adults: Inpatient: Acute State: 25 mg IM, then 25-50 mg in 1h if needed. Titrate: Increase up to 400 mg q4-6h until controlled then switch to PO. Max: 1 gm/d PO. Outpatient: 10 mg PO tid-qid or 25 mg PO bid-tid. Titrate: After 1-2d, increase by 20-50 mg BIW.	N⟨H⟩ ≋ ∨
Fluphenazine (Prolixin, Prolixin Decanoate)	Cnt: 5 mg/ml; Inj: (Decanoate) 25 mg/ml; (HCl) 2.5 mg/ml; Eli: 2.5 mg/ml; Tab: 1 mg, 2.5 mg, 5 mg, 10 mg	Adults: PO: Initial: 2.5-10 mg/d given q6-8h. Titrate: Increase up to 40 mg/d. Maint: 1-5 mg qd. Inj, HCl: Initial: 1.25 mg IM. Max: 10 mg/d. Decanoate: Initial: 12.5-25 mg IM/SC q4-6wks. Max: 100 mg/dose.	N⟨H⟩ ≋ ∨

Mesoridazine Besylate (Serentil)	Cnt: 25 mg/ml; Inj: 25 mg/ml; Tab: 10 mg, 25 mg, 100 mg	≥12 yo: Schizophrenia: PO: Initial: 50 mg tid. Maint: 100-400 mg/d. IM: Initial: 25 mg. Maint: 25-200 mg/d.	◉N ✿> QTc prolongation.
Perphenazine (Trilafon)	Inj: 5 mg/ml; Tab: 2 mg, 4 mg, 8 mg, 16 mg	≥12 yo: IM: Initial: 5 mg IM. May repeat q6h. Max: 15 mg/d if ambulatory or 30 mg/d if hospitalized. PO: Outpatients: 4-8 mg tid. Maint: Reduce to min effective dose. Inpatients: 8-16 mg bid-qid. Max: 64 mg/d.	◉N ✿>
Prochlorperazine (Compazine)	Cap,ER: 10 mg, 15 mg; Inj: 5 mg/ml; Sup: 2.5 mg, 5 mg, 25 mg; Syr: 5 mg/5 ml; Tab: 5 mg, 10 mg	Adults: Outpatients: 5-10 mg PO tid-qid. Moderate-Severe/Hospitalized: Initial: 10 mg PO tid-qid. May increase q2-3d. Severe: 100-150 mg/d PO. 10-20 mg IM, may repeat q2-4h prn. Switch to PO after obtain control or if needed, 10-20 mg IM q4-6h. Peds: PO/PR: 2-12 yo: Initial: 2.5 mg bid-tid, up to 10 mg/d on d1. Max: 2-5 yo: 20 mg/d. 6-12 yo: 25 mg/d. IM: <12 yo: 0.06 mg/lb single dose. Switch to PO after obtain control.	◉N ✿>
Thioridazine (Mellaril)	Cnt: 30 mg/ml,100 mg/ml; Tab: 10 mg, 15 mg, 25 mg, 50 mg, 100 mg, 150 mg, 200 mg	Adults: Initial: 50-100 mg tid. Maint: 200-800 mg/d given bid-qid. Peds: Initial: 0.5 mg/kg/d given in divided doses. Max: 3 mg/kg/d.	◉N ✿> QTc prolongation.

NAME	FORM/STRENGTH	DOSAGE	COMMENTS
Trifluoperazine	**Tab:** 1 mg, 2 mg, 5 mg, 10 mg	**Psychotic Disorders: Adults: Initial:** 2-5 mg bid. **Usual:** 15-20 mg/d. **Max:** 40 mg/d or more if needed. **Peds 6-12 yo: Initial:** 1 mg qd-bid. Increase gradually until symptoms controlled. **Usual:** 15 mg/d. **Non-Psychotic Anxiety: Adults:** 1-2 mg bid. **Max:** 6 mg/d or >12 wks.	◐N ❄v

THIOXANTHENE DERIVATIVES

NAME	FORM/STRENGTH	DOSAGE	COMMENTS
Thiothixene (Navane)	**Cap:** 1 mg, 2 mg, 5 mg, 10 mg, 20 mg	**≥12 yo: Mild Condition: Initial:** 2 mg tid. **Titrate:** May increase to 15 mg/d. **Severe Condition: Initial:** 5 mg bid. **Usual:** 20-30 mg/d. **Max:** 60 mg/d.	◐N ❄v

Bipolar Agents

NAME	FORM/STRENGTH	DOSAGE	COMMENTS
Divalproex Sodium (Depakote)	**Tab:** 125 mg, 250 mg, 500 mg	**Adults: Mania Associated with Bipolar Disorder: Initial:** 750 mg in divided doses. **Titrate:** Increase rapidly to clinical effect. **Max:** 60 mg/kg/d.	◐D ❄v Hepatotoxic. Teratogenic. Pancreatitis.
Lamotrigine (Lamictal, Lamictal CD)	**Chewtab:** (CD) 2 mg, 5 mg, 25 mg; **Tab:** 25 mg, 100 mg, 150 mg, 200 mg	**Bipolar Disorder: Patients not taking carbamazepine (CBZ), other enzyme-inducing drugs (EIDs) or VPA: Weeks 1 and 2:** 25 mg/d. **Weeks 3 and 4:** 50 mg/d. **Week 5:** 100 mg/d. **Weeks 6 and 7:** 200 mg/d. **Patients taking VPA: Weeks 1 and 2:** 25 mg qod. **Weeks 3 and 4:** 25 mg/d. **Week 5:** 50 mg/d. **Weeks 6 and 7:** 100 mg/d. **Patients taking CBZ (or other EIDs) and not taking VPA: Weeks 1 and 2:** 50 mg/d. **Weeks 3 and 4:** 100 mg/d (divided doses).	◐C ❄v H R Serious rashes, Stevens-Johnson syndrome reported.

		Week 5: 200 mg/d (divided doses). **Week 6:** 300 mg/d (divided doses). **Week 7:** up to 400 mg/d (divided doses). **After discontinuation of psychotropic drugs excluding VPA, CBZ, or other EIDs:** Maintain current dose. **After discontinuation of VPA and current lamotrigine dose of 100 mg/d: Week 1:** 150 mg/d. **Week 2 and onward:** 200 mg/d. **After discontinuation of CBZ or other EIDs and current lamotrigine dose of 400 mg/d: Week 1:** 400 mg/d. **Week 2:** 300 mg/d. **Week 3 and onward:** 200 mg/d.	
Lithium Carbonate (Eskalith, Eskalith CR)	**Cap:** 300 mg; **Tab,ER:** 450 mg	≥**12 yo: Mania: Acute: Cap:** 600 mg tid. **Tab,ER:** 900 mg bid. Effective serum levels of 1-1.5 mEq/L. **Mania: Long Term Control: Cap:** 300 mg tid-qid. **Tab,ER:** 450 mg bid. Effective serum levels of 0.6-1.2 mEq/L.	⬤N ❋v Lithium toxicity related to serum levels.
Lithium Citrate	**Syr:** 300 mg/5 ml	≥**12 yo: Mania: Acute:** 600 mg tid, adjust to serum level 1.0-1.5 mEq/L. **Mania: Long Term Control:** 300 mg tid-qid, adjust to serum level 0.6-1.2 mEq/L.	⬤D ❋v Lithium toxicity related to serum levels.
Olanzapine (Zyprexa, Zyprexa Zydis, Zyprexa IntraMuscular)	**Inj:** 10 mg; **Tab:** 2.5 mg, 5 mg, 7.5 mg, 10 mg, 15 mg, 20 mg; **Tab,Dissolve:** 5 mg, 10 mg, 15 mg, 20 mg	**Adults: Bipolar Mania: Acute Monotherapy: PO: Initial:** 10-15 mg qd. **Titrate:** Adjust by 5 mg/d. **Max:** 20 mg/d. **Maintenance Monotherapy:** 5-20 mg/d. **Combination Therapy with Lithium or Valproate: Initial:** 10 mg qd. **Range:** 5-20 mg/d. **Max:** 20 mg/d. **Agitation Associated with Bipolar Mania: Inj: Initial:** 10 mg IM. **Range:** 2.5-10 mg IM. **Max:** 3 doses of 10 mg IM q2-4h. May initiate PO therapy when clinically appropriate.	⬤C ❋v

NAME	FORM/STRENGTH	DOSAGE	COMMENTS
Olanzapine/Fluoxetine HCl (Symbyax)	Cap: 6 mg/25 mg, 12 mg/25 mg, 6 mg/50 mg, 12 mg/50 mg	**Adults: Depressive Episodes Associated with Bipolar Disorder: Initial:** 6 mg/25 mg qd in evening. **Range:** 6 mg/25 mg to 12 mg/50 mg.	▣C ❋ ∨
Quetiapine Fumarate (Seroquel)	Tab: 25 mg, 100 mg, 200 mg, 300 mg	**Adults: Initial:** 100 mg/day given bid. **Titrate:** Increase to 400 mg/day given bid on 4th day in increments of up to 100 mg/day given bid. Adjust doses up to 800 mg/day by 6th day by increments ≥200 mg/day. **Max:** 800 mg/day.	▣C ❋ ∨ H
Risperidone (Risperdal, Risperdal M-Tab)	Sol: 1 mg/ml; Tab: 0.25 mg, 0.5 mg, 1 mg, 2 mg, 3 mg, 4 mg; Dissolve: 0.5 mg, 1 mg, 2 mg	**Adults: Bipolar Mania: Initial:** 2-3 mg qd. **Titrate:** Increase by 1 mg qd. **Max:** 6 mg/d.	▣C ❋ ∨ H R

Migraine Therapy

5-HT₁ AGONISTS

NAME	FORM/STRENGTH	DOSAGE	COMMENTS
Almotriptan Malate (Axert)	Tab: 6.25 mg, 12.5 mg	**≥18 yo: Acute Therapy: Initial:** 6.25-12.5 mg, may repeat after 2h. **Max:** 2 doses/24h.	▣C ❋ ∨ H R
Eletriptan HBr (Relpax)	Tab: 20 mg, 40 mg	**≥18 yo: Adults: Acute Therapy: Initial:** 20 mg or 40 mg at onset of headache. If it recurs after initial relief, may repeat after 2h. **Max:** 40 mg/dose or 80 mg/d.	▣C ❋ H
Frovatriptan Succinate (Frova)	Tab: 2.5 mg	**≥18 yo: Acute Therapy: Initial:** 2.5 mg, may repeat after 2h. **Max:** 7.5 mg/d.	▣C ❋ ∨

Naratriptan HCl (Amerge)	**Tab:** 1 mg, 2.5 mg	**≥18 yo: Acute Therapy: Initial:** 1-2.5 mg, may repeat once after 4h. **Max:** 5 mg/24h.	⬤C ❄> **H R**
Rizatriptan Benzoate (Maxalt, Maxalt-MLT)	**Tab:** 5 mg, 10 mg; **Tab, Dissolve (ODT):** 5 mg, 10 mg	**≥18 yo: Acute Therapy: Initial:** 5-10 mg, may repeat q2h. **Max:** 30 mg/24h. Place ODT on tongue.	⬤C ❄> **H R** Adjust dose with propranolol.
Sumatriptan (Imitrex)	**Inj:** 6 mg/0.5 ml; **Nasal Spray:** 5 mg/spray, 20 mg/spray; **Tab:** 25 mg, 50 mg, 100 mg	**≥18 yo: Acute Therapy: Initial:** 6 mg SC, may repeat in 1h; 25-100 mg PO, may repeat in 2h; 5 mg, 10 mg, or 20 mg nasal spray, may repeat in 2h. **Max:** 12 mg/24h SC, 200 mg/24h PO; 40 mg/24h nasal spray.	⬤C ❄> **H** (Tab)
Zolmitriptan (Zomig, Zomig-ZMT)	**Tab:** 2.5 mg, 5 mg; **Tab, Dissolve (ODT):** 2.5 mg, 5 mg; **Nasal Spray:** 5 mg/spray	**≥18 yo: Acute Therapy: Initial:** PO: 2.5 mg or lower, may repeat after 2 hrs. **Nasal Spray:** 5 mg, may repeat after 2 hrs. **Max:** 10 mg/24h.	⬤C ❄> **H**

ERGOT DERIVATIVES

| Caffeine/Ergot (Cafergot, Wigraine) | **Sup:** 100 mg-2 mg; **Tab:** 100 mg-1 mg | **Adults: Initial: Sup:** 1 sup PR at start of attack, then repeat after 1h if needed. **Max:** 2 sups/attack & 5 sups/wk. **Tab:** 2 tabs at start of attack, then 1 tab q30min. **Max:** 6 tabs/attack & 10 tabs/wk. | ⬤X ❄v Life-threatening peripheral iscemia with sup & concomitant potent CYP450 3A4 inhibitors. |

NAME	FORM/STRENGTH	DOSAGE	COMMENTS
Dihydroergotamine (Migranal Nasal Spray, DHE 45)	**Inj:** 1 mg/ml; **Nasal Spray:** 0.5 mg/spray	**Adults: Initial: DHE 45:** 1 mg IV/IM/SC, repeat q1h prn up to a total dose of 3 mg IM/SC or 2 mg IV per 24h. **Max:** 6 ml/wk. **Migranal:** 1 spray per nostril, repeat in 15 min. **Max:** 6 sprays/24h or 8 sprays/wk.	▣X ✿v Life-threatening peripheral ischemia reported with potent CYP450 3A4 inhibitors.
Methysergide Maleate (Sansert)	**Tab:** 2 mg	**Adults: Usual:** 4-8 mg qd with meals. Take 3-4 wk drug-free interval q6mths of therapy.	▣X ✿v Risk of pulmonary & cardiac toxicity.

NSAIDS

NAME	FORM/STRENGTH	DOSAGE	COMMENTS
Ibuprofen (Advil Migraine, Motrin Migraine)	**Cap:** (Advil) 200 mg; **Tab:** (Motrin) 200 mg	**Adults: Advil:** 400 mg with water. **Max:** 400 mg/d. **Motrin:** Take 200-400 mg with water. **Max:** 400 mg/d.	▣N ✿>

MISCELLANEOUS

NAME	FORM/STRENGTH	DOSAGE	COMMENTS
Caffeine/APAP/ASA (Excedrin Migraine)	**Tab:** 65-250-250 mg	**Adults:** 2 tabs with water. **Max:** 2 tabs/d.	▣N ✿>
Divalproex Sodium (Depakote, Depakote ER)	**Tab:** 125 mg, 250 mg, 500 mg; **Tab,ER:** 250 mg, 500 mg	**Prophylaxis: Depakote: ≥16 yo: Usual:** 250 mg bid. **Max:** 1000 mg/d. **Depakote ER: Adults: Initial:** 500 mg qd. **Maint:** 1000 mg/d.	▣D ✿v Hepatotoxic. Teratogenic. Pancreatitis.
Isometheptene/ Dichloralphenazone/APAP (Amidrine, Duradrin, Midrin)	**Cap:** 65-100-325 mg	**Adults:** 2 caps, then 1 cap q1h until relief. **Max:** 5 caps/12h.	▣N ✿>

| Rofecoxib (Vioxx) | **Susp:** 12.5 mg/5 mL, 25 mg/5 mL; **Tab:** 12.5 mg, 25 mg, 50 mg | **Adults: Acute Therapy: Initial:** 25 mg qd. **Max:** 50 mg qd. | ⊙C ❄v H |

Muscle Relaxants

Baclofen	**Tab:** 10 mg, 20 mg	≥12 yo: **Initial:** 5 mg tid x 3d. **Titrate:** Increase q3d by 5 mg tid. **Usual:** 40-80 mg/d. **Max:** 80 mg/d.	⊙N ❄> R
Carisoprodol (Soma)	**Tab:** 350 mg	≥12 yo: 350 mg tid & qhs.	⊙N ❄>
Carisoprodol/ASA (Soma Compound)	**Tab:** 200-325 mg	≥12 yo: 1-2 tabs qid.	⊙C ❄v
Chlorzoxazone (Parafon Forte DSC)	**Tab:** 500 mg	**Adults: Usual:** 500 mg tid-qid. **Titrate:** May increase to 750 mg tid-qid.	⊙N ❄>
Cyclobenzaprine (Flexeril)	**Tab:** 5 mg, 10 mg	≥15 yo: **Usual:** 5 mg tid. **Titrate:** May increase to 10 mg tid. Do not exceed 2-3 wks of therapy.	⊙B ❄> H
Dantrolene Sodium (Dantrium)	**Cap:** 25 mg, 50 mg, 100 mg, 200 mg	**Adults: Initial:** 25 mg qd x 7d. **Titrate:** Increase to 25 mg tid x 7d, then 50 mg tid x 7d, then 100 mg tid. **Max:** 100 mg qid. **Peds: ≥5 yo: Initial:** 0.5 mg/kg qd x 7d. **Titrate:** Increase to 0.5 mg/kg tid x 7d, then 1 mg/kg tid x 7d, then 2 mg/kg tid. **Max:** 100 mg qid.	⊙N ❄v H Hepatotoxicity.
Metaxalone (Skelaxin)	**Tab:** 400 mg, 800 mg	>12 yo: 800 mg tid-qid.	⊙N ❄v

NAME	FORM/STRENGTH	DOSAGE	COMMENTS
Methocarbamol (Robaxin)	Inj: 100 mg/ml; Tab: 500 mg, 750 mg	**Adults: Tab: Initial:** (500 mg tab) 1.5 gm qid x 2-3d. **Maint:** 1 gm qid. **Initial:** (750 mg tab) 1.5 gm qid x 2-3d. **Maint:** 750 mg q4h or 1.5 gm tid. **Max:** 6 gm/d x 2-3d; 8 gm/d if severe. **IM/IV: Moderate Symptoms:** 1 gm.	●C ❋v
Orphenadrine Citrate (Norflex)	Inj: 30 mg/ml; Tab,ER: 100 mg	**Adults:** 100 mg PO bid or 60 mg IV/IM q12h.	●C ❋>
Orphenadrine/ASA/Caffeine (Norgesic, Norgesic Forte)	Tab: (Norgesic) 25-385-30 mg; (Norgesic Forte) 50-770-60 mg	**Adults: Norgesic:** 1-2 tabs tid-qid. **Norgesic Forte:** 1/2-1 tab tid-qid.	●N ❋>
Tizanidine HCl (Zanaflex)	Tab: 2 mg, 4 mg	**Adults: Initial:** 4 mg q6-8h. **Titrate:** Increase by 2-4 mg. **Usual:** 8 mg q6-8h. **Max:** 3 doses/24h or 36 mg/d.	●C ❋>

Obsessive-Compulsive Disorder

SSRIS

NAME	FORM/STRENGTH	DOSAGE	COMMENTS
Fluoxetine (Prozac)	Cap: 10 mg, 20 mg, 40 mg; Sol: 20 mg/5 ml; Tab: 10 mg	**Adults: Initial:** 20 mg qam. **Maint:** 20-60 mg/d given qd or bid, am and noon. **Max:** 80 mg/d. **Peds: ≥7 yo: Adolescents and Higher Weight Peds: Initial:** 10 mg/d. **Titrate:** Increase to 20 mg/d after 2 wks. Consider additional dose increases after several more wks if clinical improvement not observed. **Usual:** 20-60 mg/d. **Lower Weight Peds: Initial:** 10 mg/d. **Titrate:** Consider additional dose increases after several wks if clinical improvement not observed. **Usual:** 20-30 mg/d. **Max:** 60 mg/d.	●C ❋v H

Fluvoxamine	**Tab:** 25 mg, 50 mg, 100 mg	**Adults: Initial:** 50 mg qhs. **Titrate:** Increase by 50 mg q4-7d. **Maint:** 100-300 mg/d. **Max:** 300 mg/d. **8-17 yo: Initial:** 25 mg qhs. **Titrate:** Increase by 25 mg q4-7d. **Maint:** 50-200 mg/d. **Max: 8-11 yo:** 200 mg/d. **Adolescents:** 300 mg/d.	◙C ❄v H
Paroxetine (Paxil)	**Susp:** 10 mg/5 ml; **Tab:** 10 mg, 20 mg, 30 mg, 40 mg	**Adults: Initial:** 20 mg qam. **Usual:** 40 mg/d. **Max:** 60 mg/d.	◙C ❄> H R
Sertraline (Zoloft)	**Tab:** 25 mg, 50 mg, 100 mg; **Sol:** 20 mg/ml	**Initial: Adults & Peds ≥13 yo:** 50 mg qd. **6-12 yo:** 25 mg qd. **Titrate:** Adjust wkly. **Max:** 200 mg/d.	◙C ❄> H

TRICYCLIC ANTIDEPRESSANTS

| Clomipramine HCl (Anafranil) | **Cap:** 25 mg, 50 mg, 75 mg | **Adults: Initial:** 25 mg/d, increase to 100 mg/d within 1st 2 wks. **Titrate:** Increase over several wks.
Max: 250 mg/d. May give qhs. **>10 yo: Initial:** 25 mg/d, increase to 3 mg/kg/d or 100 mg/d within 1st 2 wks. **Titrate:** Increase over several wks. **Max:** 3 mg/kg/d or 200 mg/d. May give qhs. | ◙C ❄v |

Miscellaneous

| Dantrolene Sodium (Dantrium) | **Inj:** 20 mg | **Malignant Hyperthermia: Adults & Peds: Initial:** 1 mg/kg IV, until symptoms subside. **Max:** 10 mg/kg. | ◙N ❄> H Hepatotoxicity. |
| Etomidate (Amidate) | **Inj:** 2 mg/ml | **Adults & Peds >10 yo:** 0.2-0.6 mg/kg IV. **Usual:** 0.3 mg/kg IV, over 30-60 secs. | ◙C ❄> |

NAME	FORM/STRENGTH	DOSAGE	COMMENTS
Glatiramer (Copaxone)	**Inj:** 20 mg	**≥18 yo: Relapsing-Remitting MS:** 20 mg SC qd.	●B ❄>
Interferon beta-1a (Avonex)	**Inj:** 33 mcg	**Relapsing Forms of MS: Adults:** 30 mcg IM qwk.	●C ❄v
Interferon beta-1a (Rebif)	**Inj:** 22 mcg/0.5 ml, 44 mcg/0.5 ml	**Relapsing Forms of MS: Adults: Initial:** 8.8 mcg SC TIW. **Titrate:** Increase over a 4 wk period to 44 mcg SC TIW. **Maint:** 44 mcg SQ TIW. **Leukopenia/Elevated LFTs:** Reduce dose by 20-50% until toxicity resolves. Administer dose at the same time qd (late afternoon, evening) on the same 3 days/wk at least 48h apart.	●C ❄> H
Interferon beta-1b (Betaseron)	**Inj:** 0.3 mg	**Relapsing MS:** 0.25 mg SC qod.	●C ❄v
Meprobamate/ASA (Equagesic)	**Tab:** 200 mg-325 mg	**Musculoskeletal Disease: Adults & Peds ≥12 yo: Usual:** 1-2 tabs tid-qid prn for pain with tension & anxiety.	●N ❄>
Mitoxantrone (Novantrone)	**Inj:** 2 mg/ml	**Adults: Reduction of Neurologic Disability in MS:** 12 mg/m² q3mths.	●D ❄v Bone marrow suppression. Myocardial toxicity. Secondary AML. [3]
Nimodipine (Nimotop)	**Cap:** 30 mg	**Subarachnoid Hemorrhage: Adults: Usual:** 60 mg q4h x 21d. Start within 96h of hemorrhage.	●C ❄v H

[3] Give only under supervision of a physician experienced with antineoplastics.

Dermatones

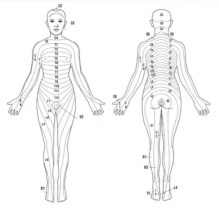

Redrawn from Keegan JJ, Garrett FD, *Anatomical Record* 102:409-437, 1948; used with permission of The Wistar Institute, Philadelphia, PA.

NAME	FORM/STRENGTH	DOSAGE		COMMENTS

PULMONARY/RESPIRATORY

Asthma/COPD Preparations

ANTICHOLINERGICS

NAME	FORM/STRENGTH	DOSAGE	COMMENTS
Ipratropium Bromide (Atrovent)	**Inhaler:** 0.018 mg/inh; **Sol,Neb:** 0.02%	**COPD: ≥12 yo: Inhaler: Initial:** 2 inh qid. **Max:** 12 inh/24h. **Sol,Neb:** 1 vial (500 mcg/2.5 ml) nebulized tid-qid, separate by 6-8h.	●B ❄>
Tiotropium Bromide (Spiriva)	**Cap, Inhalation:** 18 mcg	**Adults: COPD:** Inhale the contents of one cap qd, with the HandiHaler device.	●C ❄>

BRONCHODILATOR (BETA AGONISTS/ANTICHOLINERGICS)

NAME	FORM/STRENGTH	DOSAGE	COMMENTS
Albuterol Sulfate/ Ipratropium Bromide (Combivent)	**Inhaler:** 0.09 mg-0.018 mg/inh	**COPD: Adults:** 2 inh qid. **Max:** 12 inh/24h.	●C ❄v

BRONCHODILATOR COMBINATIONS

NAME	FORM/STRENGTH	DOSAGE	COMMENTS
Albuterol Sulfate/ Ipratropium Bromide (Duoneb)	**Sol:** 3 mg-0.5 mg/3 ml	**Adults:** 3 ml qid via nebulizer. May give 2 additional doses/d if needed.	●C ❄v
Fluticasone Propionate/ Salmeterol Xinafoate (Advair)	**Inhaler:** 100-50 mcg/inh, 250-50 mcg/inh, 500-50 mcg/inh	**Asthma: Adults & Peds ≥12 yo:** 1 inh q12h; strength depends upon previous inhaled steroid therapy. **Max:** (500-50 mcg/inh) 1 inh bid. **4-11 yo: Symptomatic on Inhaled Steroid Therapy:** (100/50 mcg only) 1 inh q12h. **COPD:** (250/50 mcg only) 1 inh q12h.	●C ❄>

Albuterol Sulfate (AccuNeb)	**Sol:** 0.63 mg/3 ml, 1.25 mg/3 ml	**2-12 yo:** 0.63 mg or 1.25 mg tid-qid via nebulizer. **6-12 yo with severe asthma or >40 kg or 11-12 yo: Initial:** 1.25 mg tid-qid.	◉C ❀v
Albuterol Sulfate (Proventil, Volmax, VoSpire ER)	**(Proventil) Inhaler:** 0.09 mg/inh, (HFA) 0.09 mg/inh; **Sol,Neb:** 0.083%, 0.5%; **Syr:** 2 mg/5 ml; **Tab:** 2 mg, 4 mg; **Tab,ER:** (Proventil Repetabs) 4 mg, (Volmax, VoSpire ER) 4 mg, 8 mg	**Adults & Peds ≥12 yo: Aerosol/HFA Aerosol:** 2 inh q4-6h or 1 inh q4h. **Sol,Neb:** 2.5 mg tid-qid by nebulizer. **Tab** 2-4 mg tid-qid. **Max:** 32 mg/d. **>12 yo: Tab,ER: Usual:** 4-8 mg q12h. **Max:** 32 mg/d. **Syr:** 2-4 mg tid-qid. **Max:** 32 mg/d. **6-12 yo: Tab,ER: Usual:** 4 mg q12h. **Max:** 24 mg/d. **Syr/Tabs: Initial:** 2 mg tid-qid. **Max:** 24 mg/d. **2-6 yrs: Syr: Initial:** 0.1 mg/kg tid (not to exceed 6 mg/d). **Max:** 12 mg/d. **≥4 yo: HFA Aerosol:** 2 inh q4-6h or 1 inh q4h. **Exercise-Induced Bronchospasm: ≥12 yo: Aerosol:** 2 inh 15 min before activity. **≥4 yo: HFA Aerosol:** 2 inh 15-30 min before activity.	◉C ❀v
Formoterol Fumarate (Foradil)	**Inhaler:** 12 mcg/inh	**Adults & Peds ≥5 yo: Asthma/COPD:** 12 mcg q12h. **Max:** 24 mcg/d. **Exercise-Induced Bronchospasm:** 12 mcg 15 min prior to exercise. Do not give added dose if on q12h schedule. Give only by inhalation with Aerolizer™ Inhaler.	◉C ❀>
Levalbuterol HCl (Xopenex)	**Sol,Neb:** 0.31 mg/3 ml, 0.63 mg/3 ml, 1.25 mg/3 ml	**Bronchospasm: Adults & Peds ≥12 yo: Initial:** 0.63 mg tid, q6-8h. **Severe Asthma:** 1.25 mg tid, q6-8h. **6-11 yo:** 0.31 mg tid. **Max:** 0.63 mg tid. Administer by neb.	◉C ❀v

NAME	FORM/STRENGTH	DOSAGE	COMMENTS
Metaproterenol Sulfate (Alupent)	**Inhaler:** 0.65 mg/inh; **Sol,Neb:** 0.4%, 0.6%, 5%; **Syr:** 10 mg/5 ml; **Tab:** 10 mg, 20 mg	**Bronchospasm: Adults & Peds ≥12 yo: Inhaler:** 2-3 inh q3-4h. **Max:** 12 inh/d. **Sol,Neb 0.4%, 0.6%:** 2.5 ml by IPPB tid-qid, up to q4h. **Syr/Tab: >9 yo or >60 lbs:** 20 mg tid-qid. **6-9 yo or <60 lbs:** 10 mg tid-qid. **Sol,Neb 5%: ≥12 yo:** Neb/IPPB: 0.2-0.3 ml (dilute in 2.5 ml saline) tid-qid. **Hand-bulb Neb:** 5-15 inh (undiluted) tid-qid. **6-12 yo:** Neb: 0.1-0.2 ml (dilute in 3 ml saline) by neb tid-qid.	▣C ❄>
Pirbuterol Acetate (Maxair, Maxair Autohaler)	**Autohaler:** 0.2 mg/inh **Inhaler:** 0.2 mg/inh	**Adults & Peds ≥12 yo:** 1-2 inh q4-6h. **Max:** 12 inh/d.	▣C ❄>
Salmeterol Xinafoate (Serevent)	**Inhaler:** 21 mcg/inh; **Diskus:** 50 mcg/inh	**Inhaler: ≥12 yo: Asthma/COPD:** 2 inh q12h. **EIB Prevention:** 2 inh 30-60 min before exercise. **Diskus: ≥4 yo: Asthma/COPD:** 1 inh q12h. **EIB Prevention:** 1 inh 30 min before exercise (do not give preventive doses if already on bid dose).	▣C ❄v Asthma-related deaths reported
Terbutaline Sulfate (Brethine)	**Inj:** 1 mg/ml; **Tab:** 2.5 mg, 5 mg	**Adults & Peds ≥15 yo: PO:** 5 mg tid. May reduce to 2.5 mg tid. **Max:** 15 mg/24h. **12-15 yo:** 2.5 mg tid. **Max:** 7.5 mg/24h. **Inj: ≥12 yo:** 0.25 mg SQ into lateral deltoid area. May repeat within 15-30 min if no improvement. **Max:** 0.5 mg/4h.	▣B ❄>

IGG1K MONOCLONAL ANTIBODY

Omalizumab (Xolair)	**Inj:** 150 mg	**Adults & Peds ≥12 yo:** 150-375 mg SQ q2 or 4 wks based on body wgt and pre-treatment serum total IgE level. **Max:** 150 mg/site. **30-90 kg & IgE ≥30-100 IU/ml:** 150 mg q4wks. **90-150 kg & IgE ≥30-100 IU/ml or 30-90 kg & IgE >100-200 IU/ml or 30-60 kg & IgE >200-300 IU/ml:** 300 mg q4wks. **90-150 kg & IgE >100-200 IU/ml or >60-90 kg & IgE >200-300 IU/ml or 30-70 kg & IgE >300-400 IU/ml:** 225 mg q2wks. **>90-150 kg & IgE >200-300 IU/ml or 70-90 kg & IgE >300-400 IU/ml or 30-70 kg & IgE >400-500 IU/ml or 30-60 kg & IgE >500-600 IU/ml:** 300 mg q2wks. **>70-90 kg & IgE >400-500 IU/ml or >60-70 kg & IgE >500-600 IU/ml or 30-60 kg & IgE >600-700 IU/ml:** 375 mg q2wks.	◐B ❊>

INHALED CORTICOSTEROIDS

Beclomethasone Dipropionate (Qvar, Vanceril)	**Inhaler:** (Qvar) 40 mcg/inh, 80 mcg/inh; (Vanceril) 42 mcg/inh	**Vanceril: Adults & Peds ≥12 yo:** 2 inh tid-qid, or 4 inh bid. **Severe Asthma:** 12-16 inh/d. **Max:** 20 inh/d. **6-12 yo:** 1-2 inh tid-qid, or 4 inh bid. **Max:** 10 inh/d. **Qvar: Adults & Adolesents: Previous Bronchodilator Only:** 40-80 mcg bid. **Max:** 320 mcg bid. **Previous Inhaled Corticosteroid Therapy:** 40-160 mcg bid. **Max:** 320 mcg bid. **5-11 yo: Previous Bronchodilator Only or Inhaled Corticosteroid:** 40 mcg bid. **Max:** 80 mcg bid. **Adults & Peds ≥5 yo: Maint With Oral Corticosteroids:** May attempt gradual reduction of oral dose after 1 wk on inhaled therapy.	◐C ❊v

NAME	FORM/STRENGTH	DOSAGE	COMMENTS
Budesonide (Pulmicort Respules, *Pulmicort Turbuhaler)	**Respules:** 0.25 mg/ 2 ml; 0.5 mg/2 ml; **Turbuhaler:** 200 mcg/inh.	**Adults & Peds ≥6 yo: Turbuhaler: Previous Bronchodilator Only/Inhaled Corticosteroid: Initial:** 200 mcg bid. [Mild-to-moderate asthma patients previously controlled on inhaled steroids may use 200-400 mcg qd]. **Max:** 400 mcg bid. **Oral Corticosteroid: Max:** 400 mcg bid. **Respules: 1-8 yo: Previous Bronchodilator Only: Initial:** 0.5 mg qd or 0.25 mg bid. Administer via jet neb. **Max:** 0.5 mg/d. **Previous Inhaled Corticosteroid:** 0.5 mg qd or 0.25 mg bid. **Max:** 1 mg/d. **Previous Oral Corticosteroid:** 1 mg qd or 0.5 mg bid. **Max:** 1 mg/d. Gradually reduce PO corticosteroid after 1 wk of budesonide.	▣B ❄> (Respules) ▣B ❄∨ (Turbuhaler)
Flunisolide (Aerobid, Aerobid-M)	**Inhaler:** 0.25 mg/inh	**Adults & Peds ≥6 yo: Initial:** 2 inh bid. **Max: Adults:** 4 inh bid.	▣C ❄>
Fluticasone Propionate (Flovent, Flovent Diskus, Flovent Rotadisk)	**Inhaler:** 44 mcg/inh, 110 mcg/inh, 220 mcg/inh; **Diskus/Rotadisk:** 50 mcg/dose, 100 mcg/dose, 250 mcg/dose	**Adults & Peds ≥12 yo: Inhaler: Previous Bronchodilator Only: Initial:** 88 mcg bid. **Max:** 440 mcg bid. **Previous Inhaled Corticosteroids: Initial:** 88-220 mcg bid. **Max:** 440 mcg bid. **Previous Oral Corticosteroids: Initial/Max:** 880 mcg bid. **Diskus/Rotadisk: Previous Bronchodilator Only: Initial:** 100 mcg bid. **Max:** 500 mcg bid. **Previous Inhaled Corticosteroids: Initial:** 100-250 mcg bid. **Max:** 500 mcg bid. **Previous Oral Corticosteroids: Diskus: Initial:** 500-1000 mcg bid. **Max:** 1000 mcg bid. **Rotadisk: Initial/Max:** 1000 mcg bid. **4-11 yo: Diskus/**	▣C ❄> (Inhaler, Rotadisk) ❄∨ (Diskus)

		Rotadisk: Previous Bronchodilator Only/Inhaled Corticosteroids: Initial: 50 mcg bid. Reduce PO prednisone no faster than 2.5 mg/d wkly; begin at least 1 wk after start fluticasone.	
Triamcinolone Acetonide (Azmacort)	**Inhaler:** 100 mcg/inh	**Adults & Peds >12 yo:** 2 inh tid-qid or 4 inh bid. **Severe Asthma: Initial:** 12-16 inh/d. **Max:** 16 inh/d. **6-12 yo:** 1-2 inh tid-qid or 2-4 inh bid. **Max:** 12 inh/d.	◉C ✿>

LEUKOTRIENE MODIFIERS

Montelukast Sodium (Singulair)	**Chewtab:** 4 mg, 5 mg; **Granules:** 4 mg/pkt; **Tab:** 10 mg	**Asthma: Adults & Peds ≥15 yo:** 10 mg qpm. **6-14 yo:** 5 mg qpm. **2-5 yo: Chewtab/Granules:** 4 mg qpm. **12-23 mths: Granules:** 4 mg qpm.	◉B ✿>
Zafirlukast (Accolate)	**Tab:** 10 mg, 20 mg	**Asthma: Adults & Peds ≥12 yo:** 20 mg bid. **5-11 yo:** 10 mg bid. Administer 1h ac or 2h pc.	◉B ✿v
Zileuton (Zyflo)	**Tab:** 600 mg	**Asthma: Adults & Peds ≥12 yo:** 600 mg qid, with meals & hs.	◉C ✿v H

MAST CELL STABILIZERS

Cromolyn Sodium (Intal)	**Inhaler:** 0.8 mg/inh; **Sol,Neb:** 10 mg/ml	**Asthma: Inhaler:** ≥5 yo: **Usual/Max:** 2 inh qid. **Sol:** ≥2 yo: 20 mg qid via neb. **Acute Bronchospasm Prevention: Inhaler:** ≥5 yo: **Usual:** 2 inh 10-60 min before precipitant exposure. **Sol:** ≥2 yo: 20 mg via neb shortly before precipitant exposure.	◉B ✿> H R
Nedocromil Sodium (Tilade)	**Inhaler:** 1.75 mg/inh	**Asthma: Adults & Peds ≥ 6 yo:** 2 inh qid. May reduce to bid-tid once desired response observed.	◉B ✿>

NAME	FORM/STRENGTH	DOSAGE	COMMENTS
XANTHINE DERIVATIVES			
Aminophylline	**Inj:** 25 mg/ml; **Sol:** 105 mg/5 ml; **Tab:** 100 mg, 200 mg	**Chronic Treatment: Adults: Initial:** 16 mg/kg/24h PO or 400 mg/24h PO of theophylline given q6-8h. **Titrate:** Increase by 25% q3d as tolerated & adjust to 10-20 mg/ml. **Peds: 1 to <9 yo: Initial:** 6.3 mg/kg. **Maint:** 1 mg/kg/h. **9 to <16 yo: Initial:** 6.3 mg/kg. **Maint:** 0.8 mg/kg/h.	◐C ❄v H R
Dyphylline (Lufyllin)	**Sol:** 100 mg/15 ml; **Tab:** 200 mg, 400 mg	**Adults:** Up to 15 mg/kg q6h.	◐C ❄> R
Theophylline (Theo-24, Theolair)	**Cap,ER:** (Theo-24) 100 mg, 200 mg, 300 mg, 400 mg; **Tab:** (Theolair) 125 mg, 250 mg	**Theolair: Initial: Adults & Peds ≥1 yo and >45 kg: Initial:** 300 mg/d divided q6-8h. **Titrate:** Increase to 400 mg/d divided q6-8h after 3d if tolerated, then to 600 mg/d divided q6-8h after 3 more days if needed and tolerated. **≥1 yo and <45 kg: Initial:** 12-14 mg/kg/d divided q4-6h. **(Max:** 300 mg/d) **Titrate:** Increase to 16 mg/kg/d divided q4-h6 (Max: 400 mg/day) after 3d if tolerated, then increase to 20 mg/kg/d divided q4-6h (Max: 600mg/d) after 3 more days if needed and tolerated. **Theo-24: Adults & Peds ≥12 yo and >45 kg: Initial:** 300-400 mg/d. **Titrate:** Increase to 400-600 mg/d after 3d if tolerated, then to >600 mg/d if needed and tolerated after 3 more days. **≥12 yo and <45 kg: Initial:** 12-14 mg/kg/d (Max: 300 mg/d). Increase to 16 mg/kg/d (Max: 400 mg/d) after 3d. May increase to 20 mg/kg/d (Max: 600 mg/d) if tolerated and needed after 3 more days.	◐C ❄> H R

Benign Prostatic Hypertrophy

ALPHA₁ RECEPTOR BLOCKERS

Alfuzosin HCl (Uroxatral)	**Tab,ER:** 10 mg	**Adults:** 10 mg immediately after the same meal qd.	⊕B ❀> **H**
Doxazosin (Cardura)	**Tab:** 1 mg, 2 mg, 4 mg, 8 mg	**Initial:** 1 mg qhs. **Titrate:** Increase q1-2wks. **Max:** 8 mg/d.	⊕C ❀>
Tamsulosin (Flomax)	**Cap:** 0.4 mg	**Initial:** 0.4 mg qd, 1/2h after same meal each day. **Titrate:** May increase to 0.8 mg qd after 2-4 wks. If therapy is interrupted, restart with 0.4 mg qd.	⊕B ❀>
Terazosin (Hytrin)	**Cap:** 1 mg, 2 mg, 5 mg, 10 mg	**Initial:** 1 mg qhs. **Titrate:** Increase stepwise to 10 mg qd. **Max:** 20 mg.	⊕C ❀>

ALPHA-REDUCTASE INHIBITORS

Dutasteride (Avodart)	**Cap:** 5 mg	**Adults:** 5 mg qd.	⊕X ❀v
Finasteride (Proscar)	**Tab:** 5 mg	**Adults:** Monotherapy/Concomitant Doxazosin: 5 mg qd.	⊕X ❀v

Enuresis Management

Desmopressin Acetate (DDAVP)	**Nasal Spray:** 10 mcg/spr; **Rhinal Tube:** 0.01%; **Tab:** 0.1 mg, 0.2 mg	**Adults & Peds ≥6 yo: Tab: Initial:** 0.2 mg PO qhs. **Titrate:** May increase up to 0.6 mg. **Max:** Up to 6 mths. **Spray/Tube: Initial:** 20 mcg intranasally qhs. **Titrate:** Decrease to 10 mcg or increase up to 40 mcg if needed. **Max:** 4-8 wks. Administer 1/2 dose per nostril.	⊕B ❀>

NAME	FORM/STRENGTH	DOSAGE	COMMENTS
Flavoxate HCl (Urispas)	Tab: 100 mg	Adults & Peds ≥12 yo: 100-200 mg tid-qid. Reduce dose with improvement.	B ☼

Erectile Dysfunction

ALPHA₂ RECEPTOR BLOCKERS

NAME	FORM/STRENGTH	DOSAGE	COMMENTS
Yohimbine HCl (Aphrodyne)	Tab: 5.4 mg	Adults: Usual: 5.4 mg tid up to 10 wks. If side effects occur, decrease to 1/2 tab tid, then gradually increase back to usual dose.	N ☼ R Do not use in pregnancy.

PHOSPHODIESTERASE TYPE 5 INHIBITOR

NAME	FORM/STRENGTH	DOSAGE	COMMENTS
Sildenafil Citrate (Viagra)	Tab: 25 mg, 50 mg, 100 mg	Usual: 50 mg qd 1h (range 0.5-4 h) before sexual activity. Titrate: May decrease to 25 mg qd or increase to 100 mg qd. Max: 100 mg qd. Concomitant CYP450 3A4 Inhibitors: Initial: 25 mg qd. Concomitant Ritonavir: Max: 25 mg q48h.	B ☼ ❤ H R Cl with nitrates.
Tadalafil (Cialis)	Tab: 5 mg, 10 mg, 20 mg	Adults: Initial: 10 mg prior to sexual activity at frequency of up to once daily. Titrate: May decrease to 5 mg or increase to 20 mg based on response. With Potent CYP3A4 inhibitors (eg, ketoconazole, itraconazole, ritonavir): Max: 10 mg/72h.	B ☼ ❤ H R Cl with nitrates, alpha-blockers (except tamsulosin 0.4 mg qd).

| Vardenafil HCl (Levitra) | Tab: 2.5 mg, 5 mg, 10 mg, 20 mg | Adults: Initial: 10 mg 60 min prior to sexual activity at frequency of up to once daily. Titrate: May decrease to 5 mg or increase to max of 20 mg based on response. Elderly: ≥65 yrs: Initial: 5 mg. Concomitant Ritonavir: Max: 2.5 mg/72h. Concomitant Indinavir, Ketoconazole 400 mg daily/Itraconazole 400 mg daily: Max: 2.5 mg/24h. Concomitant Ketoconazole 200 mg daily/Itraconazole 200 mg daily/Erythromycin: Max: 5 mg/24h. | ●B ❄v H CI with nitrates, nitric oxide donors, alpha-blockers. |

PROSTAGLANDIN E₁

| Alprostadil (Caverject, Caverject Impulse, Edex, MUSE Urethral Suppository) | Inj: 5 mcg, 10 mcg, 10 mcg/ml, 20 mcg, 20 mcg/ml, 40 mcg; Sup, Urethral: 125 mcg, 250 mcg, 500 mcg, 1000 mcg | Muse: Transurethral: Initial: 125-250 mcg. Titrate: Increase as necessary to achieve erection. Max: 2 sup/24h. Caverject, Edex: Intracavernosal: Vasculogenic/Psychogenic/Mixed Etiology: Initial: 2.5 mcg. Partial Response: Increase by 2.5 mcg, then by 5-10 mcg until desired response. No Response: Increase by 5 mcg, then by 5-10 mcg until desired response. Neurogenic Etiology (Spinal Cord Injury): Initial: 1.25 mcg. Partial/No Response: May give 2nd dose of 2.5 mcg, 3rd dose of 5 mcg, then may increase by 5 mcg until desired response. Max: 60 mcg/dose. Reduce dose if erection >1h. Give no more than TIW; allow 24h between doses. If no initial response, may give next higher dose within 1h. If partial response, give next higher dose after 24h. | ●C ❄v Not indicated in women. |

NAME	FORM/STRENGTH	DOSAGE	COMMENTS

Urinary Retention
ANTICHOLINESTERASE AGENTS

| **Neostigmine** (Prostigmin) | **Inj:** 0.25 mg/ml, 0.5 mg/ml, 1 mg/ml | **Adults: Urinary Retention:** 0.5 mg SC/IM. If urination does not occur within 1h then catheterize patient. After bladder is empty, continue with 0.5 mg q3h for at least 5 doses. **Prevention of Post-op Distention/Urinary Retention:** 0.25 mg SC/IM as soon as possible after operation; repeat q4-6h x 2-3d. **Treatment of Post-op Distention:** 0.5 mg SC/IM. |  |

PARASYMPATHETIC STIMULANTS

| **Bethanechol** (Urecholine) | **Tab:** 5 mg, 10 mg, 25 mg, 50 mg; | **Adults: Initial:** 5-10 gm. **Titrate:** May repeat q1h until satisfactory response or 50 gm given. **Usual:** 10-50 gm tid-qid. **Max:** 200 gm/d. | 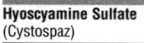 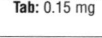 |

Urinary Tract Antispasmodics
PARASYMPATHOLYTICS

| **Hyoscyamine Sulfate** (Cystospaz) | **Tab:** 0.15 mg | **Adults:** 0.15-0.3 mg qid prn. | ⒸC ❋> |

Drug	Formulations	Dosing	
Hyoscyamine Sulfate (Levbid, Levsin, Levsinex, NuLev)	**(Levbid) Tab,ER:** 0.375 mg; **(Levsin) Drops:** 0.125 mg/ml; **Eli:** 0.125 mg/5 ml; **Inj:** 0.5 mg/ml; **Tab:** 0.125 mg; **Tab,SL:** 0.125 mg; **(Levsinex) Cap,ER:** 0.375 mg; **(NuLev) Tab,Dissolve (ODT):** 0.125 mg	**Adults & Peds: ≥12 yo:** Drops/Eli/ODT/Tab/Tab,SL: 0.125-0.25 mg q4h or prn. **Max:** 1.5 mg/24h. Cap, Tab,ER: 0.375-0.75 mg q12h; or 1 cap q8h. **Max:** 1.5 mg/24h. **2 to <12 yo:** ODT/Tab/Tab,SL: 0.0625-0.125 mg q4h or prn. **Max:** 0.75 mg/24h. Eli: Give q4h or prn. **10 kg:** 1.25 ml. **20 kg:** 2.5 ml. **40 kg:** 3.75 ml. **50 kg:** 5 ml. **Max:** 30 ml/24h. Drops: 0.25-1 ml q4h or prn. **Max:** 6 ml/24h. **<2 yo:** Drops: Give q4h or prn. **3.4 kg:** 4 drops. **Max:** 24 drops/24h. **5 kg:** 5 drops. **Max:** 30 drops/24h. **7 kg:** 6 drops. **Max:** 36 drops/24h. **10 kg:** 8 drops. **Max:** 48 drops/24h.	◉C ✿>
Oxybutynin Chloride (Ditropan, Ditropan XL)	**Syr:** 5 mg/5 ml; **Tab:** 5 mg; **Tab,ER:** 5 mg, 10 mg, 15 mg	**Adults:** Tab/Syr: 5 mg bid-tid. **Max:** 5 mg qid. Tab,ER: **Initial:** 5 mg qd. **Titrate:** Increase qwk by 5 mg. **Max:** 30 mg/d. **>5 yo:** Tab/Syr: 5 mg bid. **Max:** 5 mg tid.	◉B ✿>
Oxybutynin (Oxytrol)	**Patch:** 36 mg (3.9 mg/d)	**Adults:** 3.9 mg/d 2x/wk (q3-4d). Apply to abdomen, hip, or buttock.	◉B ✿>
Tolterodine (Detrol, Detrol LA)	**Cap,ER** 2 mg, 4 mg; **Tab:** 1 mg, 2 mg	**Adults:** Cap,ER: 4 mg qd. May decrease to 2 mg qd depending on response & tolerability. Tab: **Initial:** 2 mg bid. **Maint:** 1-2 mg bid.	◉C ✿v H R

INDEX

285